Fibrin Sealing in Surgical and Nonsurgical Fields

Volume **5**

G. Schlag P. W. Ascher
F. J. Steinkogler H. Stammberger (Eds.)

Neurosurgery
Ophthalmic Surgery
ENT

With 115 Figures, Some in Color
and 18 Tables

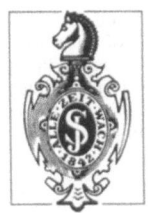

Springer-Verlag
Berlin Heidelberg New York
London Paris Tokyo
Hong Kong Barcelona
Budapest

Prof. Dr. GÜNTHER SCHLAG
Ludwig-Boltzmann-Institut
für experimentelle und klinische Traumatologie
Donaueschingenstraße 13, 1200 Wien, Austria

Univ.-Prof. Dr. PETER WOLF ASCHER
Universitätsklinik für Neurochirurgie
Auenbruggerplatz 20, 8036 Graz, Austria

Prof. Dr. FRANZ JOSEF STEINKOGLER
Universität Wien, Augenklinik
Alserstraße 4, 1090 Wien, Austria

Prof. Dr. HEINZ STAMMBERGER
Universität Graz
Universitäts-HNO-Klinik
Auenbruggerplatz 20, 8036 Graz, Austria

ISBN 978-3-540-58014-0   ISBN 978-3-642-95724-6 (eBook)
DOI 10.1007/978-3-642-95724-6

Library of Congress Cataloging-in-Publication Data. Neurosurgery, ophthalmic surgery, ENT /
G. Schlag ... [et al.] (eds.). p. cm. – (Fibrin sealing in surgical and nonsurgical fields ; v. 5) Includes index. ISBN 978-3-540-58014-0 (alk. paper). –ISBN 978-3-540-58014-0 (alk. paper) 1. Otolaryngology, Operative. 2. Nervous system – Surgery. 3. Eye-Surgery. 4. Fibrin tissue adhesive. I.
Schlag, Günther. II. Series. [DNLM: 1. Neurosurgery-methods. 2. Otorhinolaryngologic
Diseases-surgery. 3. Eye-surgery. 4. Fibrin Tissue Adhesive-therapeutic use. 5. Surgery, Plastic-
methods. 6. Biocompatible Materials. WL 368 N49517 1994] RD73.F52F53 1994 vol. 5 [RD661]
617.1'406 s–dc20 [617.48] DNLM/DLC for Library of Congress.

The use of general descriptive names, registered names, trademarks, etc. in this publication
does not imply, even in the absence of a specific statement, that such names are exempt from
the relevant protective laws and regulations and therefore free for general use.

Product liability: The publishers cannot guarantee the accuracy of any information about dosage and application contained in this book. In every individual case the user must check such
information by consulting the relevant literature.

Production: PRO EDIT GmbH, Heidelberg, FRG
Typesetting: Mitterweger Werksatz GmbH, Plankstadt, FRG
SPIN: 10428161   23/3130 5 4 3 2 1 0   Printed on acid-free paper

Preface

These eight volumes, which developed out of the international congress "Update and Future Trends in Fibrin Sealing in Surgical and Nonsurgical Fields" held in November 1992, present the state of the art in fibrin sealing. Initially, fibrin sealant played an important role in surgery. During the past few years, it has been increasingly applied nonsurgically, and we can now say that it has become an integral component of medical treatment.

The doubts which have been raised by nonusers about the efficacy of fibrin sealant are no longer valid. The correct indication and technique continue to be basic prerequisites for effective treatment. Even today – 20 years after fibrin sealant was first used – the three most prominent effects of fibrin sealant are still hemostasis, sealing of the wound, and support of wound healing.

The problems posed by the transmission of viral infections have gained substantially in importance because of the potential transmission of AIDS via fibrin sealant. Fortunately, this is so unlikely today that it no longer represents a cause for concern, which does not mean, however, that research in this field can be discontinued.

Seven years have passed since the last series of books on fibrin sealing were published. Since then many new results have been obtained and clear indications for the use of fibrin glue in neurosurgery have developed. One of the major indications is sealing of the sellar floor when a transsphenoidal surgical approach to the pituitary gland has been employed; the same applies in reconstructive operations at the frontobasal area. Due to the effect of fibrin sealant the duration of hospitalization, the number of reoperations, and the necessity of lumbar catheters have been reduced considerably. Obviously, fibrin glue can be applied both at the cranial and the spinal dura. When in doubt it should be used to secure the dural closure. Many of the publications in this book have also shown beneficial use of fibrin glue in peripheral nerve anastomoses. Fibrin glue has also been applied with some success in endovascular surgery of arteriovenous malformations and heavily vascularized tumors.

Every neurosurgeon has encountered situations in which the dura cannot be closed tightly anymore, especially after multiple reoperations in patients in whom the bone flap has already been removed. In these patients a lumbar drainage catheter combined with aspiration of subcutaneous CSF above the fistula, instillation of fibrin glue through the same needle, and a pressure bandage for 24 h may be sufficient to cause scarring between the dura and the galea and to prevent the development of further CSF fistulas.

Our experience with fibrin glue has shown only one real contraindication in neurosurgery: Application of fibrin glue inside the brain parenchyma before hemostasis is complete. In such a case the source of bleeding could not be seen by the surgeon anymore, and continued slow bleeding would physically remove this absorbable barrier and result in hemorrhage at a later time. Even so, there is no doubt that fibrin glue is a significant adjunct to modern neurosurgical techniques.

Fibrin sealing has become a standard method in various surgical specialities, also in ophthalmic surgery. There are many areas of ophthalmic plastic and reconstructive surgery and cataract and trauma surgery for utilizing fibrin sealant.

In eyelid operations the fixation of free autologous skin transplants for covering skin defects after tumor excision has proved advantageous, as early fibrovascular ingrowth into the transplant is stimulated. The treatment of severe upper eyelid entropion and special situations of trichiasis of the lower eyelid represent another special indication for fibrin sealing.

In orbital surgery the surgical management of the post-enucleation socket syndrome, mainly based on orbital volume deficit, can be improved by fibrin sealant fixation of the secondary orbital implant.

In lacrimal surgery there are also several indications for fibrin sealant. For reconstructing lacerated canaliculi lacrimales under the microscope, fibrin glue can be used to seal the microanastomosis.

In canaliculocystotomy, dacryocystorhinostomy and canaliculodacrycystorhinostomy the microanastomosis between canaliculi and lacrimal sac can be created and the lacrimal and the nasal mucosal flaps adapted with fibrin sealant.

In cataract surgery, the closure of the corneoscleral tunnel can be improved by means of fibrin sealing, thus reducing postoperative astigmatism. Traumatically perforated human lenses have been being treated successfully by fibrin sealing for years. Ophthalmic surgery has become a large and effective field of application for the fibrin sealing technique.

In modern ENT surgery fibrin sealant has become an indispensable tool. Apart from well-known and established applications in ear microsurgery, in particular, tympanoplasty with reconstructions of the ossicular chain and the tympanic membrane, plastic and reconstructive surgery with small and large grafts as well as flap plasty, the spectrum of indications has grown enormously in the past few years. Several surgical techniques have only become possible with the development of fibrin sealant. Today, endoscopic or microscopic transnasal operations of the skull base for the closure of cerebrospinal fluid fistulas, tumor excision, partial resections of the dura, and reconstruction of other defects can be safely performed, often avoiding major invasive surgery. Thus, in many cases an endonasal intervention has replaced craniotomy, which was required until recently. Endonasal surgical decompression of the optical nerve and/or orbits has also become safer thanks to the use of fibrin sealant. The sealant is also widely used in ENT tumor surgery, especially in major surgical interventions involving large reconstructions with microvascularized tissue transfer.

This volume contains a variety of examples from the broad spectrum of applications of fibrin sealant in otorhinolaryngology and head and neck surgery. We, the editors, would like to thank all the authors for their cooperation and excellent contributions and photographs. Their work has made publication of these eight volumes on fibrin sealing possible.

Special thanks are due to Dr. V. Gebhardt and his expert colleagues for efficient and constructive cooperation in the publication of these books at the Springer publishing company and Gudrun Schrodt for her untiring efforts in obtaining manuscripts, proof reading, and corresponding with the authors.

G. Schlag
P. W. Ascher
F. J. Steinkogler
H. Stammberger

Contents

I. Neurosurgery

Our Experience with Human Fibrin Glue in Neurosurgical Procedures
M. ACQUI, R. DELFINI, A. RACO, and L. FERRANTE   3

New Trends in Enlarged Middle Cranial Fossa Surgery
C. T. HAID, S. R. WOLF, and M. E. WIGAND.   8

Prevention and Treatment of Cerebrospinal Fluid Rhinorrhea
Following Transsphenoidal Surgery on Pituitary Gland Adenomas
J. EIRAS. 26

Preoperative Tumor Embolization with Fibrin Glue:
Indications and Results
E. NEUMAIER-PROBST, F. ZANELLA, M. WESTPHAL, and H. ZEUMER 32

Preliminary Observations of Local Therapy with Interferon-β
with Use of Fibrin Glue as a Carrier in Malignant Cerebral Tumor
K. MATSUMOTO, H. IZUMIYAMA, and T. IWATA 41

Frontobasal and Orbital Reconstruction Using Biological Material
P. KNORINGER 51

Fibrin Sealing in Spinal Neurosurgery
P. KNÖRINGER 59

Neurosurgical Reconstruction of Obstetric Brachial Plexus Lesions
with the Use of Fibrin Sealing
A. C. J. SLOOFF. 68

Centrocentral Anastomosis: An Elegant Alternative
in the Surgical Treatment of Painful Amputation Neuromas
J. BARBERÁ. 76

II. Ophthalmic Surgery

Fibrin Sealant in Ophthalmic Plastic and Reconstructive Surgery
F. J. STEINKOGLER and A. KUCHAR   87

Progress in Fibrin Sealing of Eye Lens and Conjunctiva
W. BUSCHMANN   97

Morphological Reactions Following Fibrin Retinopexy in Rabbit Eyes
K.-H. EMMERICH, F. J. STEINKOGLER, and G. EDEL   107

Fibrin Adhesive for Wound Closure in Small-Incision Cataract Surgery
M. RAUBER, U. MESTER, and M. ZUCHE   116

Wound Closure with Fibrin Adhesive in Cataract Surgery
U. MESTER   123

III. ENT

Rhinologic Applications of Fibrin Glue
H. STAMMBERGER, J. A. JEBELES, and W. LUXENBERGER   135

Spray Application of Fibrin Glue in Microsurgical Ethmoidectomy –
Technique and Short-Term Results
B. BERTRAND, P. ELOY, J. JAMART, A. DOYEN, and P. ROMBAUX   147

Use of Fibrin Glue in Craniofacial and Skull Base Trauma
F. X. BRUNNER and U. SCHWAB   152

Use of Fibrin Glue in Rhinoplasty
F. DISANT, A. MORGON, and J. LEBLOND   159

Use of Fibrin Glue in Intracranial Procedures Following Acoustic
Neuroma Surgery: Application in Facial Nerve Reconstruction
and Prevention of Cerebrospinal Fluid Rhinorrhea
J. KANZAKI, R. SHIOBARA, and T. O-UCHI   162

Partial and Total Reconstruction of the Auricle
H. WEERDA and R. SIEGERT   169

Mastoid Cavity Filling for Bone Reconstruction with a Mixture
of Fibrin Glue and Ceramic Granules
M. BAGOT D'ARC, P. CORLIEU, and G. DACULSI   174

Fibrin Sealing in Tympanoplasty
R. FRANK and G. STANGE.   180

Compound Prosthesis and Cartilage Layer: Two New Applications
of Fibrin Sealing in Reconstructive Middle Ear Surgery
H. SCHOBEL   186

Use of Bovine Heterologous Cartilage and Fibrin Sealant
in Middle Ear Reconstructive Surgery
F. PIRAGINE, P. BRUSCHINI, S. BERRETTINI, G. SEGNINI,
and S. SELLARI-FRANCESCHINI 193

Pharyngeal Fistulas Following Total Laryngectomy Treated
with Dilatation and Fibrin Sealant
S. SELLARI-FRANCESCHINI, G. F. MENCONI, G. SEGNINI, P. BRUSCHINI,
S. BERRETTINI, A. JANNI, C. A. ANGELETTI, and F. PIRAGINE 199

Minimally Invasive Surgery with a New Distending
Diverticuloscope and Use of Fibrin Sealing for Endoscopic Laser
Dissection of Zenker's Diverticulum
H. WEERDA and K.-H. AHRENS 206

Fibrin Sealing in Endolaryngeal Surgery
H. E. ECKEL 210

Use of Tissucol in Laryngology and in Head and Neck Surgery
M. REMACLE and G. LAWSON 218

Subject Index 225

List of Contributors

ABE, T.
Department of Neurosurgery, SHOWA University School of Medicine,
Tokyo, Japan

ACQUI, M.
Department of Neurological Sciences, Section of Neurosurgery
University of Rome "La Sapienza", Viale dell'Università 30a,
00185 Rome, Italy

AHRENS, K.-H.
Medizinische Universität zu Lübeck,
Klinik für Hals-, Nasen- und Ohrenheilkunde,
Ratzeburger Allee 160, 23562 Lübeck, Germany

ANGELETTI, A.
Unit of Thoracic Surgery, University of Pisa,
Pisa, Italy

BAGOT D'ARC, M.
E.N.T, 49 Bis Av. Franklin Roosevelt, 75008 Paris, France

BARBERÁ, J.
Department of Neurosurgery, Hospital General Universitario,
Avda. Tres Cruces s/n, 46014 Valencia, Spain

BERRETTINI, S.
Clinica Otorinolaringoiatrica,
Via Savi, 10, 56126 Pisa, Italy

BERTRAND, B.
ENT Dept., University of Louvain,
Cliniques Universitaires UCL de Mont-Godinne,
5530 Yvoir, Belgium

BRUNNER, F. X.
Universitäts-HNO-Klinik Würzburg,
Josef-Schneider-Straße 11, 97080 Würzburg, Germany

BRUSCHINI, P.
Clinica Otorinolaringoiatrica,
Via Savi, 10, 56126 Pisa, Italy

BUSCHMANN, W.
Mohnstraße 11, 97080 Würzburg, Germany

CORLIEU, P.
ENT Department, Cochin Hospital,
Paris, France

DACULSI, G.
Research Laboratory on Calcified Tissues and Biomaterials,
Nantes University, Nantes, France

DELFINI, R.
Department of Neurological Sciences, Section of Neurosurgery
University of Rome "La Sapienza", Viale dell'Università 30a,
00185 Rome, Italy

DISANT, F.
Service d'Otorhinolaryngologie et de Chirurgie Cervico-Faciale,
Pavillon U, Hôpital Edouard Herriot,
3, place d'Arsonval, 69374 Lyon, France

DOYEN, A.
ENT Dept., University of Louvain,
Cliniques Universitaires UCL de Mont-Godinne,
5530 Yvoir, Belgium

ECKEL, H. E.
Universitäts-Hals-Nasen-Ohrenklinik,
Joseph-Stelzmann-Straße 9, 50924 Köln, Germany

EDEL, G.
Gerhard Domagk-Institut für Pathologie,
Westfälische Wilhelms-Universität
Domagkstraße 17, 48149 Münster, Germany

EIRAS, J.
Neurosurgery Department, Hospital "Miguel Servet",
50009 Zaragoza, Spain

ELOY P.
ENT Dept., University of Louvain,
Cliniques Universitaires UCL de Mont-Godinne,
5530 Yvoir, Belgium

EMMERICH, K.-H.
Augenklinik, Städtische Kliniken Darmstadt,
Heidelberger Landstraße 379, 64297 Darmstadt, Germany

FERRANTE, L.
Department of Neurological Sciences, Section of Neurosurgery
University of Rome "La Sapienza", Viale dell'Università 30a,
00185 Rome, Italy

FRANK, R.
HNO-Klinik des Städtischen Klinikums Karlsruhe,
Moltkestraße 14, 76133 Karlsruhe, Germany

HAID, C. T.
Department of Oto-Rhino-Laryngology, Universität Erlangen-Nürnberg,
Waldstraße 1, 91054 Erlangen, Germany

IWATA, T.
Department of Neurosurgery, SHOWA University School of Medicine,
Tokyo, Japan

IZUMIYAMA, H.
Department of Neurosurgery, SHOWA University School of Medicine,
Tokyo, Japan

JAMART, J.
Medical Statistics Department, University of Louvain,
Cliniques Universitaires UCL de Mont-Godinne,
5530 Yvoir, Belgium

JANNI, A.
Unit of Thoracic Surgery, University of Pisa,
Pisa, Italy

JEBELES, J. A.
University ENT Hospital, Auenbruggerplatz 20,
8036 Graz, Austria

KANZAKI, J.
Dept. of Otolaryngology, School of Medicine, Keio University,
35 Shinanomachi, Shinjuku-ku, Tokyo, 160, Japan

KNÖRINGER, P.
Department of Neurosurgery,
Landeskrankenhaus, St. Veiter Straße 47, 9020 Klagenfurt, Austria

KUCHAR, A.
University Eye Clinic Vienna, Währinger Gürtel 20,
1090 Vienna, Austria

KUNII, N.
Department of Neurosurgery, SHOWA University School of Medicine,
Tokyo, Japan

LAWSON, G.
Department of O.R.L. and Head and Neck Surgery, Louvain University
Clinic at Mont-Godinne, 5530 Yvoir, Belgium

LEBLOND, J.
Service d'Otorhinolaryngologie et de Chirurgie Cervico-Faciale,
Pavillon U, Hôpital Edouard Herriot,
3, place d'Arsonval, 69374 Lyon

LUXENBERGER, W.
University ENT Hospital, Auenbruggerplatz 20,
8036 Graz, Austria

MATSUMOTO, K.
Department of Neurosurgery, SHOWA University School of Medicine,
Tokyo, Japan

MENCONI, F.
Unit of Thoracic Surgery, University of Pisa,
Pisa, Italy

MESTER, U.
Augenklinik Sulzbach der Bundesknappschaft,
An der Klinik 10, 66280 Sulzbach, Germany

MORGON, A.
Service d'Otorhinolaryngologie et de Chirurgie Cervico-Faciale,
Pavillon U, Hôpital Edouard Herriot,
3, place d'Arsonval, 69374 Lyon, France

NEUMAIER-PROBST, E.
Abteilung für Neuroradiologie, Universitäts-Krankenhaus Eppendorf,
Martinistraße 52, 20251 Hamburg, Germany

O-UCHI, T.
Dept. of Otolaryngology, School of Medicine, Keio University,
35 Shinanomachi, Shinjuku-ku, Tokyo, 160, Japan

PIRAGINE, F.
Clinica Otorinolaringoiatrica,
Via Savi, 10, 56126 Pisa, Italy

RACO, A.
Department of Neurological Sciences, Section of Neurosurgery
University of Rome "La Sapienza", Viale dell'Università 30a,
00185 Rome, Italy

RAUBER, M.
Augenklinik Sulzbach der Bundesknappschaft,
An der Klinik 10, 66280 Sulzbach, Germany

REMACLE, M.
Department of O.R.L. and Head and Neck Surgery,
Louvain University Clinic at Mont-Godinne,
5530 Yvoir, Belgium

ROMBAUX, P.
ENT Dept., University of Louvain,
Cliniques Universitaires UCL de Mont-Godinne,
5530 Yvoir, Belgium

SCHOBEL, H.
Evangelisches Krankenhaus Wien-Währing,
Wien, Austria

SCHWAB, U.
Universitäts-HNO-Klinik Würzburg,
Josef-Schneider-Straße 11, 97080 Würzburg, Germany

SEGNINI, G.
Clinica Otorinolaringoiatrica,
Via Savi, 10, 56126 Pisa, Italy

SELLARI-FRANCESCHINI, S.
Clinica Otorinolaringoiatrica,
Via Savi, 10, 56126 Pisa, Italy

SHIOBARA, R.
Dept. of Neurosurgery, School of Medicine, Keio University,
35 Shinanomachi, Shinjuku-ku, Tokyo, 160, Japan

SIEGERT, R.
Medizinische Universität zu Lübeck,
Klinik für Hals-, Nasen- und Ohrenheilkunde,
Ratzeburger Allee 160, 23562 Lübeck, Germany

SLOOFF, A.C.J.
Neurosurgical Department, Ziekenhuis DE WEVER en GREGORIUS,
Henri Dunantstraat 5, Postbus 4446,
6401 CX Heerlen, The Netherlands

STAMMBERGER, H.
Universitäts-HNO-Klinik, Auenbruggerplatz 20,
8036 Graz, Austria

STANGE, G.
HNO-Klinik des Städtischen Klinikums Karlsruhe,
Moltkestraße 14, 76133 Karlsruhe, Germany

STEINKOGLER, F.J.
2nd University Eye Clinic Vienna,
Währinger Gürtel 20, 1090 Vienna, Austria

WEERDA, H.
Medizinische Universität zu Lübeck,
Klinik für Hals-, Nasen- und Ohrenheilkunde,
Ratzeburger Allee 160, 23562 Lübeck, Germany

WESTPHAL, M.
Abteilung für Neurosurgery, Universitäts-Krankenhaus Eppendorf,
Martinistraße 52, 20251 Hamburg, Germany

WIGAND, M. E.
Department of Oto-Rhino-Laryngology, Universität Erlangen-Nürnberg,
91054 Erlangen, Germany

WOLF, S. R.
Department of Oto-Rhino-Laryngology, Universität Erlangen-Nürnberg,
91054 Erlangen, Germany

ZANELLA, F.
Abteilung für Neuroradiologie, Universitäts-Krankenhaus Eppendorf,
Martinistraße 52, 20251 Hamburg, Germany

ZEUMER, H.
Abteilung für Neuroradiologie, Universitäts-Krankenhaus Eppendorf,
Martinistraße 52, 20251 Hamburg, Germany

ZUCHE, M.
Augenklinik Sulzbach der Bundesknappschaft,
Graf-Siegfried-Straße 96, 54439 Saarburg, Germany

I. Neurosurgery

Our Experience with Human Fibrin Glue in Neurosurgical Procedures

M. ACQUI, R. DELFINI, A. RACO, and L. FERRANTE

Abstract

In the Department of Neurosurgery at La Sapienza in Rome we have been using human fibrin glue since 1986. We have always used it by simultaneously injecting the regenerated components with a thermostatic mixer. The sealant has been used in several fields of application, such as reconstruction of cranial regions, repair of cerebrospinal fluid (CSF) fistulas, sealing of vascular sutures, anastomoses of peripheral nerves, and as hemostatic adjuvant.

As to the repair of cranial regions, the product was used in transsphenoidal and transpetromastoid surgery and for the occlusion of frontal sinus, human fibrin glue being very useful to fix and amalgamate bony, fatty, and muscular tissues in the surgical procedure.

Regarding the repair of CSF fistulas, the product was utilized, after craniotomy and identification of the fistula, to reinforce the patched suture on the dural gap and to fix and amalgamate fatty, bony, and muscular tissues on the gap.

In two cases of open otoliquorrhea with serious neurosensorial hearing loss, we occluded the middle ear by filling the tympanic cavity with fibrin glue [5]. The product was also used in anastomoses of peripheral nerves after microsurgical apposition of some guiding points, thus reducing considerably the operating time for the surgical procedure. In the surgical treatment of anterior cervical myelopathy due to spondylosis we used fibrin glue in connection with heterologous bone graft.

Finally, we used fibrin glue as a hemostatic agent, particularly in cases of diffuse bleedings, which are difficult to control by bipolar coagulation.

We have used fibrin glue in about 500 surgical procedures altogether; even though we have not carried out a comparative study to evaluate its real efficacy, we believe it is very useful in the above-mentioned neurosurgical procedures, especially because of its manageability, the considerable reduction of operating time, and the reliability of the obtained seal. Moreover, we did not notice any side effects after its application. More specifically, even though we used fibrin glue made out of pools of plasma, we did not find any transfusional infections.

Introduction

Though hemostasis [2, 7] or the gluing of tissues [10, 11] with products of hematic derivation started to be reported in the literature a long time ago, the use of human fibrin glue in neurosurgical procedures has only recently been introduced [1, 8, 9]. In our department, we started using fibrin glue in 1986. It has been used in surgery of the central nervous system (particularly in the reconstruction of cranial regions) and peripheral nerves and in vascular neurosurgery.

The object of this work is to describe our experience with the intraoperative use of human fibrin glue, stressing its advantages and limitations.

Clinical Cases and Techniques

In Table 1 we list the different applications of human fibrin glue. The product, used in each case by simultaneously injecting the regenerated components with a thermostatic mixer, was employed in 520 surgical procedures. In most of the cases it was used to reconstruct cranial regions, but we also used it when diffuse bleeding occurred, in sealing the dural sutures, in surgery of CSF fistulas.

In surgery of the peripheral nerves we used human fibrin glue as a coadjuvant element of the nervous anastomoses, whereas in vascular neurosurgery we used it for sealing the vascular sutures of the neck vessels.

Discussion

Even though we did not carry out a comparative study aiming at a definite evaluation of the efficacy of human fibrin glue in the above-mentioned neurosurgical procedures, we believe this product has made an effective technical contribution to numerous fields of application in neurosurgery.

Table 1. Surgical procedures with human fibrin glue

Surgical procedure	No. of cases
Reconstruction of cranial regions	328
Transsphenoidal	210
Transpetromastoid	20
Frontal sinus	98
Neural anastomosis	44
Hemostatic coadjuvant	43
Dural closure	38
Repair of active CSF fistula	20
Use of fibrin sealant in Cloward's procedure	19
Sealing of vascular sutures	15
Miscellaneous	13

CSF, cerebrospinal fluid.

Reconstruction of Cranial Regions

In transsphenoidal and transpetromastoid surgery and in frontal approach (sinus frontalis) we employed human fibrin glue to reconstruct the bony structures which were violated in the surgical approach (sella turcica, petrosal bone, frontal bone). With this procedure it is essential to utilize bony fragments (vomer fragments are very useful in transsphenoidal surgery) and muscular and adipose tissues. Human fibrin glue, which has to be used in an operating site as dry as possible, is useful only to amalgamate the employed tissues and to promote their reactive fibrosis. In transsphenoidal surgery, human fibrin glue has helped to reduce the incidence of CSF fistulas from 9% to 1.5%.

Anastomoses of Peripheral Nerves

In nervous anastomoses we used fibrin glue (after the perineural interfascicular apposition of stitches) by applying a small quantity around the sutured surfaces. This technique allowed us to form a delicate connective pellicle around the sutured stumps, thus replacing the removed epineurium for the execution of the neurorrhaphies. In relation to the short fibrinolytic activity of the nervous tissue, we diluted the solution of aprotinin to 100 kIU/ml.

Complex Hemostasis

Human fibrin glue proved very useful in some cases of procedures involving extensive bleeding. It was very helpful as a hemostatic agent in partial resections of highly vascularized lesions. In such cases, pathological vascularization of the lesion results in considerable bleeding, and even with the help of an operating microscope it is quite difficult to identify the bleeding vessels. In such cases we applied fibrin glue to the bleeding surface, thus obtaining a more or less immediate hemostasis.

Furthermore, we used human fibrin glue during the closure of supratentorial craniotomies and subtentorial craniectomies to arrest residual extradural oozings which were still present after the application of stitches for dural suspensions.

Dural Closure

A waterproof dural closure depends mainly on a suture made with separate or continuous stitches. The use of fibrin glue seemed helpful to further reinforce the suture.

We also used it together with Surgicel and Gelfoam for cases in which a little gap remained after the closure. If this gap was larger, we used fibrin glue, alone or with a suture, to fix a patch of lyophilized dura mater sterilized by gamma rays [3].

Repair of Cerebrospinal Fluid Fistulas

In the surgical treatment of CSF fistulas we need a correct surgical approach to the fistula, good surgical visualization, and its occlusion by biological materials such as patches of lyophilized dura mater sterilized by gamma rays, vital fragments of succedanea of the dura (fragments of fascia lata, fragments of pericranium etc.), and muscular, bony, or adipose tissue.

Similar to the closure of surgical approaches, fibrin glue is utilized here to amalgamate the tissues used to occlude the fistula and to promote a fibrotic reaction.

In some specific cases, however, fibrin glue played a crucial role in closing CSF fistulas. In fact we used this product during a surgical procedure to occlude open post-surgical otoliquorrheas. This potentially life-threatening complication occurred in two patients operated on for a jugular chemodectoma and for a neurinoma of the acoustic nerve. We closed the fistula by simply filling with fibrin glue the tympanic cavity of an ear with severe neurosensorial hearing loss. Six years after the operation, we did not observe any relapses of the otoliquorrhea.

We believe that this procedure is suitable for cases of open or closed otoliquorrhea (in the latter after tympanotomy), in patients with neurosensorial hearing loss when the fistula does not have a phlogistic etiology.

Sealing of Vascular Sutures in Surgery of the Neck Vessels

In carotid endoarteriectomy, once the microsurgical sutures of the carotid have been completed, we used about 2 ml fibrin glue to reinforce the suture and to prevent any residual hematic oozing.

Conclusions

Even though the lack of a comparative study prevents us from drawing any definite conclusions about the real efficacy of human fibrin glue in neurosurgery, it has nonetheless proved very useful in reducing surgery time.

However, the efficacy of this product is directly related to the correct performance of the surgical procedure in which it is used.

The risk of transmission of diseases from blood derivatives, though remote, is a real one. However, it can be completely avoided by using autologous fibrin glue [4].

References

1 Armenise B, Montinaro A (1985) The prevention of nasal liquorrhea caused by transsphenoidal surgery for pituitary adenomas. J Neurosurg Sci 29: 57–59
2 Bergel S (1909) Über Wirkungen des Fibrins. Dtsch Med Wochenschr 35: 633–655
3 Cantore G, Guidetti B, Delfini R (1987) Neurosurgical use of human dura mater sterilized by gamma rays and stored in alcohol: long-term results. J Neurosurg 66: 93–95
4 Epstein GH, Weisman RA, Zwillenberg S, Schreiber AD (1986) A new autologous fibrinogen-based adhesive for otologic surgery. Ann Otol Rhinol Laryngol 95: 40–45
5 Ferrante L, Palatinsky E, Acqui M, Mastronardi L (1988) Endaural extracranial repair for cerebrospinal otorrhoea with human fibrin glue: technical note. Neurol Neurosurg Psy 51: 1438–1440
6 Fortuna A, Palatinsky E, Di Lorenzo N (1988) Anterior cervical arthrodesis with heterologous bone graft and human fibrin glue in the surgical treatment of myelopathy due to spondylosis. Clin Neurol Neurosurg 90: 125–129
7 Harvey SC (1916) Hemostatic glue in parenchymatous organs. Boston Med Surg J 174: 659–662
8 Liguori R, Delgazio S, Fusco G, De Bellis M (1984) "Tissucol" in spinal surgery. J Neurosurg Sci 28: 187–190
9 Parenti G, Lenzi B (1983) Use of fibrin glue in termino-lateral anastomoses for extra-intracranial by-pass. Acta Neurochir (Wien) 73: 100–101
10 Seddom HJ (1944) Early management of peripheral nerve injuries. Practitioner 152: 101–107
11 Seddom HJ, Medawar PB (1942) Fibrin suture of human nerves. Lancet 2: 87–92

New Trends in Enlarged Middle Cranial Fossa Surgery

C. T. Haid, S. R. Wolf, and M. E. Wigand

Abstract

Utilizing the enlarged middle cranial fossa approach, the authors have operated on 539 patients since 1975 until 1992. With this approach it is possible to perform different otoneurosurgical interventions, e.g., total removal of small, medium-sized, and large acoustic neurinomas (extrameatal diameter of up to 3–4 cm), neurectomy of the vestibular nerve in patients with Menière's disease, neurovascular decompression in patients with hemifacial spasm or Menière's disease, decompression or grafting of the facial nerve or repair of a cerebrospinal fluid fistula in patients with a fracture of the petrous bone, and removal of pseudotumours in patients with a cholesterol granuloma or cholesteatoma. Considering special trends such as operative techniques (e.g., fibrin glue), special microinstruments, intraoperative monitoring, and computer-assisted surgery (CAS), highly successful treatment (function-preserving surgery) with a low complication rate can be performed.

Introduction

The pioneer in micro-otoneurosurgery of the middle cranial fossa approach to the internal auditory canal was William House in the early 1960s. With the enlarged middle cranial fossa approach it is possible to perform different neurosurgical interventions [9, 10, 26, 27], e.g., total removal of small and large acoustic neurinomas, neurectomy of the vestibular nerve (e.g., Menière's disease), neurovascular decompression (e.g., hemifacial spasm, Menière's disease), decompression or grafting of the facial nerve or repair of a cerebrospinal fluid fistula (fracture of the petrous bone), and removal of pseudotumours (cholesterol granuloma, cholesteatoma). Considering special trends (e.g., operative techniques, microinstruments, intraoperative monitoring, CAS) in the enlarged middle cranial fossa surgery, a function-preserving surgery with a low complication rate is possible.

Material and Methods

From 1975 until 1992, 539 middle cranial fossa surgeries were performed at the Ear, Nose, and Throat (ENT) Department at the University of Erlangen (Table 1). In most cases patients suffering from an acoustic neurinoma were treated (355 cases, including unilateral and bilateral neurinomas). In 110 patients with Menière's disease who had no response to conservative therapy and who were suffering from intractable vertigo attacks, a neurectomy of the vestibular nerve, in many cases combined with simultaneous neurovascular decompression of the eighth cranial nerve, was carried out. There was no predominance of one sex over the other or of one side over the other. The mean age was 49 years. The youngest patient was 16 years old, and the oldest 83.

The enlarged middle cranial fossa approach, in general anesthesia, starts with a temporal skin incision forming a caudally pedicled flap over the sleeve with the root of the zygomatic arch in its center. The temporal muscle is transsected by a Y-shaped incision. An osteoplastic craniotomy of 4 × 5 cm is performed. Important landmarks can be utilized: the "grey line" of the superior semicircular canal (below the eminentia arcuata) and the superior petrosal nerve, which together form an angle of about 130°. Bisectioning of this angle usually corresponds to the axis of the internal auditory canal. Enlarged middle cranial fossa surgery consists in ample bone resection, using a diamond burr in front of, above, and behind the internal auditory canal. The otoneurosurgeon has to be very careful not to injure the cochlea, the labyrinth or the Fallopian canal with the facial nerve. It can be of great advantage to use a CAS system [22] even in middle cranial fossa surgery [11]; this is a computer-supported imaging technique which offers new possibilities of three-dimensional orientation in the surgery field in real time. This equipment (Storz, Tuttlingen, Germany) consists of a mechanical arm with a digitizer, which is easily maneuverable with an exact reliable function. Using the information processed by the CAS system and represented by images on the computer screen, a rapid intraoperative and confident recognition of anatomical landmarks in the middle cranial fossa is possible (e.g., superior semicircular canal, internal auditory canal, cochlea, cerebellopontine angle; Figs. 1–4). As a protection for the temporal lobe, it is

Table 1. Diagnosis of enlarged middle cranial fossa surgery ($n = 539$)

Diagnosis	No. of cases
Acoustic neurinoma	355
Menière's disease	110
Meningioma	14
Fracture of the petrous bone	13
Cholesteatoma	12
Facial neurinoma	8
Cochleovestibular insufficiency	7
Hemifacial spasm	5
Lipoma	2
Other diagnosis	13

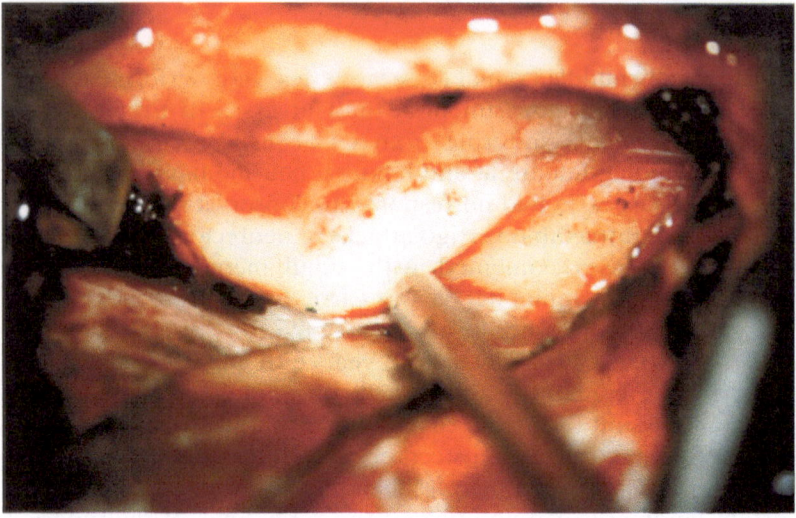

Fig. 1. Beginning of the enlarged middle cranial fossa approach of a patient (57 years, male) with an acoustic neurinoma on the left side. The digitizer of the CAS system (computer-assisted surgery) is located on the supposed superior semicircular canal. The visible petrosal nerve and the grey line are important anatomical landmarks

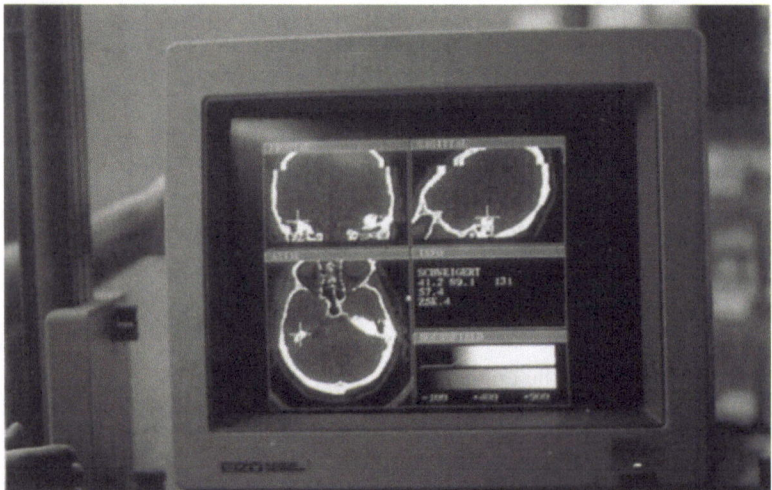

Fig. 2. Same patient as in Fig. 1; this shows the intraoperative result of the computer-assisted surgery (CAS) system on a computer screen. The tip of the digitizer shows the anatomical position (superior semicircular canal) in three dimensions (frontal, sagittal, and axial axis) in real time on the computer screen in the form of a *cross*

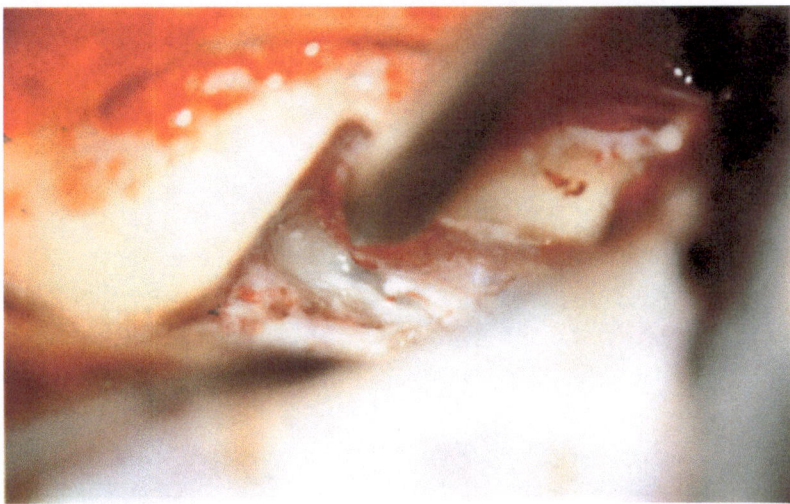

Fig. 3. Enlarged middle cranial fossa approach on the left side of the same patient as in Figs. 1 and 2 shows the digitizer of the computer-assisted surgery (CAS) system placed on the dura of the internal auditory meatus

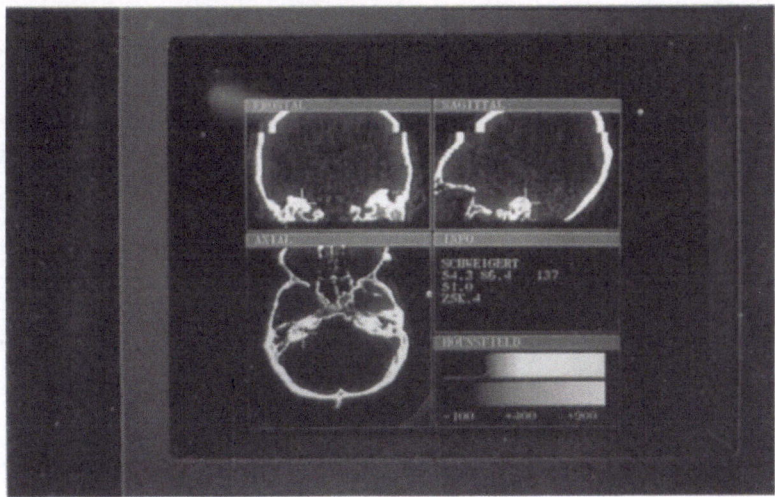

Fig. 4. Same patient as in Figs. 1–3; this demonstrates the intraoperative results of the computer-assisted surgery (CAS) system on a computer screen. The tip of the digitizer shows the anatomical position (internal auditory meatus) in three dimensions in real time on the computer screen in the form of a cross

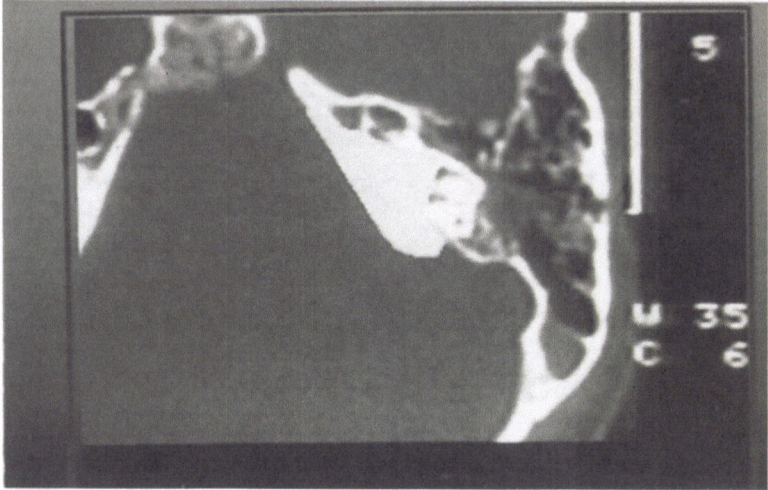

Fig. 5. Computerized tomography (CT) demonstrates the bony area which has to be removed in the enlarged middle cranial fossa approach (white field)

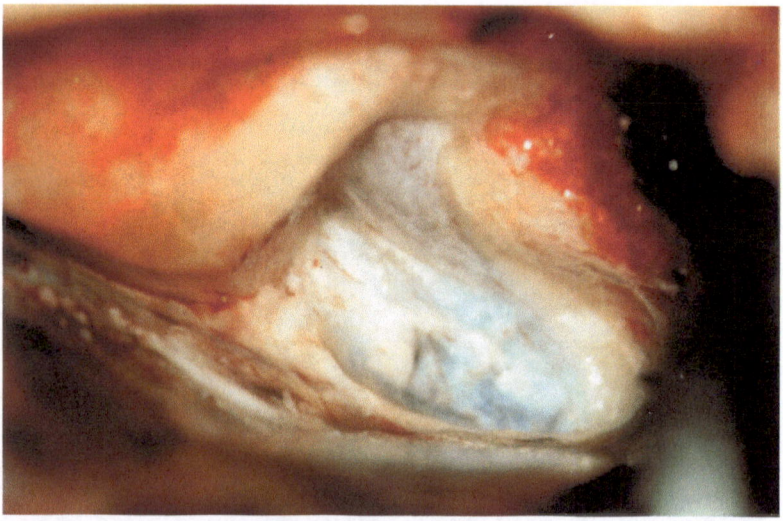

Fig. 6. Photograph taken during enlarged middle cranial fossa surgery shows the exposed dura of the internal auditory meatus and the cerebellar dura of a patient (42 years, male) with Menière's disease on the left side

advantageous to use a duraretractor with our self-developed rubber cover, which can be filled with air by the use of a syringe (Leibinger, Freiburg, Germany). Thus the mechanical pressure to the brain can be reduced. By a large excision of the petrous bone, a broad exposure into the internal auditory canal, the cerebellopontine angle, and the brain stem can be achieved (Figs. 5–7). Thus it is possible not only to remove small and medium-sized acoustic neurinomas, but also large tumours totally (Figs. 8, 9) to a size of up to 3–4 cm. The trigeminal nerve may often be visible in large acoustic neurinomas using this approach. In cases of large neurinomas, the middle meningeal artery and the superior petrosal sinus are usually resected for additional mobilization of both the temporal and the cerebellar dura blades.

In patients with Menière's disease, a neurectomy of the superior and inferior vestibular nerves and simultaneous neurovascular decompression of the eighth cranial nerve on the diseased side were usually performed by the enlarged middle cranial fossa approach (Figs. 10, 11). Frequently contacts, where considerable compression was suspected, were visualized between greater arteries (vascular loops) or veins with the eighth cranial nerve, either near the brain stem (root entry zone), in the region of the porus acusticus internus, or more laterally inside the internal auditory meatus. Such contact points were cushioned with a synthetic piece (e.g., Teflon) and/or fascia tissue [10, 16]. Strangulations of the vascular–neural bundle were also seen to be caused by

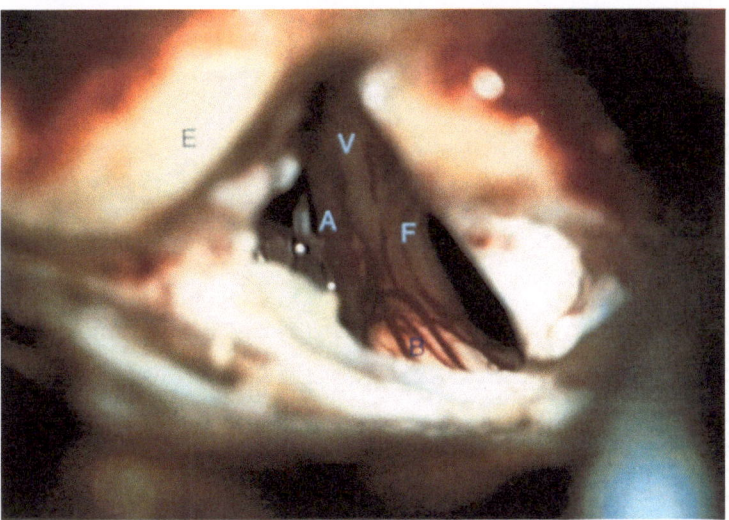

Fig. 7. Photograph taken during surgery of the same patient as in Fig. 6 demonstrates the broad surgical exposure of the enlarged middle cranial fossa approach before neurectomy of the vestibular nerve and neurovascular decompression. Excellent identification is possible of the seventh and eighth cranial nerves from the fundus of the internal auditory meatus and the cerebellopontine angle to their root entry zone in the brain stem. *A*, artery; *B*, brain stem; *E*, eminentia arcuata with the grey line of the superior semicircular canal; *F*, facial nerve; *V*, vestibular nerve (superior branch)

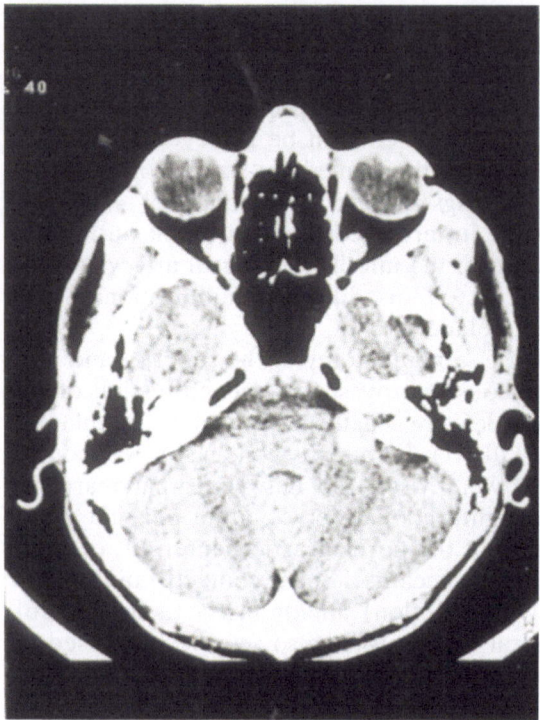

Fig. 8. Computerized tomography (CT) of a patient (27 years, male) demonstrates an acoustic neurinoma in the cerebellopontine angle on the left side

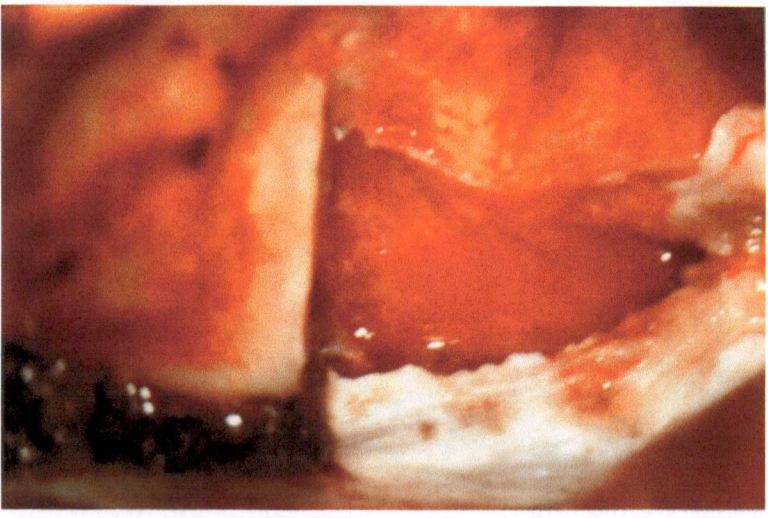

Fig. 9. Photograph taken during surgery of the same patient as in Fig. 8 shows the enlarged middle cranial fossa approach on the left side. The acoustic neurinoma has a large extension from the fundus of the internal auditory canal into the cerebellopontine angle. The tumour was removed totally. Postoperatively, the function of the facial nerve was absolutely normal (House I) and even the hearing function could be preserved

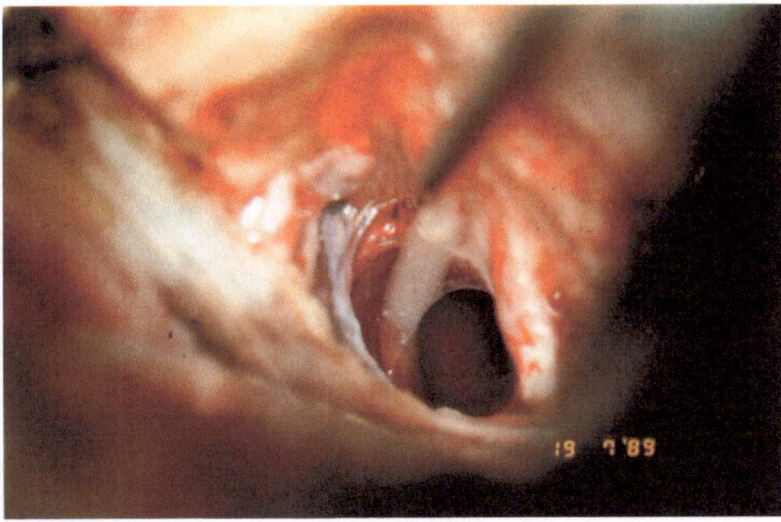

Fig. 10. Broad surgical exposure of the enlarged middle cranial fossa approach of a patient (24 years, male) with Menière's disease on the left side. With an instrument the facial nerve is carefully mobilized from the vestibular nerve. A vessel loop (artery) is located between the superior vestibular nerve and the facial nerve

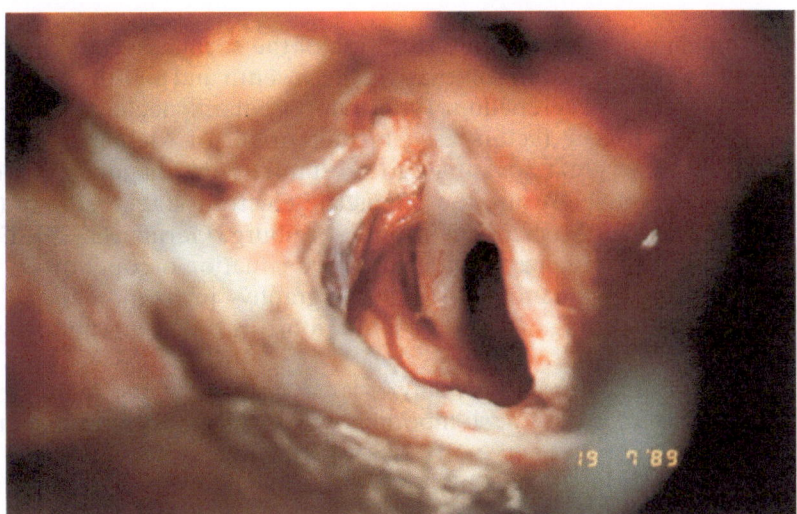

Fig. 11. Same patient as in Fig. 10; this shows the situation after neurectomy of the superior and inferior vestibular nerves and after neurovascular decompression of the eighth cranial nerve (with a piece of Teflon) by the enlarged middle cranial fossa approach on the left side. The root entry zone of the seventh and eighth cranial nerves and the brain stem are visible. The intractable vertigo attacks disappeared postoperatively

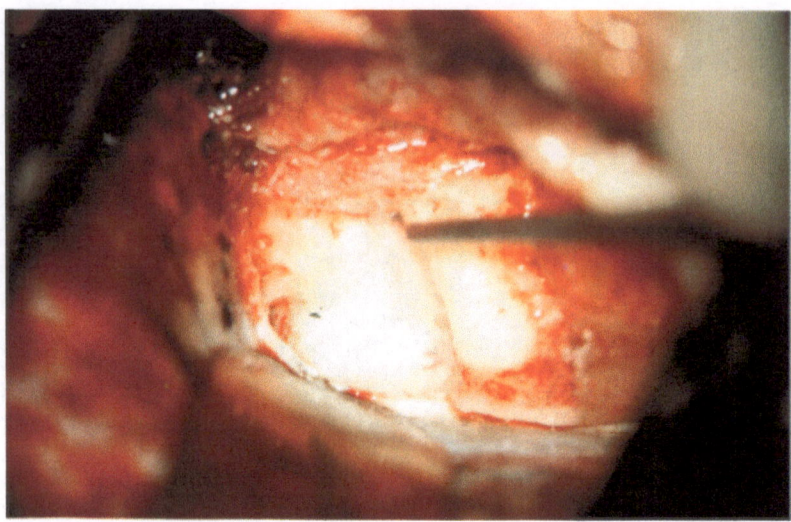

Fig. 12. By a middle cranial fossa approach a facial nerve decompression is performed on a patient (23 years, male) with a fracture of the petrous bone and a paralysis of the seventh cranial nerve (House VI) on the right side. The seventh cranial nerve has been decompressed from its tympanal course, the geniculate ganglion including the Fallopian canal and dura of the internal auditory meatus. An instrument points to the Fallopian canal. Postoperatively there was a House III 1 year after surgery

taut arachnoidal tissue with dislocation of the cochlear-vestibular nerve, which had to be eliminated. In some cases, the seventh and eighth cranial nerves were dislocated by the cerebellum (vestibulofloccular synechia). These facts could be possible trigger factors as a further origin of Menière's disease. Before surgery, it is of great advantage to substantiate the diagnosis of Menière's disease preoperatively using the telemetric electronystagmography (ENG; Nystagman, Madaus Medizin Elektronik, Freiburg, Germany) [29]. Furthermore, it is possible to visualize the neurovascular situation preoperatively with the aid of magnetic resonance (MR) angiography in combination with three-dimensional imaging without the use of ionizing radiation (noninvasive method [1]).

Moreover, even extradurally located diseases of the middle cranial fossa can be treated by the transtemporal approach, e.g., decompression (Fig. 12) or grafting of the facial nerve or repair of an extensive cerebrospinal fluid fistula in fracture of the petrous bone (Figs. 13, 14) and removal of pseudotumours (e.g., cholesteatoma; Figs. 15–17).

After finishing the surgery in the internal auditory canal and the cerebello-pontine angle, the dural flaps are replaced. One or two layers of free muscle fascia flaps together with fibrin glue (Tissucol, Immuno, Heidelberg, Germany) produce a waterproof and airproof safe reconstruction of the dural defect above the internal auditory canal and over the cerebellopontine angle. The extradural space below the craniotomy is filled with Gelfoam soaked in fibrin glue instead of fixation of the dura by sutures. A complete hemostasis

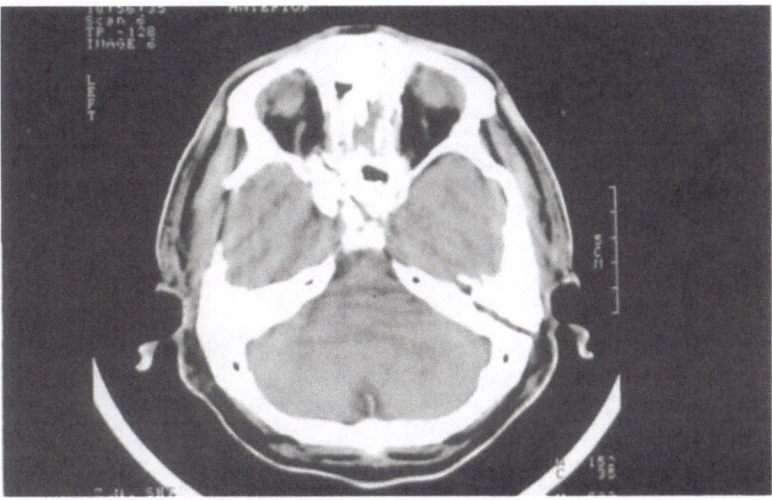

Fig. 13. Computerized tomography (CT) of a patient (35 years, male) shows an extended fracture of the petrous bone on the right side reaching the anterior fossa

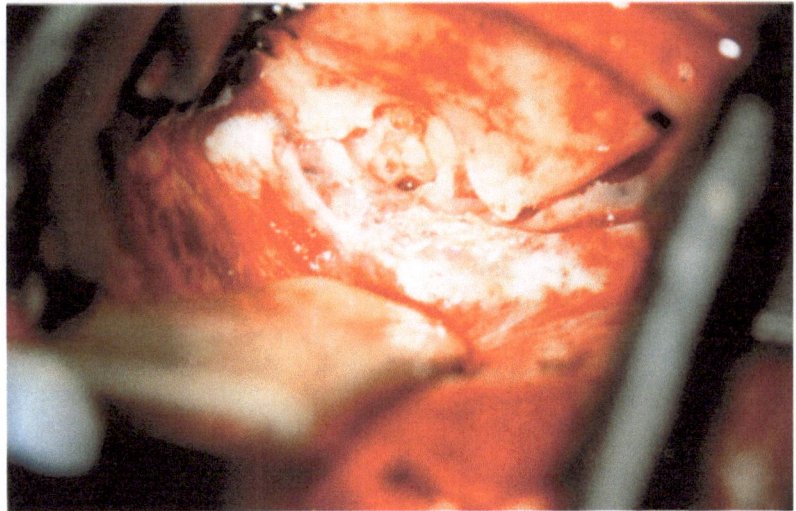

Fig. 14. Photograph taken during surgery of the same patient as in Fig. 13 via the middle cranial fossa shows in the *center* a bone fracture and on the *right side* a longitudinal fracture. In the *center*, the duraretractor with a rubber cover filled with air (on the surface next to the dura as a protection) is visible. The dura was injured. The cerebrospinal fluid fistula was covered with a piece of fascia. A waterproof and airproof closure could be achieved with fibrin glue. Furthermore, the facial nerve was grafted. The neurophysiological tests (electromyography, EMG; transcranial magnetic facial nerve stimulation) showed an early reinnervation of the ipsilateral facial muscles, which we expect to improve within another 9 months

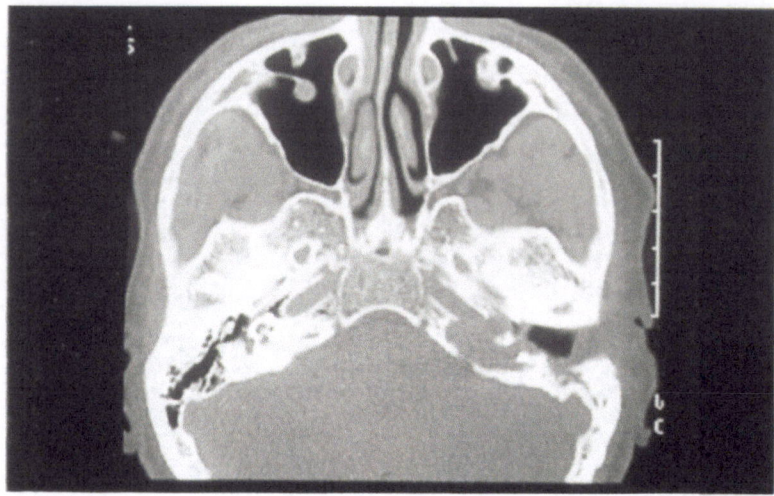

Fig. 15. Computerized tomography (CT) of a patient (36 years, male) shows a cholesteatoma in the petrous bone on the right side with an extension into the middle cranial fossa and to the cranial part of the internal carotid artery

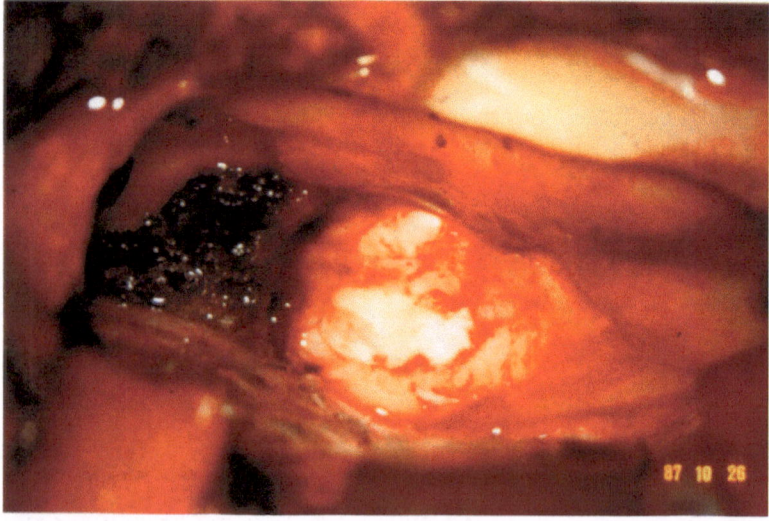

Fig. 16. Extension of the cholesteatoma *(white mass)* of the same patient as in Fig. 15 in the middle cranial fossa during surgery via the transtemporal approach on the right side is visible

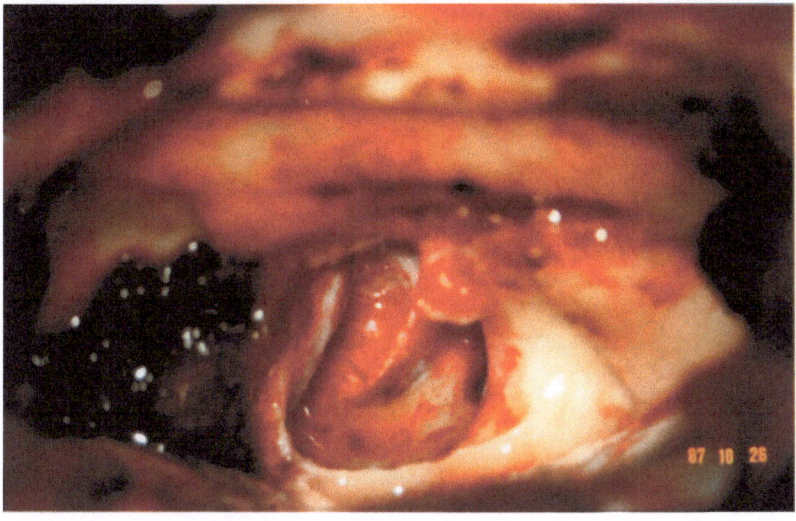

Fig. 17. Surgery in the same patient as in Figs. 15 and 16 after removal of the cholesteatoma by the middle cranial fossa approach on the right side; the cholesteatoma had a connection to the cranial part of the internal carotid artery, the geniculate ganglion, the dura of the anterior part of the internal auditory meatus, and in the depth to the jugular bulb

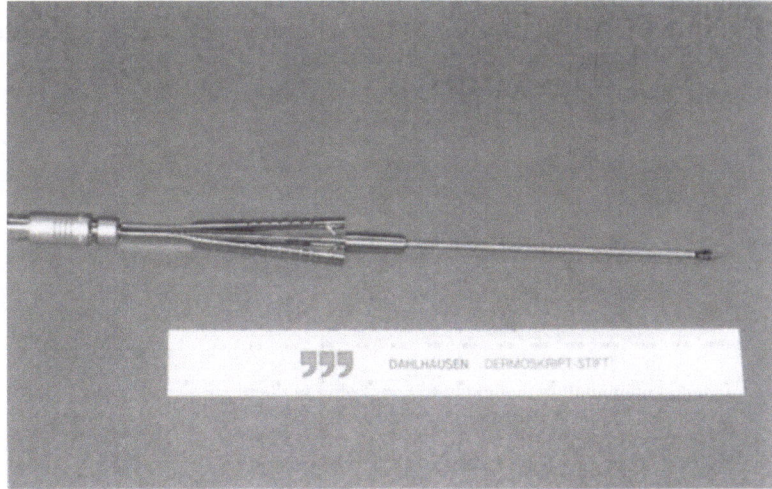

Fig. 18. A specially developed bipolar microelectrocauter, which makes it possible to deal with a hemorrhage close to important anatomical structures

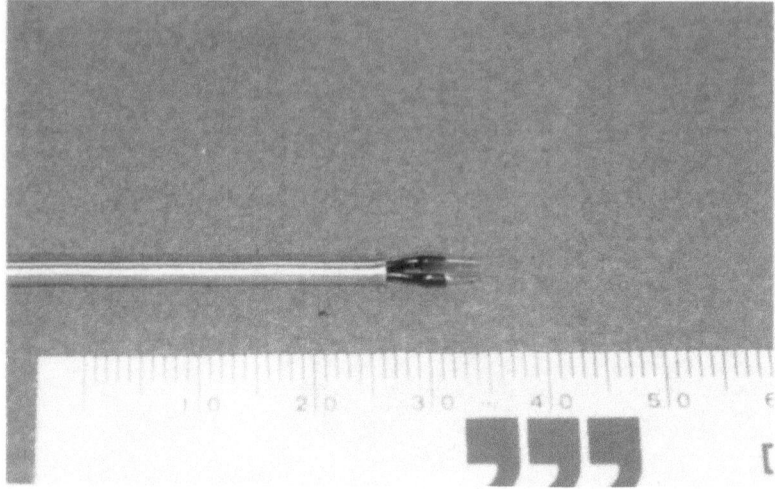

Fig. 19. Same equipment as in Fig. 18 (bipolar microelectrocauter)

during surgery is extremely important. Using Gelfoam soaked in fibrin glue or collagen fleece (Tissuvlies, Immuno, Heidelberg, Germany), hemorrhages can be controlled. In the case of a hemorrhage very close to cranial nerves (e.g., the facial nerve) or other important anatomical structures, a special microelec-trocauter has been developed ([7]; Figs. 18, 19; Leibinger, Freiburg, Germany). The bone flap is refixed by Vicryl sutures and bone paté together with fibrin glue. After the suture of the temporal muscle, a Redon drain has to be inserted. The surgery is finished by a double-layer skin suture. The patient stays for approximately 2–3 days in intensive care.

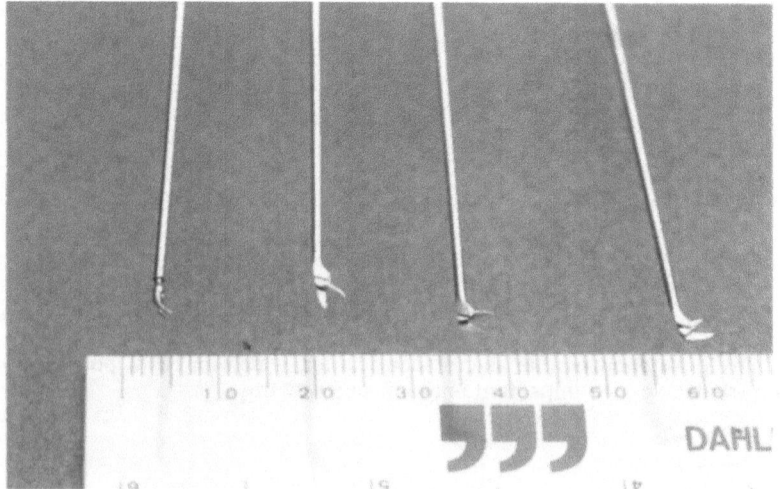

Fig. 20. Microscissors in a range of different angles

It is very advantageous to use special microinstruments (Fig. 20) and to perform intraoperative monitoring of the seventh and eighth cranial nerves (brain stem auditory evoked potentials, BAEP, for hearing preservation, and direct electrical facial nerve stimulation and transcranial magnetic facial nerve stimulation for the function of the facial nerve).

In summary, special trends (intraoperative, pre- and postoperative) in enlarged middle cranial fossa surgery can consist in usage of: (a) operative technique; (b) intraoperative monitoring; (c) special microinstruments; (d) CAS; (e) MR angiography (noninvasive method); (f) telemetric ENG.

Results

Enlarged middle cranial fossa surgery is quite a difficult approach, but the complication rate can be described as very low (Table 2). In a series of 539 surgeries, there was a mortality rate of 0.4%. Two patients with an acoustic neurinoma died, one because of an acute postoperative hemorrhage and the second because of a general anesthesia problem. Three more patients with acute hemorrhages and three intraoperative bleedings could be taken care of without any neurological disturbances. Overall, the percentage rate of meningitis (3.1%), cerebrospinal fluid fistula (1.7% requiring surgery), secondary wound healing (2.2% requiring surgery), and neurological deficits were quite low. Some patients (5.6%) developed a temporary cerebral disorientation or speech difficulty (especially in case of surgery on the left side) over a period of a few days (Table 3).

Eight patients presented with a single epileptic seizure during the first postoperative month without any recurrence (1.5%). A few patients (5.4%) complained of severe headaches after surgery. An iatrogenic lesion (Table 3) of the facial nerve occurred in four patients (0.7%) and of the inner ear or the eighth cranial nerve in nine patients (1.7%).

In the following chapter, a short comment concerning the results of acoustic neurinoma surgery, of neurectomy, and neurovascular decompression in patients with Menière's disease will be presented.

Table 2. Complications in enlarged middle cranial fossa surgery ($n = 539$)

Complication	Cases	
	(n)	(%)
Mortality[a]	2	0.4
Acute hemorrhage	6	1.1
Brain edema	11	2.0
Hydrocephalus (transitory)	2	0.4
Meningitis	22	3.1
CSF fistula (surgery necessary)	9	1.7
Secondary wound healing (surgery necessary)	12	2.2

CSF, cerebrospinal fluid.
[a] One due to acute hemorrhage and one due to general anesthesia problems.

Table 3. Possible symptoms following the enlarged middle cranial fossa approach ($n = 539$)

Symptoms[a]	Cases	
	(*n*)	(%)
Transitory stage	30	5.6
Cerebral seizure (transitory)	8	1.5
Cephalgia (severe)	29	5.4
Lesion of the trigeminal nerve	10	1.9
Lesion of the abducent nerve	0	0
Iatrogenic lesion of the facial nerve	4	0.7
Iatrogenic lesion of the inner ear or the eighth cranial nerve	9	1.7
Lesion of the caudal cranial nerves	0	0
Dryness of the eye (severe)	45	8.3

[a] Multiple occurrence of symptoms possible.

In 310 unilateral acoustic neurinomas, a total tumour removal was achieved in 97 % of the cases. The mortality rate was 0.6 %. The facial nerve could be preserved anatomically in 98.7 %. In all cases there was a House I and a House II in 78 % of the cases 1 year or more after surgery. In small and medium-sized tumours this percentage climbed to 90 %. A late poor functional and cosmetic facial nerve function occurred only in 6 % (House VI). The cochlear nerve could be preserved anatomically in 78 % of the cases. In some cases this nerve had to be sacrificed because of tumor infiltration. It was possible to preserve the hearing function in about 50 % of all patients that had a preoperative hearing function and there was a close relationship between the size of the tumor, the preoperative hearing level, and the success of postoperative hearing preservation.

Neurectomy of the vestibular nerve and especially neurectomy combined with simultaneous neurovascular decompression in patients with Menière's disease ($n = 110$) have achieved a particularly high success rate in stopping intractable vertigo attacks ($> 95 \%$). The hearing function remained mostly unchanged. A total loss of the hearing function occurred postoperatively in 8 %. In these cases the pure tone thresholds usually showed preoperatively a hearing loss of 60 dB or worse. In more than 40 % of the patients, tinnitus decreased or even disappeared and the feeling of fullness in the ear usually disappeared. The vestibular compensation after neurectomy of the superior and inferior vestibular nerves (patients with acoustic neurinoma or Menière's disease) was very satisfactory. Only 8 % of the patients showed a reduced vestibular compensation in the vestibular examination.

Discussion

There are different approaches used to treat pathological structures in the cerebellopontine angle and internal auditory meatus, e.g., the middle cranial fossa approach [13], the translabyrinthine approach [6, 14, 25], the transcochlear approach [15], the retrolabyrinthine approach [12, 23], the transotic approach [5, 17], the retrosigmoid approach [24], and the suboccipital approach [2–4, 19–21]. Using the so-called enlarged middle cranial fossa approach [9, 26], a modification of the transtemporal approach, the surgeon can achieve an excellent exposure of the middle cranial fossa, the internal auditory canal, the cerebellopontine angle, and the brain stem.

The advantages of this procedure are unique: excellent exposure of the fundus, internal auditory meatus, porus acusticus internus, cerebellopontine angle to the brain stem; good identification of the facial nerve, cochlear nerve, superior and inferior vestibular nerves, retractor in extradural position; and avoidance of compression to the cerebellum. Using the enlarged middle cranial fossa approach, it is possible to perform many different otoneurosurgical interventions (Figs. 8–17):

1. Total removal of small, medium-sized, and large acoustic neurinomas with an extrameatal diameter of up to 3–4 cm
2. Neurovascular decompression [8, 16] in patients with hemifacial spasm or Menière's disease and/or neurectomy of the vestibular nerve in patients with Menière's disease; furthermore, treatment of extradurally located diseases of the middle cranial fossa
3. Decompression or grafting of the facial nerve
4. Repair of an extensive cerebrospinal fluid fistula in fracture of the petrous bone
5. Removal of pseudotumours such as cholesterol granulomas or penetrating cholesteatomas.

The enlarged middle cranial fossa approach constitutes function-preserving surgery. Using some special developments intraoperatively, the complication rate can be quite low and the success of surgery very high. These developments consist in usage of: (a) special surgical techniques, e.g., fibrin glue (management of hemorrhage, waterproof and airproof closure of the surgery field [7]; (b) special microinstruments (microelectrocauter, microscissors in different angles); (c) intraoperative monitoring of the seventh and eighth cranial nerves [18, 28]; and (d) a CAS system [22], consisting in rapid and confident intraoperative recognition of anatomical landmarks (surgical navigation) in the middle cranial fossa [11].

Our technique of choice to treat pathological structures in the region of the middle cranial fossa, internal auditory meatus, and cerebellopontine angle is the enlarged middle cranial fossa approach. It allows function-preserving surgery of the facial nerve, cochlear nerve, and cerebral structures with an extremely low postoperative complication rate (Tables 2, 3).

Acknowledgements. This work was supported by the J. and F. Marohn Foundation.

References

1. Cidlinsky K, Stenglein C, Braun M (1992) Neurovaskuläre Kompression des VIII. Hirnnerven: direkte Darstellung durch MR-Angiographie. Klin Neuroradiol 1: 6
2. Cushing H (1917) Tumors of the nervus acousticus and the syndrome of the cerebello-pontine angle. Saunders, Philadelphia
3. Dandy WF (1925) An operation for the total removal of cerebello-pontine (acoustic) tumors. Surg Gynecol Obstet 16: 1299
4. Fahlbusch R, Strauss C, Romstöck C (1991) The advantage of intraoperative monitoring in acoustic neurinoma surgery. In: Haid CT (ed) Vestibular diagnosis and neuro-otosurgical management of the skull base. Demeter, Gräfelfing, p 37
5. Fisch U (1989) Transotic approach for acoustic neuroma. In: Fisch U, Valavanis A, Yasargil MG (eds) Neurological surgery of the ear and skull base. Kugler and Ghedini, Amsterdam, p 185
6. Glasscock ME, Kveton JF, Jackson CG, Levine SC, McKennan KX (1986) A systematic approach to the surgical management of acoustic neuroma. Laryngoscope 96: 1088
7. Haid CT (1992) Behandlung von traumatisch und operativ bedingten Liquorfisteln im Bereich der mittleren Schädelgrube. In: Freigang B, Weerda H (eds) Fibrinklebung in der Otorhinolaryngologie. Springer, Berlin Heidelberg New York, p 81
8. Haid CT, Wigand ME (1991) Experiences with neurectomy of the vestibular nerve and neurolysis of the 8th cranial nerve in Menière's disease. Annal report, sponsorship of Ministry of Health and Welfare, Japan, p 26
9. Haid CT, Wigand ME (1992) Advantages of the enlarged middle cranial fossa approach in acoustic neurinoma surgery. Acta Otolaryngol (Stockh) 112: 387
10. Haid CT, Wigand ME, Berg M (1985) Results of vestibular nerve section and neurolysis of the eighth cranial nerve in Menière's disease. Elsevier Science (Biomedical Division), Amsterdam: New dimension in otolaryngology. Head Neck Surg 2: 35
11. Haid CT, Christ P, Wolf SR, Klimek L (1992) First experiences with computer assisted surgery (CAS-System) in the middle cranial fossa. Lecture to the Prosper Menière' Society in Aspen/USA, Feb 1992
12. Hitselberger WE, Pulec JL (1972) Trigeminal nerve (posterior root) retrolabyrinthine selective section: operative procedure for intractable pain. Arch Otolaryngol 96: 412
13. House WF (1961) Surgical exposure of the internal auditory canal and its contents through the middle cranial fossa. Laryngoscope 71: 1963
14. House WF (1963) Middle cranial fossa approach to petrous pyramid: report of 50 cases. Arch Otolaryngol 78: 460
15. House WF, Hitselberger WE (1976) The transcochlear approach to the skull base. Arch Otolaryngol 102: 334
16. Jannetta PJ (1980) Neurovascular compression in cranial nerve and systemic disease. Ann Surg 192: 518
17. Jenkins HA, Fisch U (1980) Approach for resection of difficult acoustic tumors of the cerebello-pontine angle. Am J Otol 2: 70
18. Lenarz T, Ernst A, Plinkert PK (1992) Intraoperative facial nerve monitoring in the infratemporal fossa approach. Lecture, 7th international symposium on the facial nerve, Cologne 1992
19. Olivecrona H (1940) Acoustic tumors. J Neurol Neurosurg Psychiatr 3: 141
20. Rand RW, Kurze T (1967) Microneurosurgery in acoustic tumors (suboccipital transmeatal approach). Trans Am Acad Ophthalmol Otolaryngol 71: 682
21. Samii M, Penkert G (1984) Gesichtsnerven- und Hörfunktionserhaltung bei mikrochirurgischen Akustikusneurinom-Operationen. Acta Neurol 39: 11
22. Schlöndorff G, Mösges R, Meyer-Ebrecht D, Krybus W, Adams L (1987) CAS (Computer assisted surgery). Ein neuartiges Verfahren in der Kopf- und Halschirurgie. HNO 37: 187

23. Silverstein H, Norell H (1982) Retrolabyrinthine total vestibular neurectomy. In: Brackmann DE (ed) Neurosurgical surgery of the ear and skull base. Raven, New York, p 303
24. Sterkers JM (1981) Retrosigmoid approach for preservation of hearing in early acoustic neuroma surgery. In: Samii M, Jannetta PJ (eds) The cranial nerves. Springer, Berlin Heidelberg New York, p 579
25. Tos M, Thomsen J (1982) The price of preservation of hearing in acoustic neuroma surgery. Ann Otol Rhinol Laryngol 91: 240
26. Wigand ME, Haid CT, Berg M, Rettinger G (1982) The enlarged transtemporal approach to the cerebello-pontine angle; technique and indications. Acta Otorhinolaryngol (Ital) 2: 571
27. Wigand ME, Haid CT, Berg M (1989) The enlarged middle cranial fossa approach for surgery of the temporal bone and the cerebello-pontine angle. Arch Otorhinolaryngol 246: 299
28. Wolf SR, Schneider W, Hofman M, Haid CT, Wigand ME (1993) Intraoperatives Monitoring des Fazialisnervs bei der transtemporalen Chirurgie des Akustikusneurinoms. HNO 41: 179
29. Wolf SR, Christ P, Haid CT (1993) Patient use of telemetric ENG to register nystagmus in the private sphere. Laryngoscope 103, 704

Prevention and Treatment of Cerebrospinal Fluid Rhinorrhea Following Transsphenoidal Surgery on Pituitary Gland Adenomas

J. Eiras

Abstract

We used fibrin sealant in 26 cases of pituitary adenomas operated on by the transsphenoidal route to prevent or to treat cerebrospinal fluid (CSF) rhinorrheas.

In 22 cases fibrin glue was instilled in the sellar cavity after the removal of the tumor as a "preventive sealing", avoiding plugging the cavity with muscle or fat. Bone fragments were replaced and glued with fibrin. In one case, transient rhinorrhea appeared and was resolved after conservative measures. Some advantages of this technique are: (a) it avoids incisions needed to extract muscle or fat, (b) it reduces operating time, and (c) artifacts in postoperative computed tomography (CT) and magnetic resonance imaging (MRI) studies are moderate.

In four cases rhinorrhea appeared after surgery and irradiation of invasive adenomas; the sealing was then carried out percutaneously using local anesthesia and fluoroscopy (therapeutic sealing). In every case an immediate and maintained stoppage of the CSF leak was achieved with follow-up ranging from 9 to 29 months.

Introduction

Fibrin glue has been widely used in several neurosurgical procedures to fix aneurysm clips and peripheral nerve suture and to obtain waterproof sealing of dural defects [3, 7, 8, 10, 11].

The leak of CSF is an infrequent, but dangerous complication of transsphenoidal operations for pituitary adenomas. Pneumoencephalos and meningitis may be its dangerous consequences. To prevent CSF rhinorrhea, to ensure hemostasis, and also to avoid chiasmal descents, the intrasellar and sphenoidal sinus cavities are usually packed with muscle or fat obtained from a second inci-

---

Fig. 1a. Surgical field after microsurgical resection of intrasellar adenoma. **b** Bone frag- ▶ ments are placed over the intrasellar fibrin to close the sellar floor. **c** Hemostatic gauze is used to press on a second layer of fibrin

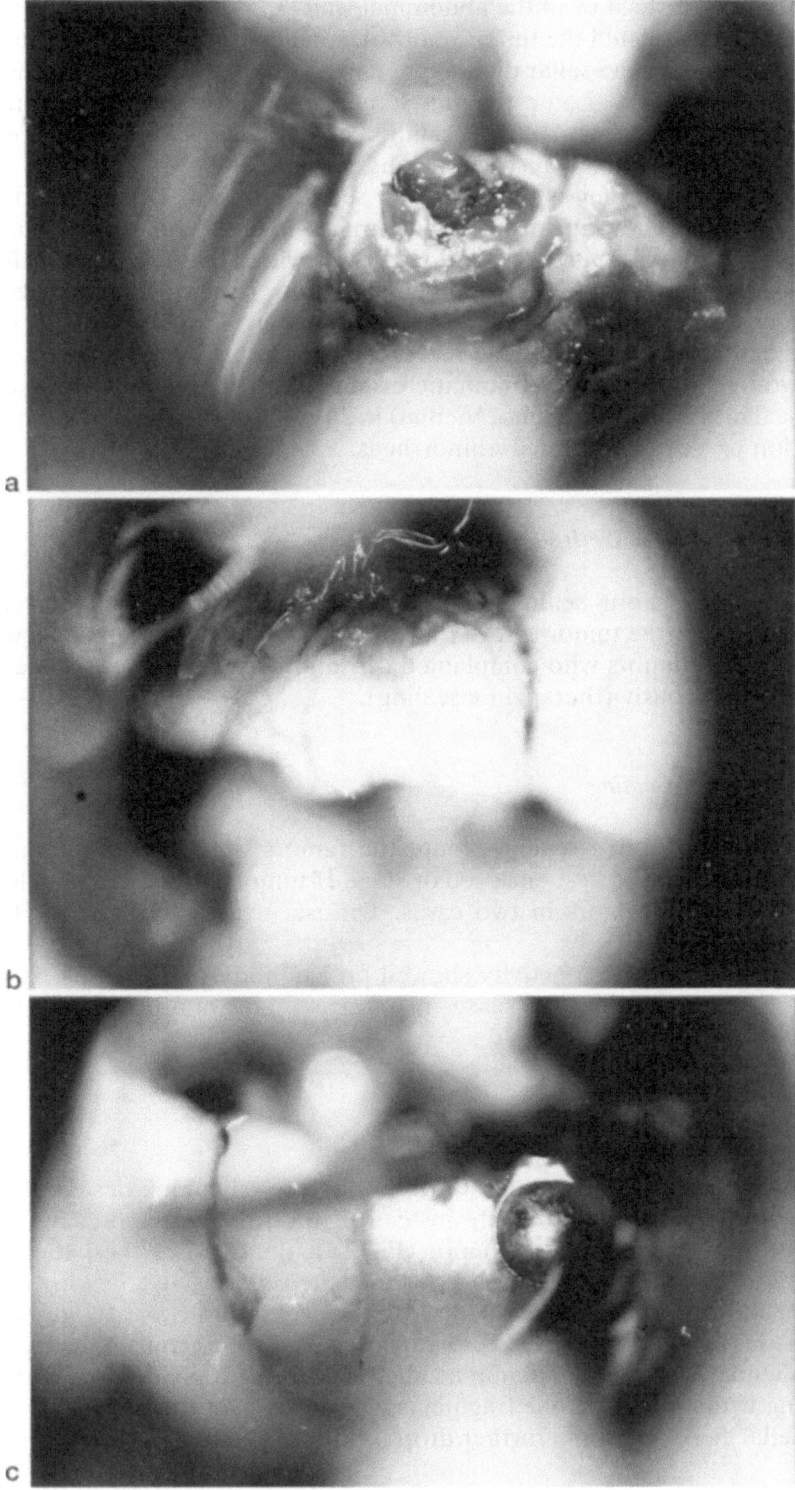

sion in the thigh or in the abdominal wall [1, 5]. When CSF is discharged after having completed the tumor removal, small pieces of fascia lata and muscle are placed under the sellar diaphragm and a continous lumbar drain is established for several days. Later, the muscle becomes fibrotic and sometimes revascularizes, obtaining an effective sealing. Postoperative CSF rhinorrheas are treated with bed rest, fluid restriction, and lumbar drain. If conservative treatment fails, a craniotomy is performed to seal the fistula. On the other hand, postoperative follow-up in adenoma surgery is based on clinical manifestations, biological hormonal tests, and images provided by the CT and MRI.

However, in some patients, granulation tissue or revascularization phenomena occurring in the muscle produces artifacts, which can lead to erroneous diagnosis. Since fibrin glue has proven to be highly effective in sealing dural wounds of surgical or traumatic origin [3, 10], the author has used the fibrin sealant Tissucol (Immuno, Vienna) in 26 cases of pituitary adenoma for prevention or treatment of CSF rhinorrheas.

Material and Methods

In 22 cases fibrin sealing was performed during transsphenoidal surgery after removal of the tumor (preventive sealing). In four other patients with invasive pituitary tumors who complained of rhinorrhea, fibrin sealing was performed percutaneously (therapeutic sealing).

Preventive Sealing

In the preventive sealing group, the tumors were microadenomas or stage I tumors in four cases, enclosed or stage II tumors in 16 cases, and local invasive or stage III tumors in two cases. Diffuse invasive or stage IV tumors were excluded.

The endocrine activity showed prolactinomas in 13 cases, acromegalia in five cases, Cushing's disease in one case, and nonfunctioning adenomas in three cases.

Intraoperative Method

All patients were operated on following the technique described by Landolt, using the right nostril route instead of the sublabial approach [5]. After the removal of the pituitary tumor (Fig. 1a), the head of the patient is hyperextended and fibrin glue is dropped into the sellar cavity. Seeking a rapid solidification, thrombin is used in a high concentration (500 IU/ml) with simultaneous application of a $CaCl_2$ solution using a double syringe (Duploject; Immuno, Vienna). A lumbar puncture needle is curved to apply the glue without interfering with the view. Bone fragments are placed over the dried fibrin to close the sellar floor and some further drops of fibrin are then placed covering the bone pieces (Fig. 1b). Small pieces of Surgicel are used to press softly on the fibrin (Fig. 1 c). The septal cartilage is replaced in its midline position and the nasal cavities are packed with gauze in the usual way.

Therapeutic Sealing

Four patients were referred to our clinic for treatment of rhinorrheas which appeared several months after surgery and irradiation of invasive pituitary tumors. Previous treatments with bed rest, dehydration, and continuous lumbar drain had proved to be ineffective.

Percutaneous Technique

Nasal cavities were cleaned and prepared as for a transsphenoidal approach. The patient lay awake with the head hyperextended. Local anesthesia and vasopressin were injected in the mucosa over the cartilaginous septum. Under fluoroscopic control a lumbar tap needle was directed to the sphenoid sinus cavity. The caudal surface of the tumor was delineated by air in the sphenoidal sinus or by using radiological contrast. Air was intermittently aspirated from the residual sphenoidal cavity until the tumor surface had been penetrated. Rapidly solidifying fibrin glue was injected under pressure at several points 2–4 mm below the tumor surface. A layer of glue was left in the sphenoid sinus. No nasal package was carried out, but a continuous lumbar drain and antibiotic protection was maintained for 4 days.

Results

The sealing was effective in the preventive sealing group, with the exception of one patient of invasive adenoma who presented with rhinorrhea 2 days after intervention; this resolved after bed rest and lumbar drain. No other complications were detected. The mean operative time was shortened.

Radiological checking on days 2 and 5 after intervention showed fibrin in the CT scans as a moderate hyperdense image, which faded out in the following scans. Contrast enhancement appeared in several cases after the second month, very inconstantly, sometimes as a patchy image and sometimes as a peripheral enhancing ring. Fibrin appeared in the MRI in the first postoperative week as a medium intensity signal. Gadolinium did not enhance the fibrin, but it did enhance the peripheral tissues.

Discussion

Although Grey [2] used fibrin tampons as early as 1916 to control bleeding and Young and Medawar [11] tried to seal peripheral nerves in 1940, it was not until 1973 that Matras and colleagues developed the two-component fibrin glue that is now extensively used in a wide field of application [7]. Dural waterproof closure, epineural suture, and aneurysm clip fixation are the most common neurosurgical uses [10].

Spinal fluid rhinorrhea is a well-known complication of transsphenoidal surgery [1, 5]. It can be followed by pneumoencephalos and meningitis.

Sellar plugging with muscle from the thigh or fat from the abdominal wall is usually performed to prevent rhinorrhea and chiasmal descents. Although the procedure is highly effective, artifacts resulting from muscular revascularization may hinder the diagnosis of tumor recurrence in postoperative radiological controls. In cases of nonfunctioning tumors, when the serum hormonal determinations are lacking, the final therapeutic decision relies on radiological data [4, 6]. Dural defects in all locations have been repaired successfully with fibrin sealant [3, 10]. In our group of 22 patients submitted to transsphenoidal resection of intrasellar adenomas, the sealing with fibrin proved to be effective and long-lasting. In one of the two patients with local invasive adenomas, spinal fluid drops were observed on the second postoperative day. In both patients, a wide opening of the sellar floor was carried out and more than 3 ml rapidly solidifying fibrin was applied to obtain thorough sealing. In cases of invasive macroadenomas, in which we are dealing with a wide destruction of the sellar floor or in which rhinorrhea appears during the tumor removal, the use of fibrin as the sole plugging material might be suggested.

The application of fibrin glue saved the time needed to obtain muscle from the thigh and close the wound.

The results from the evaluation of radiological artifacts provided by fibrin are not homogeneous and therefore no final conclusion can be drawn. The mixed components of intrasellar contents, different volumes of fibrin, and probably different degrees of revascularization may explain the diversity of images obtained in both CT and MRI. For Perrin and coworkers [9], intrasellar fibrin appears in CT and MRI scans as a nonenhanced adenoma. In our patients fibrin glue provided less radiological artifacts than muscle, but a detailed analysis is currently underway.

References

1. De Divitis E, Spaziante R, Stella L (1981) Empty sella and benign intrasellar cysts. In: Krayenbühl H (ed) Advances and technical standards in neurosurgery, vol 8. Springer, Vienna New York, pp 3–69
2. Grey EG (1915) Fibrin as a haemostatic in cerebral surgery. Surg Gynecol Obstet 21: 452–454
3. Hadley MN, Martin NA, Spetzler RF et al. (1988) Comparative transoral dural closure techniques: a canine model. Neurosurgery 22: 392–397

4. Kucharczyk W, Smith ML (1990) Magnetic resonance imaging of sellar and parasellar lesions. In: Wilkins RH, Rengachary SS (eds) Neurosurgery update, vol I (2, 5). McGraw-Hill, New York, pp 57–68
5. Landolt AM, Strebel P (1980) Technique of transsphenoidal operation for pituitary adenomas. In: Krayenbühl H (ed) Advances and technical standards in neurosurgery, vol 7. Springer, Vienna New York, pp 167–185
6. L'Huilier, Combes C, Martin N, Leqlerc X, Pruvo JP, Gaston A (1989) MRI in the diagnosis of so-called pituitary apoplexy. J Neuroradiol 16: 221–237
7. Matras H, Dinges HP, Mamoli B, Lassmann (1973) Non-sutured nerve transplantation: a report on animal experiments. J Maxillofac Surg 1: 37–40
8. Mickey BE, Samson D (1980) Neurosurgical applications of the cyanoacrylate adhesives. Clin Neurosurg 28: 429–444
9. Perrin G (1991) The use of fibrin sealant in transsphenoidal surgical removal of pituitary micro- or large macroadenomas: an experience of 194 cases. In: Schlag G (ed) Update and future trends of fibrin sealing in surgical and non-surgical fields. Abstract book, p 67
10. Rossitch E Jr, Wilkins RH (1990) The use of fibrin glue in neurosurgery. In: Wilkins RH, Rengachary SS (eds) Neurosurgery update I (3, 17). McGraw-Hill, New York, pp 195–196
11. Young JZ, Medawar PB (1940) Fibrin suture of peripheral nerves: measurement of the rate of regeneration. Lancet 2: 126–128

Preoperative Tumor Embolization with Fibrin Glue: Indications and Results

E. NEUMAIER-PROBST, F. ZANELLA, M. WESTPHAL, and H. ZEUMER

Abstract

The goal of the preoperative embolization of tumors is the distalmost loading of the vascular bed. A fibrin glue preparation is presented as an easy to handle and safe material which causes confluent tumor necroses within the injected vascular territory. Between 1991 and 1992, 42 patients underwent preoperative embolization with this fibrin glue mixture with excellent results. Of the 42 patients, 33 had a meningioma, five a glomus tumor, three an angiofibroma, and one 2-month-old child a rapidly growing hemangioma.

Introduction

Preoperative embolization of tumors such as meningiomas, angiofibromas, or glomus tumors is now mostly done using PVA (polyvinylalcohol) particles [1]. Nevertheless, even with the newer preparations of this type of embolic material, a careful and successful embolization is extremely time-consuming, since premature clumping of particles leading to proximal vessel occlusion has to be avoided. In these cases, the result will only be "pretty pictures" without clinical effect. We tested fibrin glue as an alternative in order to achieve capillary embolization and to avoid premature vascular occlusion.

Material and Method

Following the basic ideas of Richling [4] and Solymosi et al. [3, 5], presented at an interventional neuroradiologic meeting in Salzburg in 1990, we performed laboratory tests in order to find a mixture of components which:

1. Can be continuously injected through a 165-cm-long microcatheter at 37 °C
2. Does not precipitate too early inside the catheter or proximal vessels
3. Is radiopaque in order to control injection
4. Produces a stable occlusion for at least 3–4 days

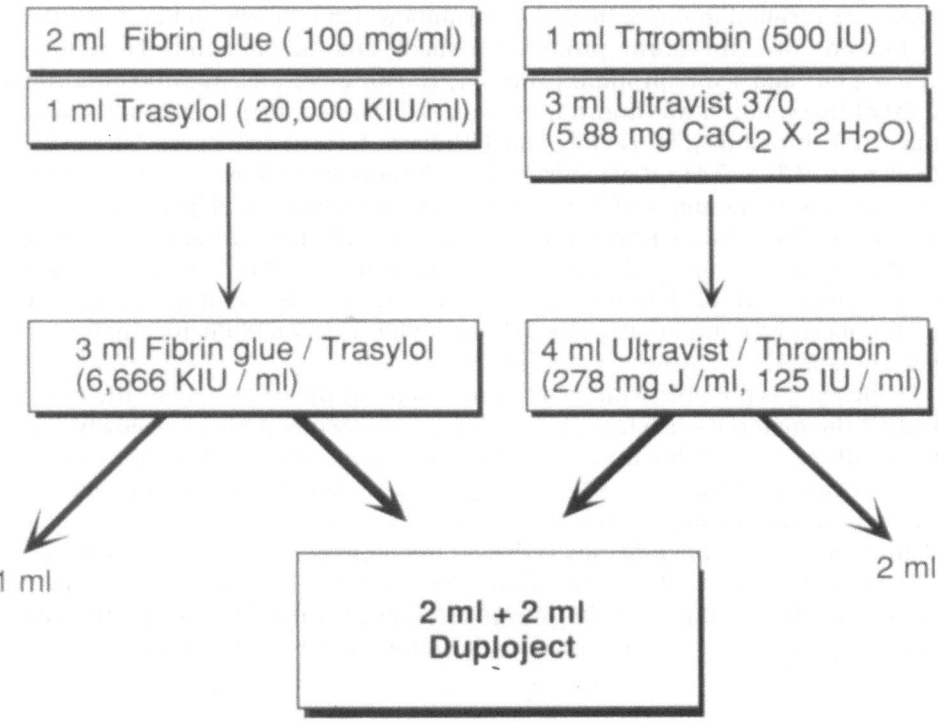

Fig. 1. Preparation formula for the fibrin glue mixture. Final concentrations: 139 mgJ + 62.5 IU thrombin + 33.25 mg fibrin glue + 3333 kIU Trasylol/ml

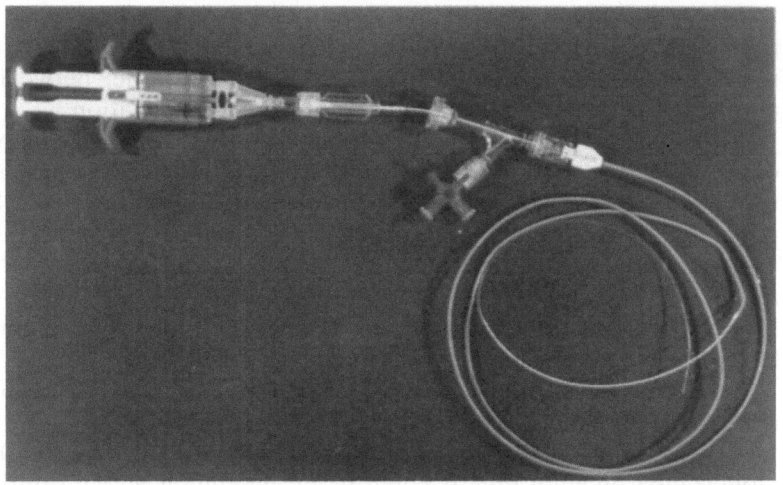

Fig. 2. Embolization set, ready for fibrin glue injection. The Tracker 18 catheter is guided by a flushed 5 French angiocatheter. The two components of glue are put together via a "y" connector into the hub of the tracker catheter

Our tests resulted in the preparation formula which is shown in Fig. 1. We used a mixture of 2 ml fibrin protein (Tissucol Duo S, Immuno, Heidelberg; 100 mg/ml) and 1 ml aprotinin (Trasylol, Bayer, Leverkusen; 20 000 kIU/ml); 2 ml of this solution was drawn into one of the two syringes, while in the other one 2 ml thrombin (500 IU/ml) and Ultravist (Schering, Berlin; 370 mgJ/ml, 5.88 mg $CaCl_2 \times 2\ H_2O$/ml), mixed in a 2:3 ratio, were drawn up. The mixture of Ultravist containing $CaCl_2$ was made by the pharmacy department at the University Hospital in Eppendorf. The concentration of fibrin protein in the double syringe was 33.25 mg/ml, of Trasylol 3333 kIU/ml, of thrombin 62.5 mg/ml, and of Ultravist 139 mgJ/ml. Using the double syringe, the material can be continuously injected through a Tracker-18 microcatheter (Target Therapeutics, San Jose, CA; Fig. 2).

Flushing is possible with contrast medium. At the beginning of the embolization the material is slightly visible under fluoroscopy if injected slowly. With intermittent small bolus injections, the continuous reduction of the capillary blush within the tumor is easily monitored. When the column of glue becomes stagnent in the feeding vessel, this is always recognized under fluoroscopy or digital substraction angiography (DSA) roadmapping. Even in large tumors we seldom needed more than 6 ml fibrin glue mixture. The material was mixed freshly just before injection, but never used longer than 2 h after preparation. Surgical treatment was performed in all tumor cases within 4 days.

Results

A total of 42 patients underwent embolization with fibrin glue. As was to be expected, the successful preoperative treatment of meningiomas ($n = 33$) strongly depended on the type of vascularization (Fig. 3a, b). If more than two thirds of the tumor was fed by embolized meningeal branches, the surgeons reported large parts of the tumor which did not have to be cut, but could be removed by suction. Figure 3c demonstrates the border between tumor cells and necrotic areas within the tumor following embolization.

Figure 4a shows the angiography of a 40-year-old women with a carcinoma of the breast and a progressive gait disturbance due to a tumor mass in the right cerebellopontine angle. The anterior part of this tumor was a histologically proven central necrotic metastasis, and the posterior part was a meningioma. The angiography demonstrates the supply of the meningioma by the right ascending pharyngeal artery and the progression of embolization. The computed tomography (CT) after embolization of the meningioma shows the hyperdense posterior part of the tumor mass (Fig. 4b).

To demonstrate the necrotic development we performed magnetic resonance imaging (MRI; Fig. 4c, d).

In the glomus jugulare and tympanicum tumors ($n = 5$), the small and monocompartimental tumors could be nicely embolized with fibrin glue alone. In the larger ones, however, we observed a network of feeding arteries connected to small A–V shunts which appeared only after embolization of the tumor parenchyma. These residual vessels were packed with PVA particles afterwards.

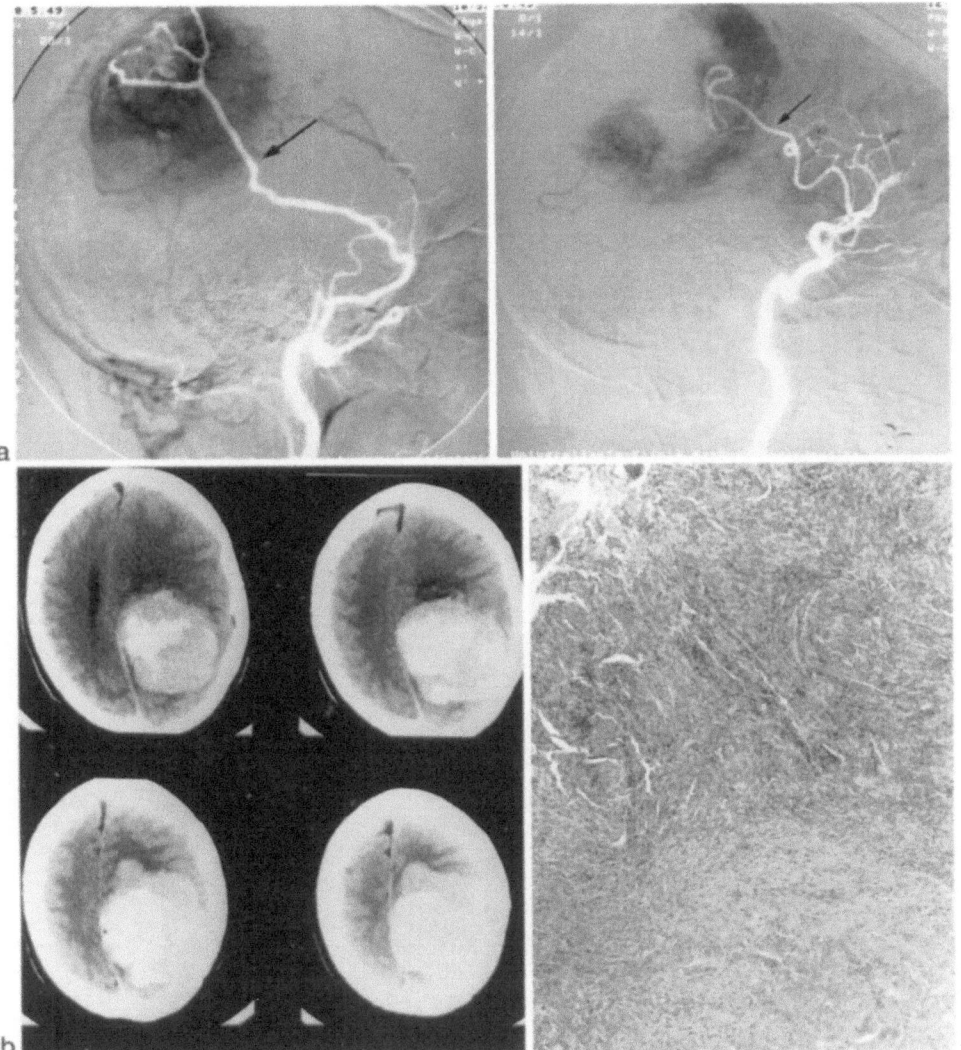

Fig. 3a. Vascular compartments of tumor supply in a meningioma. The *large arrow (left)* shows the feeding middle meningeal artery; the *small arrow (right)* demonstrates the part of the tumor supplied by the middle cerebral artery. **b** CT of the same patient after embolization of the tumor core fed by the middle meningeal artery. Considerable hyperdensity due to fibrin glue homogeneously dispersed in this supply area. Less hyperdensity within the nonembolized areas (from the internal carotid artery) caused by contrast medium alone. **c** Histologic specimen demonstrating the clear-cut borderline between necrotic meningeal *(lower right side)* and vital arachnoidal *(upper left side)* supply areas after embolization. Hematoxylin and eosin (H & E) stain; × 40

Fig. 4a. The angiography demonstrates the supply of the meningioma by the right ▶ ascending pharyngeal artery *(top left)*. The *upper right* and the *lower* pictures show the progression of embolization. **b** The CT after embolization of the meningioma demonstrates the hyperdense posterior part of the tumor mass (to be continued on page 38)

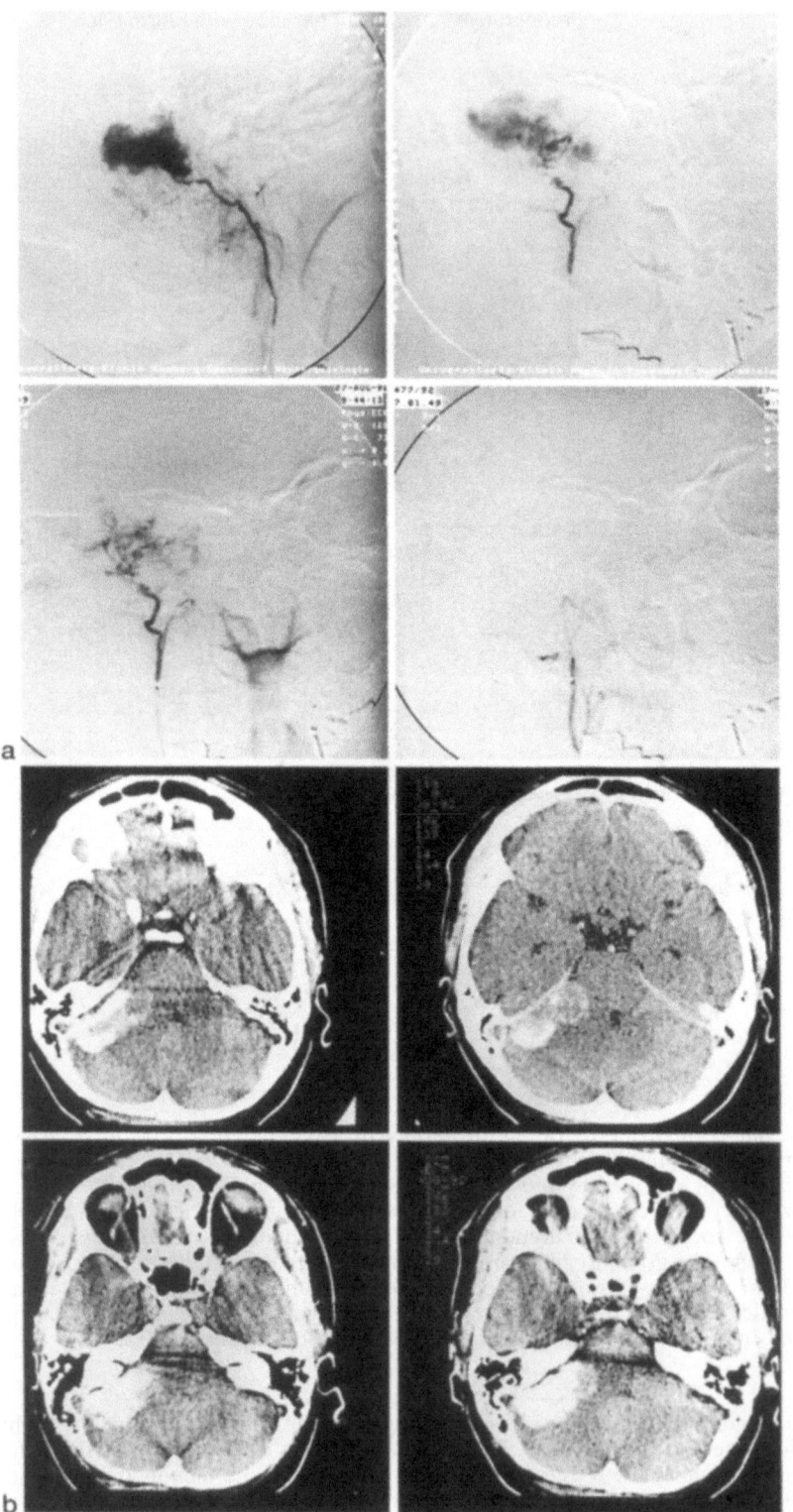

a

b

Fig. 4a, b

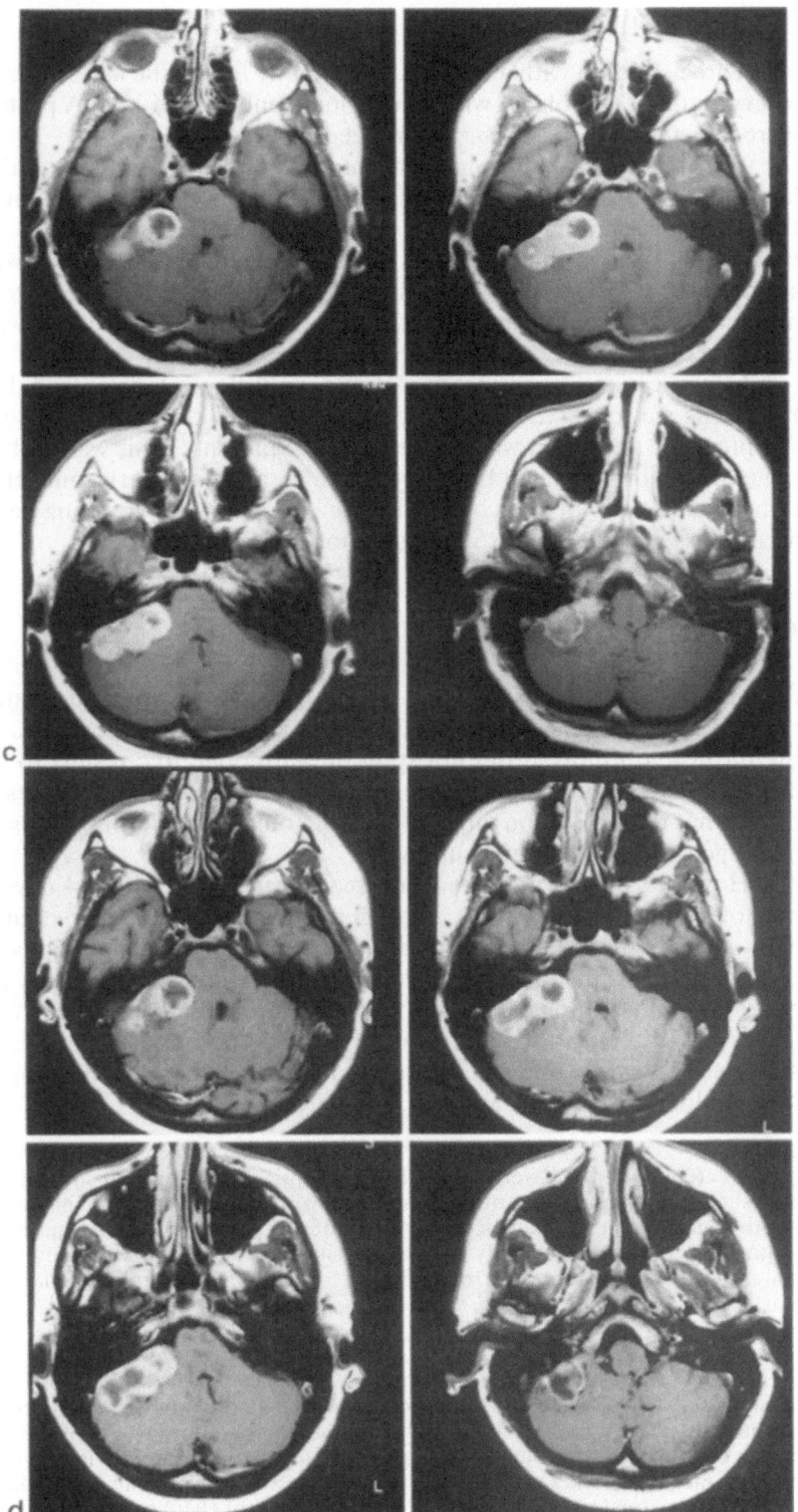

Fig. 4c, d

Three children with angiofibromas mainly fed by the ascending pharyngeal artery were all embolized with fibrin glue combined with PVA particles, which were injected into the stump of the feeding vessel.

We treated one 2-month-old infant suffering from a rapidly growing hemangioma obstructing the respiratory pathways (Fig. 5a, b). Due to the life-threatening situation, surgery was unavoidable and urgently necessary. The day before surgery, we injected 6 ml fibrin glue and packed the proximal vessel stumps with PVA particles. At surgery, the hemangioma was removed with only minimal loss of blood and the vascular tumor mass dissected without only bleeding at all.

Complications resulting in definite neurological deficits did not occur. Headache was observed in most patients, and headache and nausea requiring symptomatic treatment was noticed in three patients. This was probably due to the embolization of small branches of the meningeal artery connected with the tumor that could not be avoided. In one patient severe vomiting occurred, and hoarseness worsened after glomus tumor embolization.

Discussion

Fibrin glue is in our experience an easy to handle and safe material if the embolization of a parenchymatous tumor is required. Recanalization due to the intrinsic fibrinolysis did not spoil the intraoperative results to any reasonable degree. On the contrary, the material induces tumor necroses to such an extent that recanalization might play a role only in borderline zones with mixed meningeal and arachnoidal supply.

However, all our patients were treated surgically within 4 days. Thus, the risk of recanalization of the large feeding meningeal arteries and possible hemorrhage into the necroses was unlikely. If, however, a palliative embolization is undertaken, this possible complication should be borne in mind and a packing of the stump vessels with particles should be considered. We have had no serious complications either in relation to the mode of application of the material or to the composition of the mixture containing fibrinogen protein. Immunological reactions are rare, but may occur [2].

◀ **Fig. 4. c.** (continued) T1-weighted axial images prior to the embolization of the meningioma show the enhancement of the tumor following administration of gadolinium–DTPA (diethylenetriaminepentaacetic acid). The anterior part shows central necrotic areas corresponding to the histologically proven metastasis. **d** T1-weighted axial images following embolization demonstrate the regressive areas within the meningioma part of the tumor mass

Fig. 5a. Contrast enhanced CT of the face and neck of a 2-month-old infant. Large ▶ hemangioma of the right soft tissues of the neck compressing the respiratory pathways. **b** Selective angiogram (i.e. digital substraction angiography, DSA) of the hemangioma before embolization and successful surgery (*upper left side*, lateral view; *upper right side*, posteroanterior view). The *lower left side* demonstrates the result after additional packing of the proximal vessel stump with polyvinylalcohol (PVA) particles

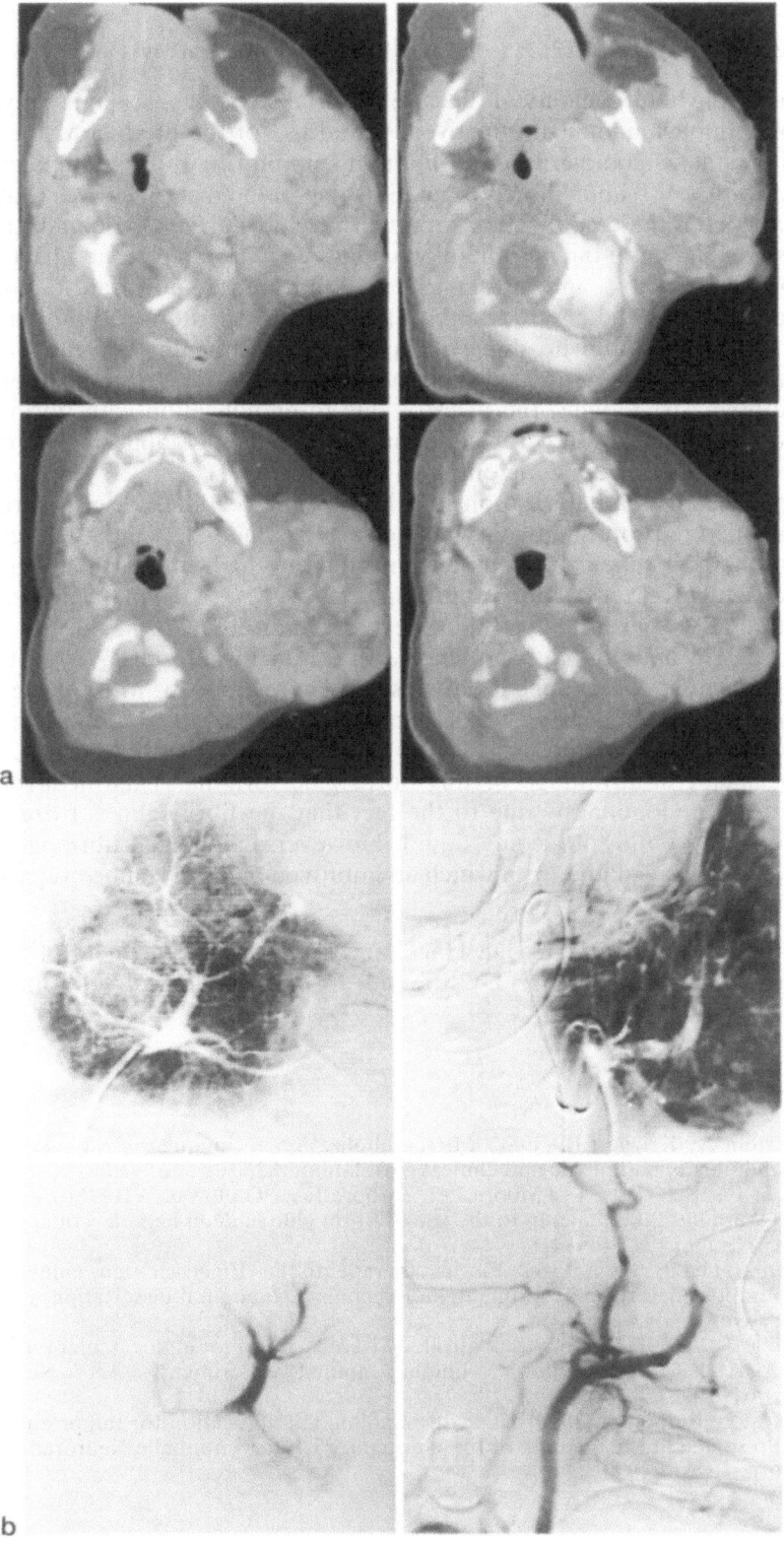

a

b

Due to the heterogeneity of the case material (type of vascular supply, site of lesion), the evaluation of effectiveness and use of the preoperative embolization cannot be standardized. Continuous monitoring during embolization together with a CT immediately after finishing embolization proves that the technical goal of the embolization is regularly achieved. The CT demonstrates the massive loading of the peripheral vascular bed with radiopaque fibrin glue. Intraoperative findings and histological work-up both demonstrate tumor necrosis in the embolized areas. Another, less objective, criterion is the opinion of our neurosurgeons, who directly experience the benefits of preoperative embolization of meningiomas, angiofibromas, and glomus tumors. For the neuropathologists, though, the necrosis due to embolization with fibrin glue might at some time cause confusion concerning tumor grading, if material is provided from the border zone only.

Superselective catheterization of all accessible feeding vessels is crucial, since the mixture proposed by us would dissolve immediately in larger vessels. Dissolution also happens if the glue is injected into high-flow fistulae and it is also not useful for arteriovenous malformation (AVM). In comparison with our results using PVA particles, the tumor necroses induced by fibrin glue are often more extensive and confluescent than with optimally infused PVA particles, where the necroses often appear only insufficient and patchy. Most of the time used for the procedure is spent on superselective catheterization. The glue injection itself is completed within a few minutes, including the controls.

One major disadvantage of this fibrin glue formula is its inconvenient preparation, predominantly due to the fact that the fibrinogen is frozen and needs at least 15 min to become liquid. However, lyophilized fibrinogen has recently become available, with which an improved mixture can be prepared in the future.

Acknowledgement. We thank Dr. Hagel and Dr. Laas (Department of Neuropathology under Professor Dr. Dr. Stavrou) for the histological work-up.

References

1. Berenstein A, Kricheff II (1981) Microembolization techniques of vascular occlusion: radiologic, pathologic and clinical correlation. AJNR 2: 261–267
2. Berguer R, Staerkel RL, Moore EE, Moore FA, Galloway WB, Mocklus MB (1991) Warning: fatal reaction to the use of fibrin glue in deep hepatic wounds. Case report. J Trauma 31: 408–411
3. Reipen A (1990) Homologes Fibrin, therapeutische Eigenschaften eines neuen Embolisationsmaterials, experimentelle Ergebnisse. Inaugural dissertation, Medical Library University Bonn
4. Richling B (1982) Homologous controlled-viscosity fibrin for endovascular embolization, part 2. Catheterization technique, animal experiments. Acta Neurochir (Wien) 64: 109–124
5. Solymosi L, Reipen A (1990) Tissucol: handling and indication for tumor embolization. Presented at the meeting of the German AG-Interventionelle Neuroradiologie, Salzburg, 20 Apr 1990

Preliminary Observations of Local Therapy with Interferon-β with Use of Fibrin Glue as a Carrier in Malignant Cerebral Tumor

K. Matsumoto, H. Izumiyama, and T. Iwata

Abstract

In our hospital, the intravenous administration of interferon-β (IFN-β) to patients with malignant cerebral tumors has been practiced for a long time; however, the efficacy of this therapy has proved to be insufficient. Therefore, we tried applying IFN-β packed into fibrin glue to the cavities of extirpated tumors. First, we analyzed the activity of fibrin glue and observed that the fibrin glue material (0.3 ml) dissolved completely within 3–4 weeks. Secondly, we investigated the activity of IFN-β packed into fibrin glue. We inserted fibrin glue-packed IFN-β into the brains of ten dogs by needle and compared sampling times and IFN-β titers (IU/g) in tissue at a distance from the site of infusion after 1 day to 4 weeks following the intervention.

We conclude that this method of using IFN-β packed into fibrin glue is effective against malignant tumors, since the chemotherapeutic substance is gradually released into the surrounding tissue. Therefore, we have been using this method clinically since 1990. We clinically used IFN-β packed into fibrin glue in 20 cases of malignant cerebral tumor. The patients were aged between 30 and 70 years (12 men and eight women); there were ten cases of glioblastoma multiforme, four cases of grade III astrocytoma, three cases of grade II astrocytoma, and three others. Regrettably, pathological tissue and physiological activity of these cases after operation cannot be investigated.

Introduction

This is the first report of a fundamental study of the clinical applications of fibrin mass (F) as carrier of interferon-β for the local treatment of malignant cerebral tumor. Intravenous administration or local injection from an Ommaya reservoir does not always result in good intratumor penetration of IFN-β; however, it is thought that the utilization of F as carrier of IFN-β enables sustained action of IFN [8, 10, 12, 14, 15].

Method

Biological tissue adhesive (Tisseel, Nippon Zoki) and IFN-β (Mochida Pharmaceutical Co.) were mixed (F–IFN-β; Fig. 1).

First, the time course of the activity of IFN-β in F–IFN-β was measured. A total of 3 mIU/g IFN-β was dissolved in 0.15 ml thrombin solution of Tisseel and was mixed with 0.15 ml fibrinogen solution of Tisseel to make 0.3 ml stabilized fibrin mass (F–IFN-β). The latter was further preserved in thermostat at 37 °C and was measured for the time course activity of IFN-β (0, 3, 6, 24, 48, 72, 168, 336, and 672 h later). The homogenate and the operational methods of activity measurement are as follows (requested by the Special Reference Laboratory, Inc.).

1. About 0.4 g aliquot of the sample is taken and put into the 10 ml Eiken tube.
2. Add buffer (phosphate buffer, pH 7.0, containing 0.05 % Tween 20).
3. Put homogenate in icewater for 15 s.
4. Let it stand for 45 s.
5. Repeat steps 3 and 4 three times (1 min homogenation in total).
6. Centrifuge at 3000 rpm for 10 min.
7. Transfer the supernatant into another tube.
8. Perform enzyme immunoassay (EIA) using the supernatant.

Second, F–IFN-β (3 mIU/g) thus prepared was fixatively injected into the brain of mongrel dogs and was measured for the time course of the intratissue activity of IFN-β. Cerebral histological changes were also examined. Ten mongrel dogs weighing 8–12 kg were used. Under intravenous anesthesia with pentobarbital, F–IFN-β was manually injected slowly from the cerebral surface of a decapitated mongrel dog into a depth of 7–10 mm stereotactically, using a 25-gague Teflon indwelling catheter. At 24, 72, 96, 168, 336, 404, and 672 h, the animals were killed with an overdose of barbiturate, decerebrated immediately after perfusion with physiological saline, and cut in coronary section at the injection site. As shown in Fig. 1, tissue was collected from four points at a dis-

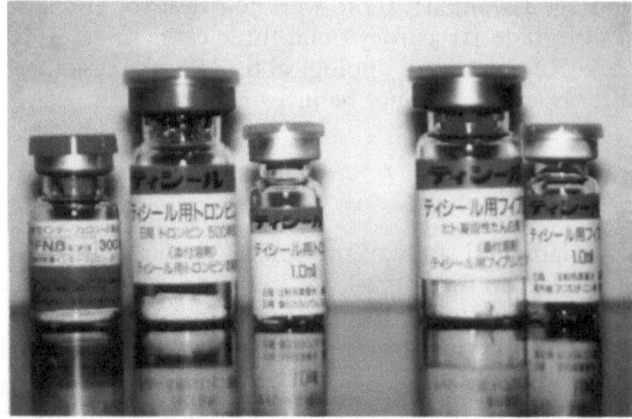

Fig. 1. Biological tissue adhesive (Tisseel, Nippon Zoki) and interferon-β (IFN-β, Mochida) were mixed (F–IFN-β)

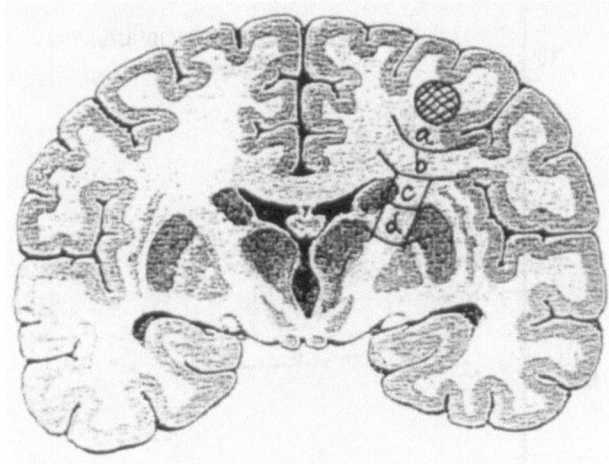

Fig. 2. Method of sampling. Distances from infusion site: *a* 0–5 mm; *b* 5–10 mm; *c* 10–15 mm; *d* 15–20 mm

tance, from the injection site (Fig. 2) up to 20 mm in depth and in the cerebellum and brain stem to measure the intratissue activity of IFN-β. Partial sections (0- to 5-mm sections 336 and 672 h later) were H&E stained for preparation and observed through a light microscope.

Results

Table 1 and Fig. 3 show the time-course of IFN-β activity in F–IFN-β and Table 2 the time course of intratissue IFN-β activity.

Microhistopathological Findings

Figure 4 shows a coronary-cut, cerebral tissue section of F–IFN-β after 336 h (2 weeks). F–IFN-β still definitely persists.

Table 1. Time course of interferon-β (IFN-β) activity in fibrin mass (F)–IFN-β

Time (h)	IFN-β (IU/g)
0	710 000
3	270 000
6	160 000
24	43 000
48	28 000
72	38 000
168	16 000
336	13 000
672	4 800

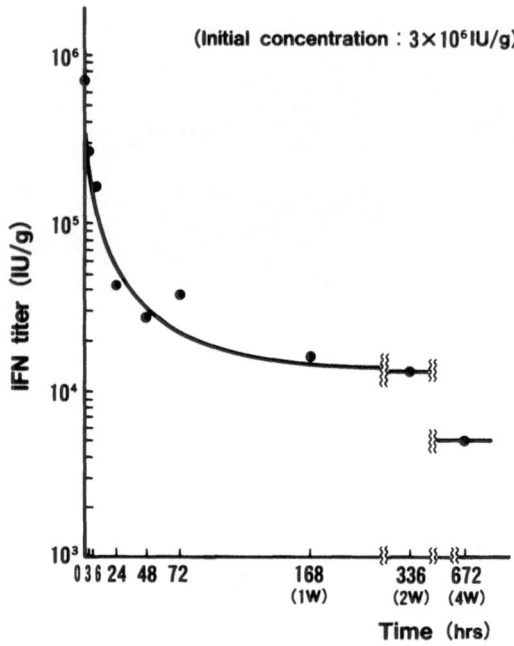

Fig. 3. Declination curve of IFN-β concentration in fibrin mass (F)–interferon-β (IFN-β)

Figure 5 shows a coronary-cut, cerebral tissue section of F–IFN-β after 672 h (4 weeks). F–IFN-β became fused and did not appear.

Table 2. Time course of interferon-β (IFN-β) activity in tissue

Sampling time (h)	IFN-β titer (IU/g tissue)					
	Distance from infusion site (mm)					
	0–5	5–10	10–15	15–20	Cerebellum	Brain stem
24	1100	1200	23	19	19	120
72	9400	280	240	85	140	36
96	4900	1100	280	130	21	21
96	1800	1100	170	70	27	120
168	200	39	21	21	21	21
168	21	20	19	19	19	19
336	250	29	28	26	21	24
336	120	93	49	43	19	50
404	21	33	25	19	20	20
672	38	21	23	22	21	30

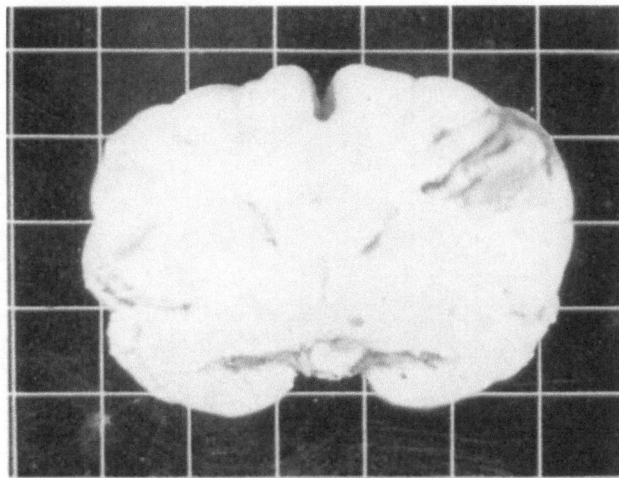

Fig. 4. Coronary-cut, cerebral tissue section of fibrin mass–interferon-β (F–IFN-β) after 336 h

Macrohistopathological Findings

Figures 6 (small magnification) and 7 (large magnification) show H & E stained cerebral tissue specimens after 336 h (2 weeks). F and softening foci due to compression therapy are seen as well as a round cellular infiltration of macroglia, lymphocyte etc. in focus.

Figures 8 (small magnification) and 9 (large magnification) show H & E stained cerebral tissue specimens after 672 h (4 weeks). Cystic formation, fused diminution of F, thinner round cellular infiltration than that after 336 h, and subsequent compression-free, larger softening foci can be seen. Foreign matter-type giant cells are also visible, representing a vital reaction of the histiocyte line.

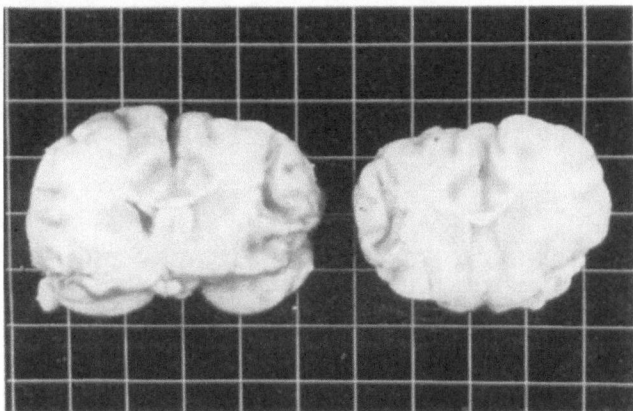

Fig. 5. Coronary-cut, cerebral tissue section of fibrin mass–interferon-β (F–IFN-β) after 672 h

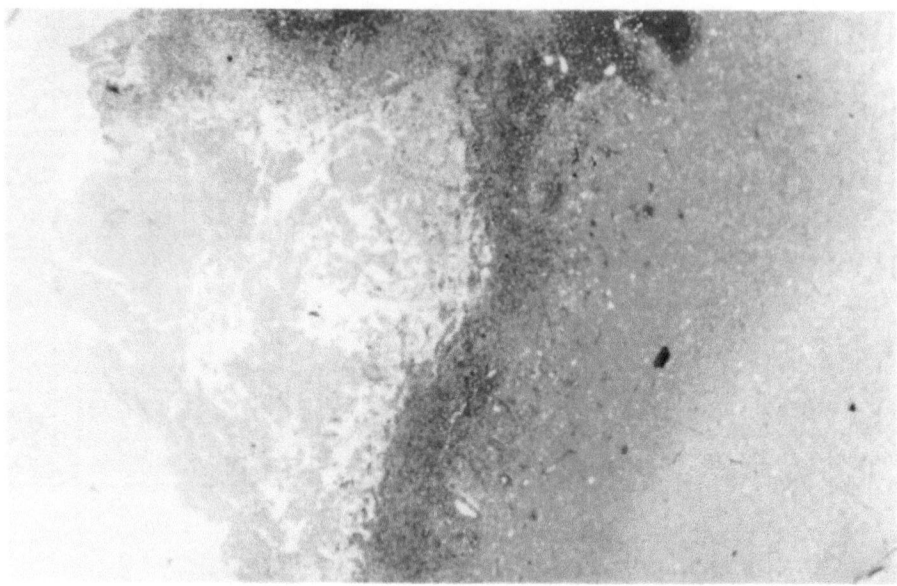

Fig. 6. Hematoxylin and eosin (H & E) stained cerebral tissue specimens after 336 h (small magnification)

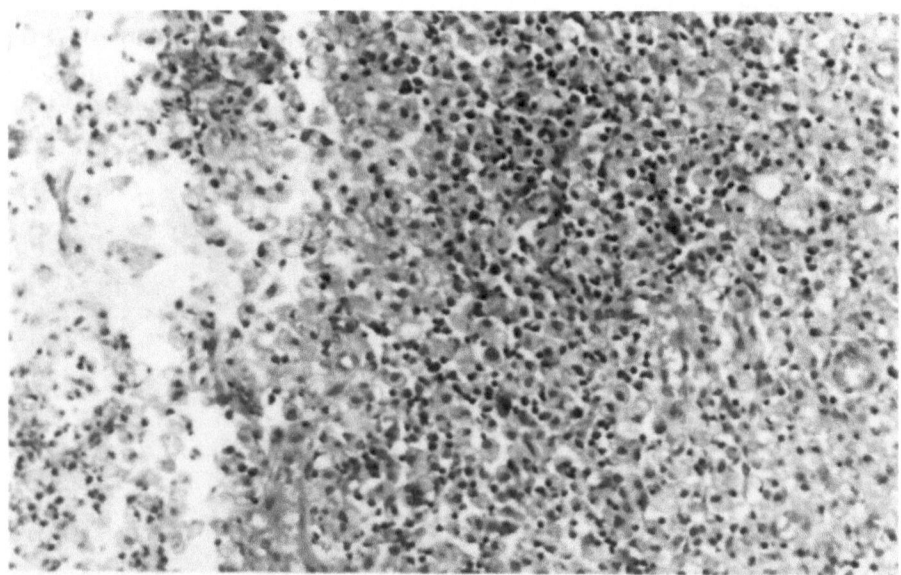

Fig. 7. H & E stained cerebral tissue specimens after 336 h (large magnification)

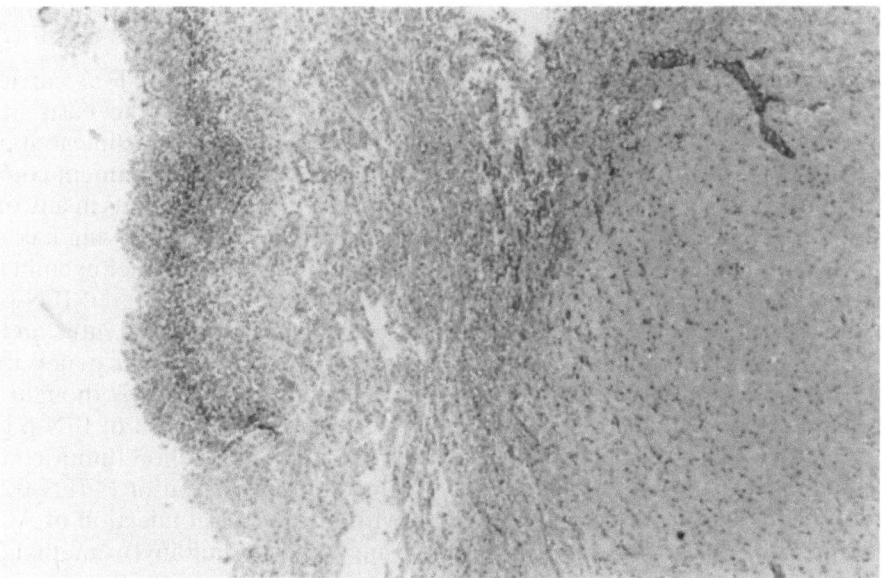

Fig. 8. H & E stained cerebral tissue specimens after 672 h (small magnification)

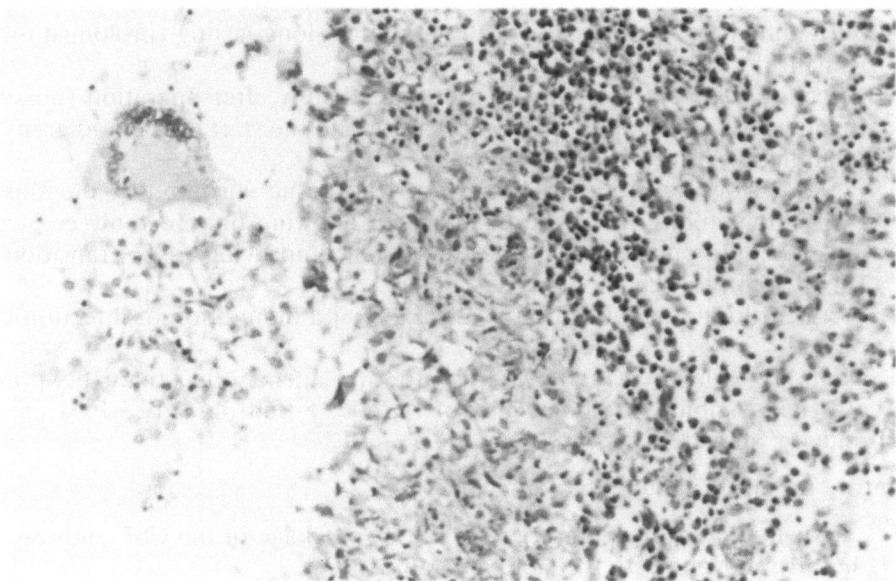

Fig. 9. H & E stained cerebral tissue specimens after 672 h (large magnification)

Discussion

In the present study, we examined the clinical application of F as carrier of IFN-β for local therapy of malignant cerebral tumors. On the basis of the results of the above examination, we are now engaged in the clinical application of F–IFN-β in 20 cases and the observation of their posttreatment courses; very good results are being obtained. There were no complications in any of the cases, and we have had better results than usual. We are now trying a control study and, here too, very good results are being obtained. Further examination of the intratumor penetrability of generally or locally administered IFN-β has to be carried out [10, 13, 15]. Intravenous administration or local infusion from an Ommaya reservoir does not always result in good intratumor penetrability of IFN-β. With the method of our present device, however, it is thought that the utilization of F as carrier of IFN-β enables sustained action of IFN-β [15].

Our present basic plan of treatment for malignant cerebral tumor consists of the most extensive possible tumorectomy, administration of F–IFN-β, and subsequent synchronized chemotherapy with intra-arterial injection of ACNU [Nimustine hydrochloride, (4-amino-2-methyl-5-pyrimidinyl) methyl-3-(2-chloreothyl)-3-nitrosourea hydrochloride] following administration of vincristine and nicardipine, together with about 60 Gy irradiation.

The advantages and future possibilities of F–IFN-β are as follows:

1. Sustainment of IFN-β action makes its effect long-lasting (prolongation of its half-life, Fig. 10).
2. Effective availability of IFN-β from immediately after operation (possible treatment at a blank period of 1–2 weeks up to the start of chemotherapy or radiotherapy.
3. Possible slow transition of IFN-β into the tissue surrounding the site of extirpation (filling up of the dead space following tumorectomy creates a pressure difference between the tumor cell, improving tissue transition of IFN-β; Fig. 11).
4. Frequent local administration is avoidable and diminution of infection risk possible.
5. Multidrug combined therapy with antitumor agents other than IFN-β may also be possible. Combined use of ACNU, 5-fluorouracil (5-FU) etc. is under examination.

Future problems include the following:

1. Intraventricular injection of IFN-β causes blockage of the CSF pathway, so that the above injection is not preferable.
2. Although the optimal dose of IFN-β is a matter of some uncertainty, even a dose as large as 6 mIU/g may be possible.

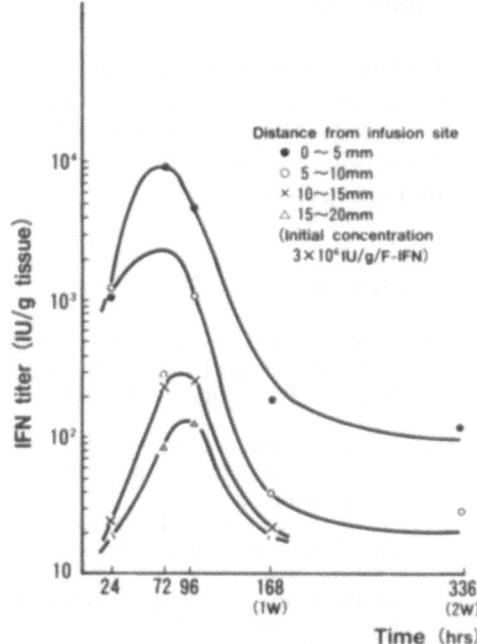

Fig. 10. Time-dependence of interferon-β (IFN-β) concentration

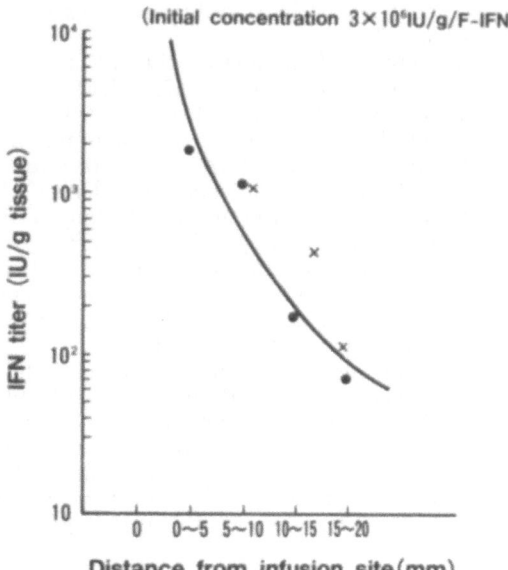

Fig. 11. Histological transition of interferon-β (IFN-β) after 4 days of infusion

Conclusion

We believe F–IFN-β to be a new treatment which is effective for the prevention of postoperative recurrence of malignant cerebral tumor. F–IFN-β, which is a sustained action drug, is to be administered upon tumorectomy and prior to the formation of a barrier between the drug and the tumor. We intend to make further case studies.

References

1. Kintomo Takakura (1988) An intermediary report of phase III study on treatment of malignant glioma by a concomitant therapy with feron, ACNU and radiation (IAR therapy). Proceeding of the 2nd interferon therapy symposium. Medical Tribune, pp 36–45
2. Nobuyuki Shitara et al. (1988) A long-term maintenance therapy of glioma by feron drip infusion. Proceeding of the 2nd interferon therapy symposium. Medical Tribune, pp 46–53
3. Teruyuki Mori et al. (1988) A local treatment of malignant glioma by interferon therapy. Proceeding of the 2nd interferon therapy symposium. Medical Tribune, pp 54–67
4. Akifumi Oda et al. (1989) Treatment of malignant glioma and β-interferon. Effectiveness of Interferon-β and its adverse reaction. J Jpn Soc Cancer Ther 24 (10): 2411–2417
5. Takashi Nishihara (1988) An experimental study on a new immunotherapy of malignant glioma by transduction of extrinsic interferon-Y gene. Arch Jpn Chir 58(1): 18–42
6. Nobuyuki Shitara et al. (1987) Cytokinase therapy of malignant glioma. Jpn J Cancer Chemother 14(12): 3235–3244
7. Yasunobu Miyao et al. (1987) A basic study on antitumor effect of recombinant interferon-β on human malignant tumor. Jpn J Cancer Chemother 14(2): 490–494
8. Hiromata Miki (1987) Antitumor effect of human fibroblast interferon on human malignant glioma. Neurol Med Chir (Tokyo) 22: 785–796
9. Kiyoshi Aoyagi et al. (1988) Study on intracerebral transfer on IFN-β after local injection. Biotherapy 2(1): 99–103
10. Akifumi Oda et al. (1985) Basic study on a slow releasing anticancer agent-pellet with a silicon base. J Jpn Soc Cancer Ther 20(10): 2236–2242
11. Masahiro Nobuhara et al. (1986) Basic study on interferon-β I–IV. Jpn J Cancer Chemother 13(6): 2100–2122
12. Tomokatsu Hori et al. (1989) Local effect and mechanism of interferon on human malignant glioma. Brain Nerve 41(9): 911–917
13. Shiro Kubo et al. (1982) Basic and clinical study on application of a fibrin adhesive (Tisseel) in the area of oral surgery. J J Stomatol Soc 28(9): 1577–1584
14. Masakatsu Nagai et al. (1988) Immunological feature of patients with malignant glioma and its change after interferon treatment. Biotherapy 2: 242–247
15. Tsukasa Fujimoto et al. (1984) J Showa med Assoc 44: 91–94

Frontobasal and Orbital Reconstruction Using Biological Material

P. KNÖRINGER

Abstract

A total management approach in initial surgical interventions has proven highly successful and has become generally accepted for the treatment of frontobasal cerebrocranial injuries, bone-destroying tumors of the frontal basis, and after removal of orbital neoplasms. After treatment of secondary brain damage involving the orbital and cranial nerves and after extirpation of the tumor, reconstruction measures are performed on the dura mater, in the area of the base of the skull, and on the calotte. At the same time plastic surgery is performed to close the skin, if necessary.

Biological material is preferable because its active incorporation prevents late sequelae. This consists of bone fragments, bone meal obtained by trepanation, periost from the pericranium, small fat patches from the temporal fossa, muscle and fascia fragments of the temporalis muscle, and pediculate periost galea patches. These tissues are obtained from the operating field, and surgical intervention in other areas of the body is therefore necessary only in exceptional cases. Fixation is performed by tissue sealing, which additionally plays an important role in the sealing of the subarachnoid space and absorbable suture material and in osteosynthetic measures.

For restoration of the damaged bone, the orbital roofs, lateral orbital walls, and frontorhinal basis are sealed with an antibiotic bone-meal fibrin adhesive graft. The contour of the orbital borders is reconstructed using orbital fragments connected and refixated by osteosynthetic procedures. Defects of the calotte are covered by applying miniature scales of calotte fragments for fixation and, if necessary, alloplastic materials such as Refobacin-Palacos or Ionocem. Alloplasts may be applied rather generously since they do not come into contact with the external environment and therefore prevent late infections.

Restoring the bone structures of the orbitofrontal basis is easy using the bone-meal fibrin adhesive graft. The fibrin sealant maintains a given shape in the area not subject to mechanical strain. The instantaneous watertightness of the reconstructed osseous layer significantly improves the seal of the subarachnoid space since it creates a tissue barrier in addition to the dura mater. The admixing of an antibiotic provides effective local prophylaxis against infection in the critical posttraumatic stage. As a result, an endogenous bone develops that prevents late infections, in contrast to alloplasts that are in contact with the paranasal sinus and with which infections have been observed. This also helps to prevent ascending infections which may lead to meningitis and brain abscess whenever open frontobasal bone defects are not closed.

Introduction

The total management approach has proven itself successful in the treatment of cerebrocranial injuries and after the removal of tumors of the posterior orbita and frontobasis [3, 7]. In the initial stage, particularly reconstruction of bone structures is easier and can be performed more accurately, thus providing the most favorable results. Another advantage is the prevention of follow-up interventions, which generally serve reconstruction purposes and are performed under more complicated technical conditions. Moreover, typical late complications after frontobasal injuries, such as cerebrospinal fluid leak, pneumocephalus, pneumatocele, meningitis, and brain abscess, can be prevented with a high degree of certainty due to conclusive repair at an early stage [9]. In the reconstruction stage of the intervention preference should be given to biological material. This includes the use of endogenous tissue, the sealing of the subarachnoid space and tissue sealing by means of fibrin glue, and the use of absorbable suture material and osteosynthetic material, which in future will be biodegradable.

Material and Methods

Periost Patch

After the frontobasis is exposed by coronary incision, for cosmetic reasons, periost patches are obtained from the pericranium and preserved in physiological saline solution, to which an antibiotic may be added. These patches are secure and actively incorporated and therefore highly suitable for free grafting and covering of dural defects. The fixation is carried out by means of tissue sealing and, if required, an additional suture. Alternatively, a pediculate galea periost patch [2] may be prepared. Compared to the pediculate galea periost patch which is rather difficult to obtain, the freely grafted periost patch has the advantage that its application requires less material, and its removal is unproblematic. Additionally, it does not destroy the galea layer of the scalp.

Bone Meal

There is a significant difference between the freely grafted autogenous spongy part of bone and the cortical part regarding reliability and speed of adaption to the implant site [7]. Freely grafted spongy bone generally adapts itself more safely, quickly, and actively to the implant site than does isolated cortical bone. However, the adaption rate of finely ground cortical bone approximates that of spongy bone and may therefore also be used.

Bone tissue obtained by trepanation is referred to as bone meal. Depending on the structure of the skull bone, it consists of two-thirds finely ground cortical bone and one-third spongy bone. In terms of adaption it is similar to isolated spongy bone and is therefore suitable as bone graft material. Thermal damage of the bone tissue due to drilling is prevented by a permanent sprinkle of cool physiological saline solution. Only finely ground tissue is collected; coarse pieces are not used. The bone meal thus obtained is mixed with an antibiotic solution and stored in a dish until use. Immediately before grafting excess solution is squeezed from the bone meal, which is mixed with 1–2 ml Tissucol (Tissucol DuoS, human fibrinogen, human thrombin, steam-treated). Both components of the fibrin glue are applied simultaneously either by hand using Duploject or by Tissumat and nozzle. Since processing requires a considerable amount of time, a slowly acting adhesive must be used.

The mixture of bone meal, antibiotic and fibrin glue is then ready for the modeling process, which takes 3–4 min. After the glue becomes solid (approximately 5 min after application) a viscous graft forms which closes bone defects, resists deformation, remains watertight, and seals bone defects [6]. The admixed antibiotic protects against infection in the adaption stage. If necessary, the procedure can be divided into several steps. In this case the bone-meal fibrin adhesive graft is produced by modeling freshly prepared portions which are then combined. This allows several sites to be closed one after the other, and complex structures can be formed in succession; in addition, there is the possibility for correction.

Frontobasal Trauma Procedure

The cranial wound is repaired after the removal of possible hematoma, foreign bodies, and bone splinters, followed by microsurgical revision of the frontorhinal basis. The pterioneal approach is used to maintain an undamaged bulbus olfactorius. If the revision is to be performed on both sides, two bone lids are formed, and a handlelike bone bridge is left above the center of the superior sinus sagittalis to protect it from damage. If the frontal sinus and/or ethmoid cells are extensively damaged, cranialization must be performed. A lesser degree of damage to the sinuses preserves the mucous membrane and therefore spares the sinuses from treatment. If the orbitae are also affected, the procedure is similar, and the crushed fragments of the orbital roof and/or lateral walls are removed. The optic nerve in the optic canal and the orbital muscle nerves in the cranial orbital fissure are decompressed if necessary.

The reconstruction stage begins with careful closure of the dura mater performed either intradurally, extradurally, or in extensive injuries in a combined manner. If single olfactory nerves are torn but the bulbus olfactorius is undamaged, this should be maintained since partial olfaction can be expected [5]. In this case the empty passages of the torn nerves, which may cause a cerebrospinal fluid leak, are sealed with tiny fat patches and fibrin glue. In addition, the bulbus olfactorius may be covered with a periost patch which overlaps it rostrally and on both sides. If the dura mater cannot be closed by means of a primary suture, a periost patch is added, which may be fixated by suture. The sealing of a site with a number of minor lacerations by means of intra- and extradural periost patches has proven to be of value.

In the bony area the reconstruction measures begin at the frontal basis. If cranialization of the frontal sinus and/or ethmoid cells has been performed, the respective passages are closed with added fat, muscle, and periost patches, and an osseous layer in the area of the frontorhinal basis is built up (Figs. 1–4) using the bone-meal fibrin adhesive graft. If the paranasal sinus is mostly or partly preserved, the bone defects in this area are closed with a bone-meal fibrin adhesive graft. The orbital roofs and lateral walls are remodeled in the same manner. If sufficient bone meal is not available, further material can be obtained from drilling, in addition to trepanation. Additional bone tissue can be obtained by grinding bone fragments derived from depression fractures.

The orbital borders and dorsum of the nose should be reconstructed with endogenous fragments and fixated, if possible, by means of miniature scales. A bony defect in the area of the frontal calotte caused by the lifting of a depression fracture should be reconstructed with endogenous fragments. With such miniature-scale osteosynthesis even large areas can be treated in a short time. Gaps are filled with Refobacin-Palacos [4] or Ionocem (Fig. 5).

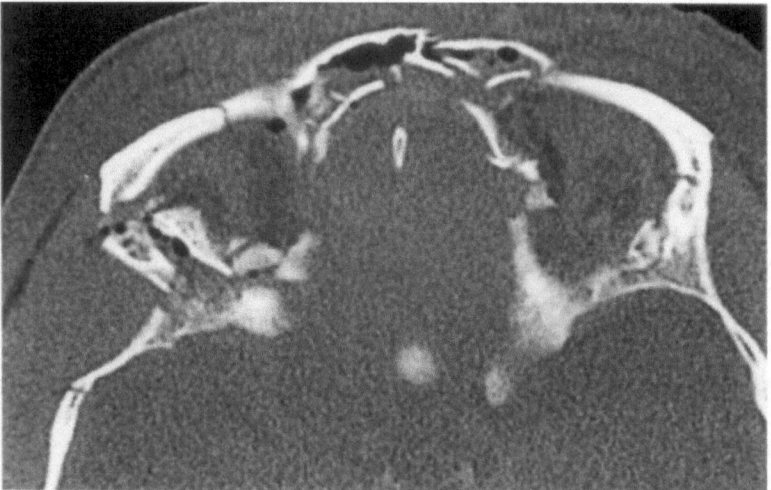

Fig. 1. Axial computed tomography of a frontobasal cerebrocranial trauma. Extensive damage to the frontal sinus and anterior ethmoid cells leading to both orbitae, which are partly covered by bone fragments

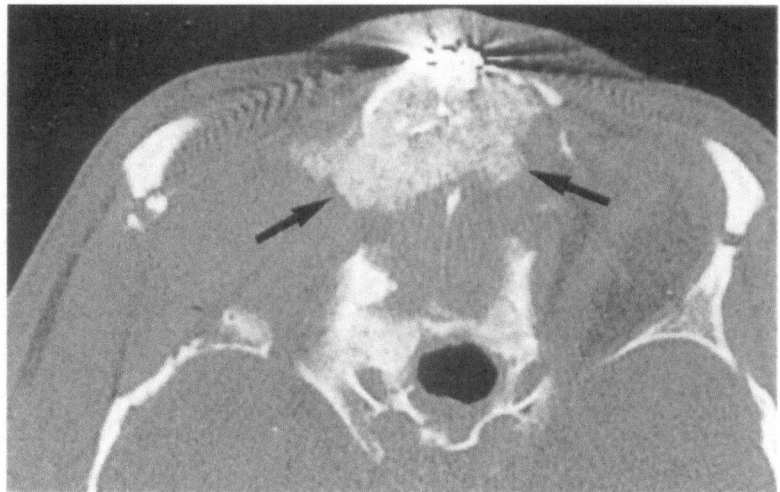

Fig. 2. Comparative view of postoperative axial computed tomography. The frontal sinus and anterior cellulae ethmoidales are cranialized, and both orbitae are entirely decompressed. *Arrows*, bone-meal fibrin adhesive graft in the area of the frontobasis and rostral half of the rhinobasis

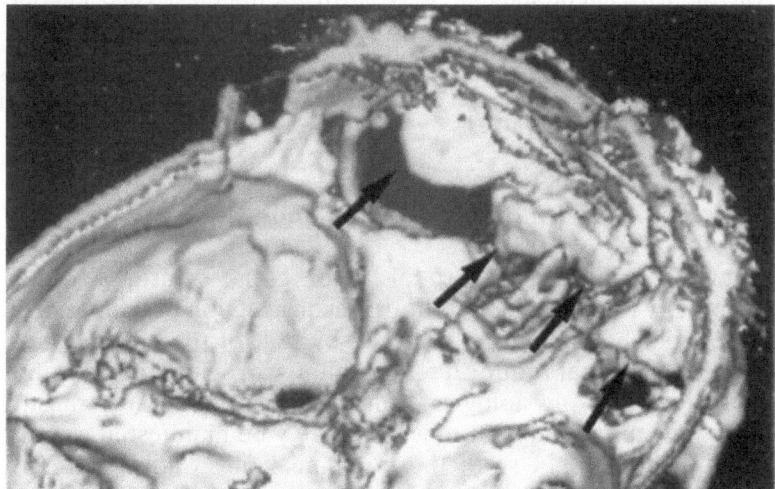

Fig. 3. Three-dimensional reconstruction illustrating the restored frontobasis, anterior rhinobasis, and orbital borders by means of the bone-meal fibrin adhesive graft. *Four arrows*, dorsal end; *between the two arrows (middle)*, crista galli

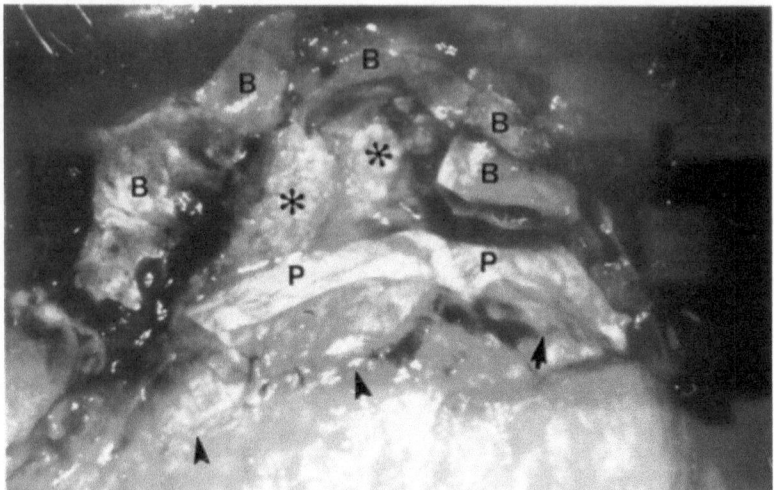

Fig. 4. Operative field with an illustration of the left and right anterior base of the skull and both frontal poles. The intradural revision for the cranial wound repair on both sides is terminated; *three arrows*, suture of the dura mater. Multiple minor lacerations of the dura mater on both sides (frontobasal) are sealed with two free grafted periost patches from the pericranium and Tissucol. *P (left)*, area of the left basal and convex frontal pole; *P (right)*, area of the right one. Frontobasis, rhinobasis, and both orbital roofs are reconstructed by means of a bone-meal fibrin adhesive graft containing an antibiotic. *Asterisk (left)*, left orbital roof; *asterisk (right)*, frontobasis and anterior rhinobasis. The right orbital roof is covered by a bone fragment from the frontal sinus where the mucous membrane has been removed. *B*, bone fragments, which refer to the superior orbital borders and root of the nose. These were left in situ; this facilitates the subsequent precise anatomical reconstruction of the structures of the remaining fragments by means of miniature-scale osteosynthesis

Procedure After Removal of Orbital Tumor

After the removal of an orbital tumor, either subfrontally, at the pterion, or temporally (Krönlein's operation), reconstruction of the periorbita by means of periost patches should be followed by that of the osteoclastical defect in the area of the orbital roof or lateral orbital wall. This stabilizes the content of the orbita, restores physiological conditions, and prevents transmission of brain pulsations to the bulbus oculi, which may be manifested as pulsating exo- and enophthalmos [8]. Use of the bone-meal fibrin adhesive graft permits good reconstruction as the endogenous bone tissue can take almost any shape. In this case the fibrin glue maintains the shape until the osteoplasty is completed.

Discussion

Biological material should be used in reconstruction of the frontal base of the skull and the orbitae due to its active adaption. For the closure of defects of the dura mater free grafts taken from the periost of the pericranium, fascia of the

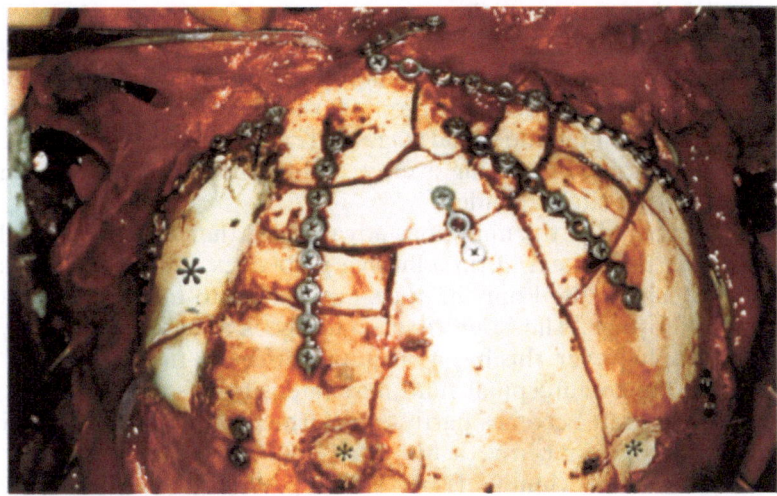

Fig. 5. Operative field after reconstruction of the orbital borders, root of the nose, and frontal calotte by means of a stabilized bone mosaic due to osteosynthetic measures. A remaining bone defect (left temporal; *) and two drilling holes (*) are covered with a Refobacin-Palacos osteoplasty. The bone meal has been obtained for the osteoplasty of the frontal base of the skull from drilling holes and the ground bone fragment (left temporal; extension, see Fig. 3). *Dissector,* left superior orbital border which was reconstructed by osteosynthetic means with remaining bone fragments. The miniature scale *(upper corner, center)* stabilizes the bony root of the nose. *Lower left corner,* probe measuring the cranial pressure

temporal muscle, and fascia lata have proven successful. This type of tissue is incorporated rapidly, safely, and actively whereas a patch of Tutoplast or Lyodura is covered only by a thin layer of connective tissue and is vascularized at best at the peripheral section.

Sclerosis of the paranasal sinus that is permanent can be filled with the bone-meal fibrin adhesive graft; alternatively, fat patches can be added after resection of the mucous membrane. If late repneumatization is required, this should be sealed with muscle patches. Over the course of 1 year the muscle tissue in the center is usually absorbed while that at the wall becomes organized in a connective manner and thus maintains the sealing of the walls.

The bone-meal fibrin adhesive graft allows endogenous, vital bone tissue to be built up which prevents late rejection caused, for example, by late infection such as is seen in alloplasts. The mixture of bone tissue and fibrin glue provides an easily formed, shape-retaining material as well as a watertight closure even in the area of the osseous layer. The double sealing in the dura mater and osseous layers significantly increases the watertightness of the closure [6, 7]. Active incorporation of the grafted bone tissue helps to restore the physiological barrier of the dura mater and osseous layers between the subarachnoid space and the external environment (paranasal sinus), which prevents the ascending infections that may occur in open bone gaps.

Admixing of an antibiotic provides an effective prophylaxis against infections at the critical stage after grafting [1]. This is important because the grafted tissue may extend into the paranasal sinus and hence communicate with the external environment. Such prophylaxis against infection enables osteoplasty to be carried out in the initial stage of treating directly and indirectly open frontobasal injuries. Processing is easy, and the need for further removal of tissue from another site is avoided.

Compared to the numerous advantages, there are only few disadvantages. Since the bone-meal fibrin adhesive graft does not provide instantaneous stability, it can be used only in areas not subject to mechanical strain, at least in the initial stage. The bone tissue undergoes a certain shrinking during incorporation; however, this has no negative effect on the indications. Strong pulsations in the cerebrospinal fluid may intensify this physiological shrinking. At worst, the graft becomes partly transformed into a firm connective tissue, but even then the aim can be achieved.

When this technique is performed precisely, the rate of infection is minimal. In approximately 70 osteoplasties on the frontal base of the skull and orbitae no infections or long-term complications have been reported so far.

References

1. Braun (1986) Preparation and application of fibrin-antibiotic complex. In: Schlag G, Redl H (eds) Fibrin sealant in operative medicine, vol 7. Springer, Berlin Heidelberg New York, pp 171–182
2. Dietz H (1970) Die frontobasale Schädelhirnverletzung. Monographien aus dem Gesamtgebiet der Neurologie und Psychiatrie, no 130. Springer, Berlin Heidelberg New York
3. Knöringer P (1979) Sofortdeckung von Schädellücken bei offenen und geschlossenen Impressionsfrakturen des Hirnschädels mit Acrylharzkunststoff. Ein klinischer Vergleich zwischen Palacos K und Refobacin-Palacos R. Neurochirurgia 22: 18–23
4. Knöringer P (1979) Langzeitergebnisse der Schädelplastik mit Acrylharz. Zentralbl Neurochir 40: 197–202
5. Knöringer P (1986) Use of fibrin glue for sealing and prophylaxis of cranial and spinal CSF fistulae. In: Schlag G, Redl H (eds) Fibrin sealant in operative medicine, vol 2. Springer, Berlin Heidelberg New York, pp 148–156
6. Knöringer P (1986) Bone meal-fibrin sealant plasty in the neurocranium: technique and indications. In: Schlag G, Redl H (eds) Fibrin sealant in operative medicine, vol 2. Springer, Berlin Heidelberg New York, pp 157–167
7. Knöringer P (1987) Frontobasal and orbital reconstruction following trauma and tumor removal using a compound of bone meal, antibiotic, and fibrin sealant. Neurosurg Rev 12: 31–39
8. Knöringer P (1992) Pterionale, subfrontale und temporale Entfernung von Orbitatumoren mit Rekonstruktion der knöchernen Orbita. Videotape, Immuno V 0
9. Rath StA, Knöringer P (1989) Late brain abscess years after severe cerebro-cranial trauma with frontobasal fracture. Childs Nerv Syst 5: 121–123

Fibrin Sealing in Spinal Neurosurgery

P. KNÖRINGER

Abstract

Considerable importance is now being attached to fibrin sealing both in cerebral interventions and in operations on the spinal column and spinal cord. The most frequent indication remains the sealing of the subarachnoid space and treatment of spinal CSF fistulas. Primary dura mater sutures or patches are sealed, and traumatic or iatrogenic dura mater defects are sealed at sites which are inaccessible to sutures, or at which a suture would excessively narrow the intradural space. When there is no other indication for revision, postoperative subcutaneous CSF fistulas can be sealed percutaneously, and, as the high success rate demonstrates, reoperation is unnecessary. Fibrin sealing also plays an important role in duroplasty for the treatment of defects (meningocele, lipomyelocele, diastematomyelia). Fibrin sealing is now an integral part of operative medicine and is used to treat arachnoid cysts and pseudomeningoceles, whether by sealing after cyst shunting or by sealing the cyst cavity with adipose tissue.

A high success rate is obtained using the combined suture and adhesive technique to reconstruct transsected cauda fibers by end-to-end coaptation or autologous suralis transplantation. An established procedure is the use of a spongiosa fibrin adhesive graft to fill defects in the vertebral body after excision of benign, expansively growing tumors, or to perform intercorporeal fusion after removal of a spondyoldiscitic focus. Control of hemorrhages by the use of fibrin adhesive and collagen sponges during surgery of hyperemic spinal tumors (e.g., vertebral angiomas or metastatic tumors) may be absolutely vital. At all events, the adhesive plays a considerable part in stemming the flow of blood. The use of fibrin adhesive and sponges to control hemorrhages at the site of bone chip removal can also be beneficial and helps to reduce the incidence of secondary complications. After removal of intramedullary tumors small oozing hemorrhages are controlled safely and completely atraumatically by spraying the resection bed.

A further indication for the use of fibrin adhesive is during epidural fat graft, most frequently after the removal of recurrent herniated disks, to reconstruct the epidural sheath to prevent cicatrization. Sealing not only allows accurate fixation of the small transplants but additionally prevents the formation of a hematoma between the transplant and dura mater, the cicatrization of which would raise doubts about the value of reconstructing the epidural sheath.

Introduction

Matras et al. [7] were the first to demonstrate experimentally and histologically the possibility of using fibrin sealant as a watertight seal for the spinal dura mater. They not only observed rapid physiological healing of the sealed dural incision but also demonstrated that the constituents of the sealant have no neurotoxic effects, at least in animal experiments. Since then the frequency and indication spectrum of histoanastomosis with fibrin adhesive during neurosurgical intervention in the spinal column and spinal cord have increased considerably. The most important indications for fibrin sealing in the spinal region are addressed and the technical procedure outlined.

Materials and Methods

Sealing of the Subarachnoid Space

The most frequent indication for the use of fibrin adhesive (Tissucol DuoS, human fibrinogen, human thrombin, steam-treated) is sealing of dural sutures and patches. The risk of a CSF leak is undoubtedly reduced, even when a dural suture has been performed accurately, when a collagen sponge or autologous transplant is glued over [5]. Traumatic and iatrogenic dura mater defects or lesions at sites which are inaccessible to patch or suture treatment can be tightly sealed by adhesive. Autologous tissue (adipose lobules, muscle and fascial pieces) or collagen gauze can serve as transplant. Autologous tissue is obtained from the operating field, precluding the necessity of surgical removal of tissue from another part of the body. Adipose tissue can be extracted from the subcutis, muscle tissue from the ecektor trunci muscular system, and fascia from one of the two layers of the erector trunci. Dural lesions in the root canal or the ventral dural sac should be sealed in the way described, rather than with a suture, which tends to narrow the dural space and thus leads to compression of the radicular filaments [4]. An additional advantage of dura mater sealing in this region is that there is no danger of the type of injury to the radicular filaments which may occur when using a needle or inaccurately placing a suture. Of course, it is essential when applying the suture and adhesive to reduce herniated filaments so that they are completely tension free after intradural intervention. Slowly acting adhesive should be applied to ensure sufficient time to place a transplant accurately, also under difficult spatial conditions. Appropriate positioning during the sealing process should prevent a CSF leak at the site to be treated.

If subcutaneous or open CSF fistulation occurs after intradural intervention, despite all care taken, and if there are no other reasons for open revision, such as radicular pain and protuberance of incarcerated radicular filaments in a dural lesion which went unnoticed during an operation, the CSF fistula can be glued percutaneously with a good chance of success [2]. This procedure spares the patient revisionary intervention or lengthy conservative treatment, which usually includes lumbar drainage. This procedure involves percutaneous cannulization of the CSF cavity after spinal computed tomography to determine the topographical position and extension of the CSF cavity. It is useful to place an adapter with a tap between the cannula and the syringe. The tap is closed before the cannula is deposited to prevent air from entering the cavity. After the CSF cavity has been completely drained 2–4 ml fibrin adhesive is injected with Duploject through the cannula, which is still positioned, and a compression dressing is applied immediately. Slowly acting adhesive must be applied to allow sufficient time to distribute the adhesive on the surfaces of the tissue and to position the compression dressing. This should be followed by bed rest of 1–2 days. In the event of a relapse renewed percutaneous sealing can permanently seal the CSF fistula. It is important that the decision to seal percutaneously is made in time as the CSF cavity is usually endothelialized within 3–4 weeks, which considerably lessens the chances of success of conservative fistula treatment.

Physiological tissue sealing with fibrin greatly contributes to the construction of a dural layer in the operative treatment of defects, such as meningoceles, myeloceles, lipomyeloceles, and diastematomyelias [3]. The same applies to the treatment of spinal cysts (e.g., caudal sac cysts, arachnoid cysts, pseudomeningoceles). The valvular mechanism is removed from the caudal sac cyst prior to its being plastically reduced. Although the cyst walls can usually be doubled by imbrication, they are often so thin that the puncture holes for the suture become small fistula openings, thus making watertight sealing impossible by suture alone. Additional sealing of sutures with fibrin adhesive and autologous tissue, as in the method described above, usually prevents the formation of CSF fistulas. The shunted cyst wall is strengthened at the same time. Large cysts whose chronic pressure has already caused local osteanabrosis frequently communicate extensively with the spinal subarachnoid space. Sealing in the remaining cavity with a fat graft after cyst shunting has proven successful here. This decreases the possibility of a relapse and renewed growth of the cyst, which would ultimately lead to local instability of the affected segment of the vertebral column. Osteoplastic laminotomy always helps to maintain local stability, and, if required, a spongiosa fibrin adhesive graft can also be performed to strengthen the dorsal osseous section. The required osseous tissue can be taken from the operating field from the spina iliaca posterior superior. Figures 1–4 show the purposeful, simple, and elegant elimination of a large cyst extending over a whole section of the vertebral column.

Fixation of Transplants

In a limited number of trauma cases transsected cauda fibers have been reconstructed using the suture and adhesive technique. One of these patients was suffering from intradural transsection of the right sensory and motor radicular

62   P. Knöringer

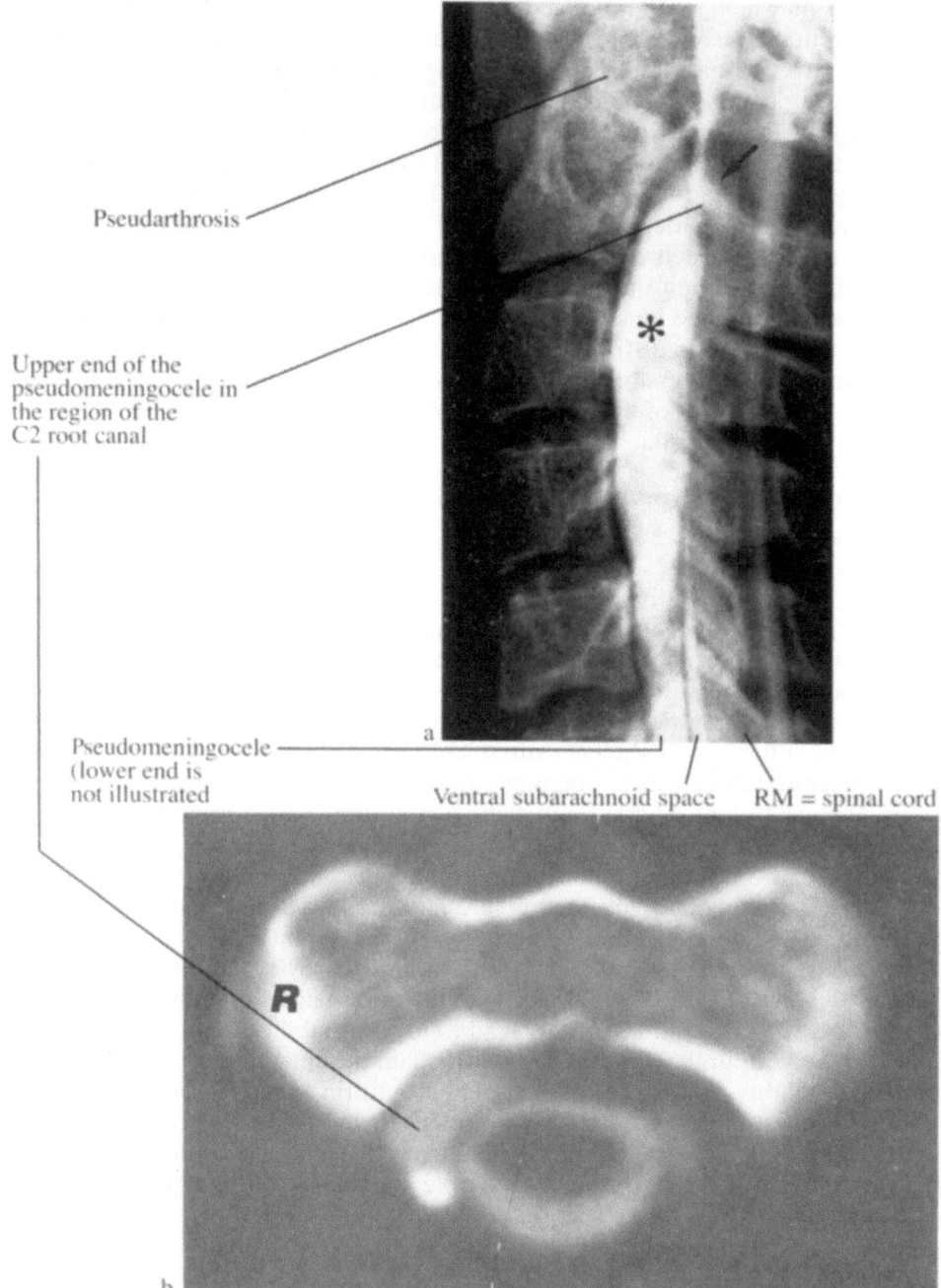

Pseudarthrosis

Upper end of the
pseudomeningocele in
the region of the
C2 root canal

Pseudomeningocele
(lower end is
not illustrated

Ventral subarachnoid space   RM = spinal cord

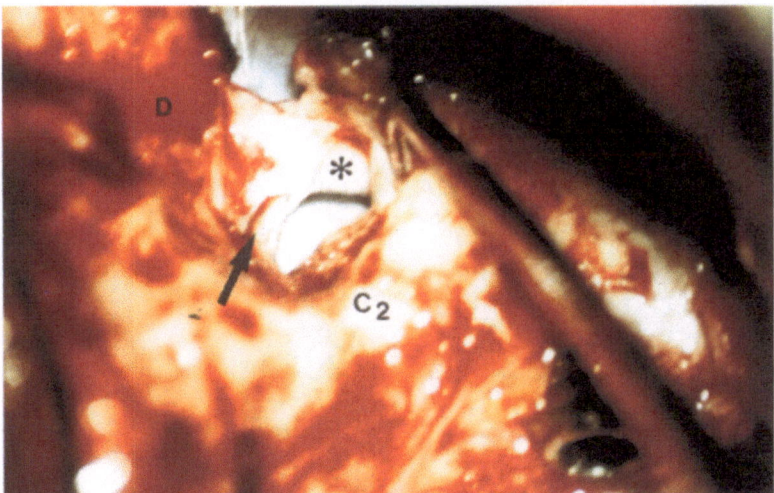

Fig. 2. Operation site. The pseudarthrosis has been stabilized by transarticular screwing (basal thread of the double-threaded screw as referred to by Knöringer is visible, *lower right edge*). A dorsal view of the pseudomeningocele which was opened via a passageway between the C1 and C2 laminae (*C2*, C2 lamina on the right). The C2 root (*) runs through the pseudomeningocele; its filaments are intact, but it shows a dural lesion *(arrow)* at the root axil from which fluid continually pulsates (*D*, dural tube). The pseudomeningocele is the consequence of this traumatic dural lesion. Resection of the cyst walls is made impossible by its enormous expansion and its ventral position. Therapy therefore consists of watertight sealing of the dural lesion with a fat graft and fibrin adhesive and draining the fluid out of the cyst with a catheter pushed to T1

◀ **Fig. 1.a** Lateral myelography shows a compressive pseudomeningocele (*) in a ventral position stretching from the middle of the second cervical vertebra to the caudal end of the first thoracic vertebra (not illustrated). The compressive effect of the pseudomeningocele is most pronounced at C3 and C4. Not only is the subarachnoid space consumed and the spinal cord incisure thinned (spinal cord compression), but compression on the vertebral body has also caused lesions. **b** Myelographic computed tomography of the second cervical vertebra in the region of the C2 root canals suggests that the pseudomeningocele is connected to the C2 root canal on the right *(R)*. It can be recognized in the myelogram in **a** at the same height after a contrast medium cupula (*arrow* in **a**) administered at the dorsal region. The patient ran into the path of a car while playing ball at the age of 11 years and was seriously injured. Among other injuries he contracted a dens fracture, which was not recognized, however. His condition was finally neuroradiologically clarified by progressive myelopathy. On the basis of his case history and results of examinations the patient was diagnosed as having pseudarthrosis with C2–T1 compressive pseudomeningocele with injury to the dura mater at the C2 root

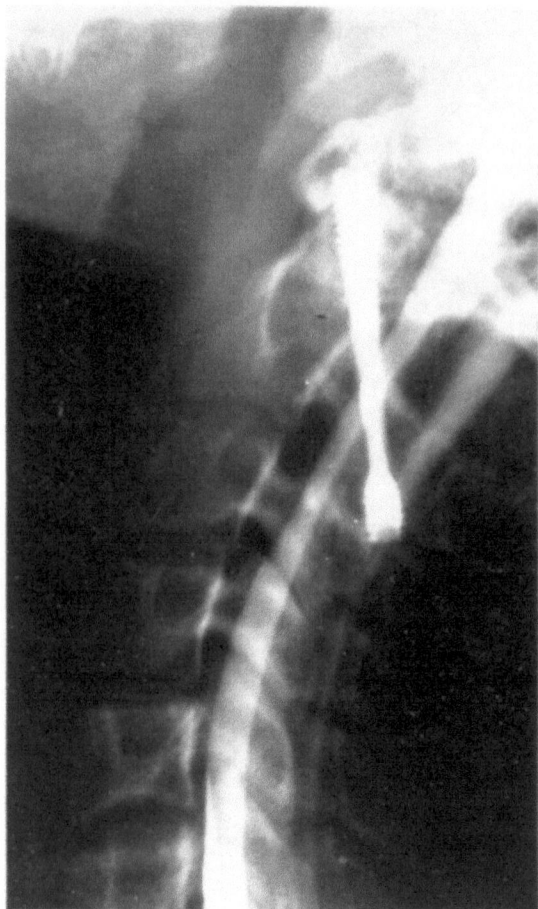

Fig. 3. Control myelogram 6 weeks postoperatively. The cyst has been completely eliminated, the ventral subarachnoid space has developed, and there is no more pressure on the spinal cord. The pseudarthrosis is now C1/2 stable through transarticular screwing and interarcual fusion and has healed in a reduced position. The myelopathy has clinically retrogressed surprisingly well

filament with additional loss of substance caused by crushing. This was reconstructed using a combined suture and adhesive technique with two 3.5-cm-long autologous suralis transplants. Regular check-ups were carried out over a period of 4 years and 7 months with accurate intraoperative documentation. Considerable results were achieved. The sensitive L5 dermatome was almost completely restituted; the motor function was partially restored as the proximal L5 musculature was very well reinnervated (m gluteus medius 5/5), and the distal only slightly owing to the large distance (elevation of foot 1–2/5, elevation of great toe 1/5) [6].

The spongiosa fibrin adhesive graft [9] for filling defects of the vertebral body after resection of benign vertebral tumors is an excellent method to prevent a postoperative spontaneous fracture with the collapse of the vertebral body. After removal of a spondylodiscitic focus even rather large and unclearly delimited spaces which are unsuitable for implanting formed bone chips can be relatively easily filled with a spongiosa fibrin adhesive graft. Slowly acting

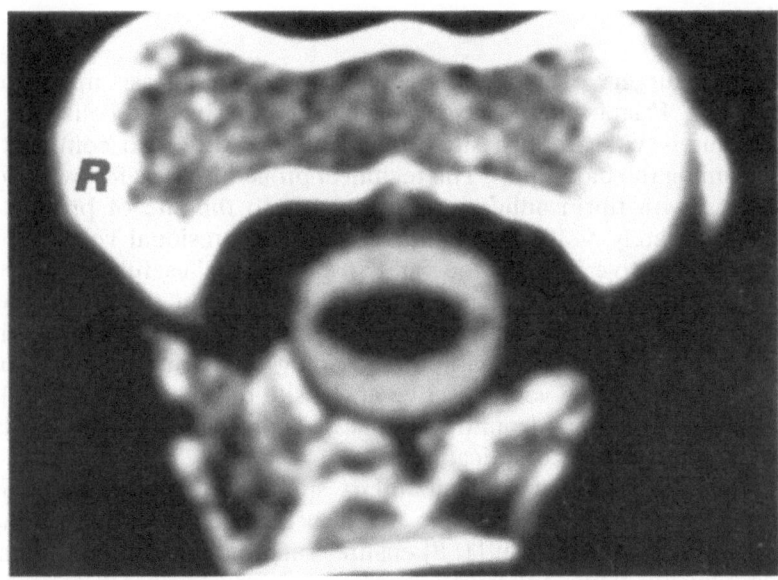

Fig. 4. Myelographic computed tomography in C2 region of the root canal confirms the watertight sealing of the dural corner of the C2 root on the right *(R)* and shows the actively healed interarcual fusion C1/2 which has been carried out with corticospongiosa chips and a spongiosa fibrin adhesive graft

adhesive is indicated. The malposition is corrected with a transpedicularly anchored fixation of the vertebral column, and the achieved correction is maintained until the graft takes and stabilizes in the bone.

All operative steps can be performed by the dorsal approach alone. Thus, even seriously ill patients who can no longer cope with the considerable strains of ventral or dorsoventral therapy can be helped.

Another important indication for the use of fibrin adhesive is the graft of epidural fatty tissue. This procedure restores the epidural sheath by transplanting fatty tissue after removal of a recurrent herniated disk and prevents cicatrization. On the one hand. the sealant allows highly accurate fixation of the small transplants on the dorsal, lateral, and if necessary ventral structures of the dural tube and roots. On the other hand, the risk of hematoma formation between the transplant and the dura mater is considerably less than when transplants are merely superimposed. The formation of a hematoma at this site would lead to increased cicatrization and reduce the chances of the fat graft actively taking, which would cast doubt on the value of a reconstruction of the epidural myelin sheath. The operative steps proceed more smoothly when both constituents of the adhesive are administered separately and quickly acting adhesive is applied. When one constituent of the adhesive is applied to the dura mater and the other to the transplant, the transplant adheres immediately to the desired location, and the next transplant can be fitted without delay.

Hemostasis

During surgery of hyperemic spinal tumors hemostasis may prove extremely difficult. Primary hemostasis using fibrin adhesive and collagen gauze may be absolutely vital in such situations. This measure also contributes greatly to stemming the blood flow. The technical procedure is as follows. Collagen gauze coated with fibrin adhesive is pressed onto the site of profuse bleeding for approximately 5–10 min in the region of the residual vertebral body. Slowly acting adhesive is indicated, and it has proven useful to apply the collagen gauze with a slightly moistened spherical swab. The bioelectrical energy, which would cause the spherical swab and the gauze to adhere, can thus be eliminated and the swab removed without loosening or tearing off the gauze. This procedure can also be very effective at the site of bone chip removal in the pelvic crest when bleeding from the spongiosa is profuse and can contribute to reducing the secondary complication rate.

After removal of intramedullary spinal cord tumors small oozing hemorrhages often remain. Spraying the resection bed with fibrin adhesive using a nozzle and the Tissumat [1, 8] ensures safe and complete atraumatic hemostasis. Quickly acting adhesive is applied.

Discussion and Conclusion

Histoanastomosis by the application of physiological fibrin adhesive is of great significance and has become an integral part of the neurosurgical treatment of diseases of the spinal column and spinal cord. It helps to simplify and thus accelerate operations by tightly sealing the spinal subarachnoid space through the fixation of transplants and hemostasis. Intervention is considerably safer, i.e., the complication rate is reduced. A valuable addition to other advances made in operative medicine is the contribution to the increased atraumatic and physiological [10] treatment of sensitive tissue such as bone marrow, cauda fibers, and radicular filaments. The neurological result is thus improved, and increasingly complicated surgical interventions can be carried out successfully.

References

1. Habison G, Kaspar R, Redl H (1985) Fibrinklebung mit Sprühkathetern. Die Ellipse 12 (5): 49–52
2. Knöringer P (1985) Perkutane Fibrinklebung bei subkutanen Liquorfisteln nach Operationen am Gehirn und Rückenmark. Zentralbl Neurochir 46: 256–262
3. Knöringer P (1986) Therapie und Prophylaxe kranialer und spinaler Liquorfisteln durch Fibrinklebung. Chir Praxis 36: 157–169
4. Knöringer P (1986) Use of fibrin glue for sealing and prophylaxis of cranial and spinal CSF fistulae. In: Schlag G, Redl H (eds) Fibrin sealant in operative medicine. Springer, Berlin Heidelberg New York, pp 148–156
5. Knöringer P (1986) Abdichtung der spinalen Dura mittels Fibrinklebung. Videotape, Immuno V 039

6. Knöringer P (1993) Autologous transplantation of cauda fibers: results of a recon-
    struction of transsected L5 filaments in a luxation fracture L 4/5. In: Lorenz R,
    Klinger M, Brock M (eds) Advances in neurosurgery 21. Springer, Berlin Heidel-
    berg New York, pp 232–345
7. Matras H, Jesch W, Kletter G, Dinges HP (1978) Spinale Duraklebung mit Fibrin-
    kleber. Eine experimentelle Studie. Wien Med Wochenschr 90 (12): 419–425
8. Redl H, Schlag G (1986) Fibrin sealant and its modes of application. In: Schlag G,
    Redl H (eds) Fibrin sealant in operative medicine. Springer, Berlin Heidelberg New
    York, pp 13–26
9. Stübinger B (1984) Klinische Erfahrungen mit der Spongiosa-Fibrinkleber-Plastik.
    In: Scheele J (ed) Fibrinklebung. Springer, Berlin Heidelberg New York,
    pp 201–204
10. Schlag G, Redl H, Turnher M, Dinges HP (1986) The importance of fibrin in
    wound repair. In: Schlag G, Redl H (eds) Fibrin sealant in operative medicine.
    Springer, Berlin Heidelberg New York, pp 4–12

Neurosurgical Reconstruction of Obstetric Brachial Plexus Lesions with the Use of Fibrin Sealing

A. C. J. SLOOFF

Abstract

Our series of 655 brachial plexus lesions of various types included only recently a relatively important number of obstetric cases ($n = 240$). Erb's paralysis is a C_5C_6 and sometimes a $C_5C_6C_7$ lesion; Klumpke's paralysis with a severe lesion of the lower spinal nerves is always associated with an upper spinal nerve lesion of varying severity. The results of neurophysiological and radiologic investigations are often disappointing in regard to the evaluation of the severity of the lesion. For the surgical treatment we follow the criterium of Gilbert, i.e., the lack of clinical recovery of the biceps at the end of the third month. Other criteria indicating an unfavorable prognosis and constituting an indication for surgery are a Horner syndrome, persistent hypotonic paralysis, persistent phrenic nerve paralysis, and skin ulcers. Intra- and/or extraplexal neurotizations were performed in 94 children. Although the follow-up period of 2 years is too short, some general conclusions are justified, based upon 28 operated children. We achieved good to very good results in all children with an upper plexus lesion born in a cephalic presentation ($n = 10$). Breech presentation ($n = 7$), often associated with an avulsion, has less good results. Total or subtotal lesions ($n = 11$) form a prognostically unfavorable group, but some gain, even in hand function, is possible. The reconstruction is worthwhile.

Introduction

Deep medical interest in birth palsy first developed toward the end of the nineteenth century, especially following the pulications of Duchenne in 1861 [3] and Erb in 1874 [4]. In 1903, operative intervention was reported by Kennedy [13]; later reports on surgical treatment were presented by Wyeth and Sharpin [23] in 1917 and by Taylor [21] in 1920. However, in about 1930, surgical intervention fell into disfavor because of the high mortality rate and dubious results. It took 50 years of conservative treatment before interest in surgical treatment was revived; this was due to the application of microsurgical techniques and the experience in microsurgical reconstructions in adults with traumatic bra-

Table 1. Etiology of brachial plexus lesions

Lesion	No. of patients	No. of patients operated on
Traumatic lesions	582	
Traction/crush lesions lacerations, gunshot wounds	315	161
Obstetric lesions	240	94
Iatrogenic lesions	27	–
Tumors	30	19
Entrapment syndromes	12	8
Lesions due to irradiation	10	–
Others	21	–
Total	655	282

chial plexus lesions. The publication by Tassin [20] (based on Gilbert's clinical material) on obstetric lesions formed a real breakthrough.

These were followed by papers from several other authors including Alanen [1], Boome [2], Hidehiko Kawabata [10], Laurent [14], Narakas [15], Solonen [17], Sztonak [19] and Terzis [22]. Our series of 655 brachial plexus lesions of various types (Table 1) has only recently been expanded with a relatively important number of obstetric cases ($n = 240$).

Special features in older patients with an obstetric brachial plexus lesion were the retardation of growth of the affected arm, as well as severe contractures, skeletal deformities, and sensory disturbances, which in younger patients could even cause ulcerations and automutilation.

Clinical Features

The incidence of obstetric brachial plexus injuries varies between 0.5 and 3 per thousand live births in a hospital population. Recovery rates of 80%–90% have been reported. Recent publications suggest important improvements in conservative treatment through intensive physical therapy as well as better obstetric care.

The traumatic origin of the lesion at birth is generally accepted. It is a stretch injury caused by a mechanism combining lowering of the shoulder with opposite inclination of the cervical spine. Two situations seem to predispose to this birth injury: large infants in cephalic presentation with shoulder dystocia and small, often asphyctic, infants in breech presentation. In some cases, however, a quite normal delivery is described and it has been presumed that the palsy is caused by an intrauterine maladaptation [12]. A birth palsy is also mentioned after cesarean section [16].

The diagnosis is usually readily apparent. After a difficult delivery, the upper limb is flaccid.

After some days, weeks, or months, two different types of palsy can be identified. Erb's paralysis, with a C5C6 and sometimes a C7 lesion, is a paralysis of the upper spinal nerves with a limb held in internal rotation and pronation. There is no abduction or external rotation; the wrist is flexed, and sometimes the fingers and wrist will not extend. Flexors of the wrist and fingers are active, as is the pectoralis major. This is the so-called waiter's tip position.

Klumpke's paralysis with a severe lesion of the lower spinal nerves is always associated with a upper spinal nerve lesion of varying severity, or the lesion is a manifestation of a complete lesion of the plexus with a Horner syndrome and sometimes dystrophic changes in the upper limb.

When compared to the traumatic lesions in adults, the obstetric plexus injury has some typical features. It is more uniform and situated supraclavicularly. There is never a double lesion or a vascular lesion, and a pain syndrome is very rare. This, together with the disappointing results of the neurophysiological, radiologic, and histologic investigations, indicates that the obstetric brachial plexus lesions form a specific entity among the brachial plexus lesions.

Unfavorable signs are neglect of the upper limb, persisting hypotonia, persisting phrenic nerve palsy, contractures, dystrophy, growth retardation, and skeletal deformities.

The associated lesions in 94 operated children are shown in Table 2. In the literature, the incidence of phrenic nerve palsy is reported as 5%–9%, of facial nerve palsy as 5%–14%, and of a bilateral lesion as 8%–22% [18]. Also accessory and hypoglossal nerve lesions are described.

The obstetric phrenic nerve palsy can be present as an isolated lesion, but is associated with a brachial plexus lesion in more than 70% of patients, mostly in children with an upper plexus lesion who were born in a breech presentation [5, 16]. The injury of the phrenic nerve can be either an avulsion or an extraforaminal lesion.

Special Investigations

Neurophysiological investigations such as electromyography (EMG), sensory nerve action potentials (SNAP), somatosensory evoked potentials (SSEP), and radiologic investigations including cervical myelography and CT myelography are carried out preoperatively in order to map the severity and extent of the lesion, to make an evaluation, and finally to assist in the decision-making process.

Table 2. Associated lesions in 94 operated obstetric brachial plexus lesions

Lesion	No. of patients	No. of patients born in breech presentation
Sternocleidomastoid muscle	9	4
Clavicle fracture	9	1
Humerus fracture	6	1
Persistent phrenic nerve palsy	8	6
Bilateral plexus lesion	6	6

We studied the results of these investigations in 94 operated children in relation to the operative and histologic findings and concluded that there were important discrepancies in approximately 50 % of the cases. Nevertheless, these investigations still have some value. An EMG generally gives too optimistic an impression. The combination of denervation signs with absent action potentials is a severe and unfavorable prognostic sign, as well as the absence of roots and a meningocele formation outside the vertebral foramen on the CT myelography.

Indications for Surgical Treatment

Gilbert's [6] most important indication for surgical treatment was the lack of clinical recovery of the biceps muscle at the end of the third month. The biceps function was used as the key function because of the difficulty involved in testing the deltoid muscle.

The selection of this criterion was based upon the thesis by Tassin [20].

Comparison of the results in Gilbert's series of operated children [7, 10, 11] with those obtained following nonoperative measures as assessed by Tassin is also convincing and shows better results in Gilbert's operatively treated children.

Other criteria indicating an unfavorable prognosis and sustaining an indication for surgical treatment are a Horner's syndrome, persistent hypotonic paralysis, persistent phrenic nerve palsy, persisting skin ulcers, severe pathological CT myelography, persistent denervation, and no action potentials during EMG investigation. They are the clinical expression of lesions which are histologically characterized by axonotmesis with laceration of perineurium, neurotmesis, avulsion or severe fibrosis (stage IV or higher according to Sunderland [18]).

Although controversies continue [13] we are strongly convinced by these criteria. Moreover, we had the same experience with children who were only surgically exploted or in whom only a neurolysis was performed and with children who were deliberately conservatively treated against our advice to intervene surgically.

Patients

According to these criteria, 94 children underwent surgical treatment during the period from April 1986 to November 1992. Their age at operation varied from 2.5–29 months, with an average age of 7 months. Some 75 children presented cephalically with a birth weight of between 2980 and 6000 g (mean 4340 g), while 19 children were breech deliveries with a birth weight of 1830–4000 g (mean, 2806 g). The anatomical lesion consisted of 15 C5C6 lesions, 49 C5C6C7 lesions, and 30 subtotal or total lesions. There were 32 injuries on the left side and 62 on the right side. The series consisted of 46 female and 48 male neonates.

Surgical Policy and Procedures

The operation is performed under general anesthesia with special measures to facilitate perioperative neurophysiological investigations. A supraclavicular approach is generally used, but in some cases, for example, with total or subtotal lesions, an additional infraclavicular approach is necessary, sometimes combined with an osteotomy of the clavicle. The dissection and reconstruction is conducted with the aid of a magnifying glass or an operating microscope.

In most cases a neuroma in continuity is found in the spinal nerves and/or trunks. Sometimes a rupture is found or a flaccid spinal nerve makes one suspect an avulsion. The neuroma can be limited to the upper trunk, but in severe cases can extend to the lower trunks or even further down as far as the cords. The phrenic nerve, which can be ruptured as well as avulsed, is more frequently involved in adhesions and tightly fixed on the spinal nerve C5 and the scalenic muscle.

The assessment of the severity and extension of the lesion can be supported by perioperative neurophysiological and histologic investigations.

Depending on the clinical signs and the operative findings, the neuroma is excised and reconstructive procedures are planned, bearing in mind the priorities for functional recovery: external rotation of the shoulder, flexion of the elbow, extension of the wrist, and flexion of the digits. A direct suture (coaptation) is seldom possible, and after resection of the neuroma grafting procedures (intraplexal neurotizations) are almost always necessary. The number of grafts and their length depends on the extension and severity of the lesion. A reconstruction from C5 to the upper trunk as a whole or other intraplexal combinations can be performed, e.g., with the aid of the long thoracic, thoracodorsal, or pectoral nerves. The sural nerves are mostly used as donor nerves. With the presence of avulsions, the reconstruction must always be tailor-made according to the local situation and priorities. The accessory nerve, the cervical plexus, the intercostal nerves, and sometimes the hypoglossal nerve or the contralateral plexus can be used as proximal stumps for the so-called extraplexal neurotizations.

There is only limited space for neurolysis and, moreover, neurolysis as the only procedure for treating a neuroma surgically is apparently not successful.

For coaptation, we bring the proximal and distal nerve stumps together without any tension. With a cutting device the stumps are sharply cut and fibrin glue is placed at the coaptation site, but we nearly always need a grafting procedure with several sural nerves grafts. The grafts are bundled at both ends and glued together. The ends are sharply cut and the graft is placed inbetween the corresponding proximal and distal nerve stumps. Fibrin glue is then placed at the coaptation site. Sometimes the coaptation is reinforced by 10/0 sutures.

In nearly all 94 cases, the lesions found at exploration were impressive with wide-spread neuromas and/or signs of avulsion. Sometimes a few fasciculi were found in the neuroma. These histologic findings might perhaps explain the weak motor responses which were sometimes elicited perioperatively and the overoptimistic preoperative neurophysiological findings.

Table 3. Surgically treated obstetric brachial plexus lesions

Type	Number	Presentation	
		Cephalic	Breech
C5C6	15	2	13
Avulsion	12	1	11
Rupture	3	1	2
C5C6C7	49	44	5
Avulsion	12	8	4
Rupture	37	36	1
(Sub)total	30	29	1
Avulsion	17	17	0
Rupture	13	12	1
Total	94	75	19
Avulsion	41		
Rupture	53		

After the operation, the child is immobilized in a plastic cast for 3 weeks. After this period, physical therapy can be started gradually.

The first signs of recovery depend on the level, severity, and extension of the lesion and the reconstructions performed, but cannot be expected before 4–6 months. We wait at least 4 years before making a final evaluation.

An overview of our first 94 operated children shows 15 with a pure C5C6 lesion; breech presentations ($n = 13$) prevail, often with avulsion of one or both roots ($n = 11$). The C5C6C7 lesions ($n = 49$) are more extraforaminal lesions ($n = 37$); avulsions are less frequent ($n = 12$) in this type. The frequency of total and subtotal lesions is relatively high ($n = 30$); breech presentation in this group is rare, and an avulsion is somewhat more frequent ($n = 17$). In the total series of 94 operated cases, 41 children had one or more root avulsions. Indeed, the upper plexus lesions C5C6 and C5C6C7 were more frequent than the severe (sub)total lesions (ratio, 64:30; see Table 3).

Follow-Up and Prognosis

The follow-up period in this series of 94 operated children varied between 1 month and 5 years. Most patients were operated on in the last 2 years. For a complete evaluation, we need at least 4 years, as Gilbert's results have shown [6, 7], but after 2 years we can nevertheless obtain an impression of a certain rate of recovery.

In the first group of 28 children with a follow-up of 2 years, the lesions were only explored or partially reconstructed in eight patients, because of the risk to the apparently still functioning nerves (perioperative motor stimulation). The results in these children were disappointing and served as an additional argument for a more aggressive policy.

The frequency of total and subtotal lesions was relatively high (11 out of 28). The possibilities open for reconstruction in these cases are clearly fewer and these children form a prognostically unfavorable group. Nevertheless, as Gilbert demonstrated, in these cases some gain, even in hand function, is possible and the procedure is therefore worthwhile.

The results are better in lesions of the upper plexus (17 out of 28) – Erb's type C5C6(C7) – unless this is associated with an avulsion, as is often seen in breech presentation (seven out of 17). We achieved good to very good results – a Mallet score of at least IV – in all children with an upper plexus lesion born in a cephalic presentation (ten out of 17).

In addition, the worse results can be upgraded by the results of secondary surgical interventions such as muscle or tendon transfers.

Also remarkable for this obstetric palsy is the observation that some infants, especially with late interventions, have apparently good return of neuromuscular function and sensation, but are not able to use the affected upper limb or a specific function of it. It is likely that a transitory sensory/motor deprivation in early life impairs normal development of the use of the arm.

Conclusion

It is extremely important to improve our understanding and gain further knowledge; this will only be acquired when every obstetric brachial plexus lesion is presented at an early stage, at the age of 3–6 weeks, to a team specialized in this field. Such a multidisciplinary team consists, for example, of a pediatric neurologist, a rehabilitation physician, neurosurgeons, and orthopedic and plastic surgeons. A pediatric physiotherapist also plays an important role. This policy is crucial for early and total, conservative as well as primary or secondary surgical treatment.

Until different criteria have been defined, based upon further developments of standardized methods and intervals for evaluation of the children, we have decided to adhere to the indications for operative treatment as formulated by Gilbert.

Sometimes secondary surgery such as tendon or muscle transfers is required to treat contractures and to supplement unsatisfactory results of conservative or surgical treatment. It is important to make a decision in time, before neuroplasticity is damaged and contractures have developed; however, we should not forget that these improvements of therapeutic measurements, based upon further studies and research, need to be supplemented by preventive measures.

References

1. Alanen M, Halonen JP, Katevuo K, Vilki P (1986). Early surgical exploration and epineural repair in birth brachial palsy. Z Kinderchir 41: 335–337
2. Boome RS, Kaye JC (1988) Obstetric traction injuries of the brachial plexus. J Bone Joint Surg 70 B: 571–576
3. Duchenne G (1861) Diagnostic différentiel des paralysies cérébreale de l'enfance d'avec la paralysie atrophique graisseure de l'enfance et d'avec certaines paralysies

traumatiques congénitales. In: De l'electrisation localisée et de son application à la pathologie et à la therapeutique, 2nd edn. Baillière, Paris

4. Erb W (1874) Uber eine eigenthumliche Localisation von Lahmungen im Plexus Brachialis. Verh. Naturhist Med 2: 130–136

5. France NE (1954) Unilateral diaphragmatic paralysis and Erb's palsy in the new-born. Arch Dis Childhood 64: 357–359

6. Gilbert A (1989) Indications et resultats de la chirurgie du plexus brachial dans la paralysie obstetricale. In: Alnot J, Narakas A (eds) Les paralysies du plexus brachial. Expansion Scientifique Franciase, Paris

7. Gilbert A (1991) Surgical treatment of brachial plexus birth palsy. Clin Orthop Relat res 264: 39–49

8. Hentz VR, Meyer RD (1991) Brachial plexus microsurgery in children. Microsurgery 12: 175–185

9. Hentz VR (1991) Operative repair of the brachial plexus in infants and children. In: Gelberman RH (ed) Operative nerve repair and reconstruction. Lippincott, Philadelphia

10. Hidehiko Kawabata, Kazuhiro Masada, Yuichi Tsuyuguchi, Hideo Kawai, Keiro Ono, Koichi Tada (1987) Early reconstruction in birth palsy. Clin Orthop Relat Res 215: 233–242

11. Hoffer HM (1991) Assessment and natural history of brachial plexus injury in children. In: Gelberman RH (ed) Operative nerve repair and reconstruction. Lippencott, Philadelphia

12. Jennet RJ, Tarby TJ, Kreinick CJ (1992) Brachial plexus palsy: an old problem revisited. Am J Obstet Gynecol 166: 1673–1677

13. Kennedy B (1903) Suture of the brachial plexus in birth paralysis of the upper extremity. Br Med J 1: 298–301

14. Laurent JP (1990) Upper brachial plexus birth injuries. A neurosurgical approach. Concept Pediatr Neurosurg 10: 156–164

15. Narakas A (1986) Injuries to the brachial plexus. In: Bora W (ed) The pediatric upper extremity. Saunders, Philadelphia

16. Painter MJ (1988) Brachial plexus injuries in neonates. Int Pediatr 3: 120–124

17. Solonen KA, Teleranta T, Ryoppy S (1981) Early reconstruction of birth injuries of the brachial plexus. J Pediatr Orthop 1: 367–378

18. Sunderland S (1978) Nerves and nerve injuries. Churchill Livingstone, London

19. Sztonak L, Warnke JP (1987) Die operative Versorgung der perinatalen Schädigung der Plexus brachialis. Zentralbl Neurochir 48: 162–167

20. Tassin JL (1983) Paralysies obstetricales du plexus brachial. Evolution spontanée; resultats des interventions reparatrices precoces. Thesis, Paris

21. Taylor AS (1920) Brachial birth palsy and injuries of similar type in adult. Surg Gynecol Obstet 39: 494–502

22. Terzis J (1987) Microreconstruction of nerve injuries. Saunders, Philadelphia

23. Wyeth JA, Sharpe W (1917) The field of neurological surgery in a general hospital. Surg Gynecol Obstet 24: 29–39

Centrocentral Anastomosis:
An Elegant Alternative in the Surgical Treatment
of Painful Amputation Neuromas

J. Barberá

Abstract

Centrocentral anastomosis (CCA), as defined by Samii [16], is the surgical connection between the proximal fascicles of a sectioned nerve by means of interposed nerve grafts. In previous experimental work, we observed that CCA prevents the painful induced autotomy due to the neuroma after sciatic nerve section in rats. The present clinical study was designed to evaluate the results of CCA in 43 patients suffering pain due to an amputation neuroma (sciatic nerve in 31 cases, cutaneous branches of the femoral nerve in one case, peroneal nerve in two cases, and digital nerves in nine cases). CCA was not used to treat phantom pain. When operating on major nerves, the neuroma was excised and four to eight fascicular groups were isolated proximal to it. Then the stumps of each pair of fascicular groups were anastomosed between them, interposing a fascicular nerve graft taken from the sectioned nerve itself. In the case of finger amputation, CCA is carried out between the two digital nerves of the same side. Fibrin glue (Tissucol) was used to unite the nerve ends to avoid foreign body reactions, increasing the potentially terminal neuroma. The mean postoperative follow-up is 5 months (ranging from 3 to 24 months). Total and immediate suppression of pain was achieved in 90% of cases. The previous phantom sensations, when present, were unchanged. We think that the success of this technique is due to avoiding a new neuroma production by arresting definitively the nerve fiber regeneration inside the graft, as has been experimentally demonstrated.

Painful Amputation Neuroma

The amputation neuroma is a typical reactive fibrous structure which invariably results from peripheral nerve section This structure stretches out from the transected area at the central, proximal end of the nerve. Its most significant histological feature is the presence of bare axonal sprouts deprived of their normal endoneural lining. The axonal growth accounts for regenerative activity taking place at the injured neuron and since it lacks distal endoneural tubes, axons grow into an adverse environment formed by a synchronic reactive fibroblastic proliferation.

In 1974, Wall and Gutnick [22] described the presence of spontaneously generated ectopic and abnormal activity in the axon sprouts of the neuroma. Later studies [4, 6, 7, 11, 17] confirmed the above condition to be characterized by spontaneous electric discharges which appear to be related to a special sensitivity to mechanical and chemical (alpha-sympathetic agonists) stimuli, to the presence of ephaptic (cross-talk) synapsis between the fibers themselves, and to a relative excess in the number of unmyelinated fibers. However, this abnormal activity of nerve fibers at the neuroma is not unique. Abnormal electric activity has also been observed in the dorsal horn neurons of sectioned peripheral nerves [21], and it is probably responsible for the chronicity and centralization of the pain whenever the primary physiopathological situations they derive from last for longer periods of time [8, 26].

Neuroma formation results invariably from the section of any nerve. However, painful neuroma is quite an exceptional complication. No significant histological differences can be observed between normal and painful neuroma. This being the case, the presence of pain should be attributed to factors external to the neuroma. Clinical phenomena associated with painful amputation neuromas are clearly defined and present themselves in an unmistakable form. The most characteristic sign is the sudden perception of intense pain, regarded by the patient as an electric discharge spreading towards the sensitive anatomical area, which depends on the sectioned nerve. Such discharges can occur spontaneously, but they have often been associated with mechanical stimulation of the cutaneous area next to the neuroma [20]. This allows us to suggest the hypothesis that the mechanical irritation to growing axons does indeed cause a remarkable electric discharge to occur, which is interpreted by the central nervous system as a typical sudden pain episode [23]. Pain can sometimes be so intense that patients carefully avoid any mechanical stimuli to the area and refuse the use of prosthetic supports on the zone of neuroma location, thus restricting their everyday life activity.

Superficial sensitive nerves, such as digital nerves, are constantly exposed to mechanical stimuli in normal life activity. It is precisely because of this that the presence of painful neuroma at this level is much more frequent. Major mixed nerves of the limbs are normally well protected by the muscles which cover them, so preventing direct mechanical stimulation of the nerve. Nevertheless, pathological circumstances that are actually indications for limb amputation can favor the presence of painful neuroma. Indeed, chronic ischemia resulting from irreparable artery disease is still a frequent cause for amputation. This usually occurs in elderly patients, with scarce muscular mass, in which the tissues located at an amputation level are insufficiently irrigated, probably due to the disease itself. Hypoxia has been shown to increase the ectopic hypersensitivity at the neuroma [14]. On the other hand, the larger fibrous scar proliferation resulting from ischemia can trap the neuroma by attaching it to the neighboring tissues and, therefore, rendering it more accessible to compressive mechanical and traction stimuli.

Treatment of specific neuroma pain is a difficult task. Conservative treatments have failed most times [5] and surgery does not yield consistent success. This can be demonstrated by the fact that more than 100 surgical techniques have already been described [19]. Whipple and Unsell [24] systematized the current surgical possibilities in two groups: (a) those intended to translocate the nerve, trying to move it away from harmful stimuli, and (b) those intended to inhibit axonal growth. Among the latter, a distinction can be made between those which are intended to provide physical contention (ligature, cauterization), synthetic contention (capping with inert materials), or physiological contention (end-to-end suture) of the neuroma.

In any case, given the difficulty of arresting axonal growth by means of physical or synthetic procedures and taking into account the local conditions of development of the painful neuroma, it becomes evident that the best solution to avoid the genesis of pain in the neuroma would be, in theory, to prevent the formation of the neuroma itself, i.e., the physiological contention.

Centrocentral Anastomosis

CCA is the anatomical connection, surgically performed, between the fascicular groups of the central stump of a severed nerve via an interposed nerve graft. The aim of the operation is to divert the regenerative axonal sprouts of each fascicular group towards the inner part of the graft, where they can grow freely in a normal physiological environment, as is achieved following reconstruction of a sectioned nerve provided with a distally accessible part. CCA should be distinguished from direct end-to-end centrocentral connection, without grafting, used by other authors [1, 25].

The procedure was described by Samii in 1981 [16]. Later on, Gorkisch et al. [10] reported excellent results obtained by means of CCA in the treatment and prevention of painful neuroma in severed digital nerves. In 1983 our group embarked upon laboratory research of the technique. CCA has proved to be a remarkable method for the prevention of autotomy that occurs following experimental section of the sciatic nerve in rats [2, 9]. Histological studies of the interposed graft, carried out several weeks postoperatively, showed that regenerative growth in the proximal stumps of the nerve usually takes place within the interposed graft. Most remarkable, too, is the fact that regenerative growth is limited, so that axonal sprouts never cross the second suture [3]. This spontaneous arrest of axonal growth within the graft prevents the formation of neuroma. These findings confirm those obtained by Gorkisch et al. [10].

Several reasons have been suggested in order to explain the arrest of axonal growth inside the graft [10, 18, 24]. First the penetration of axons into the endoneural tubes of the graft, without a peripheral purpose, prevents target point-dependent neurotrophic factors from having an effect upon them. The absence of these stimuli could explain the arrest of axonal growth. Second, central, neuronal suppression of the axonal growth could occur due to the biochemical identification with neighboring normal axons belonging to another central stump and housed in the same endoneural tube within the graft. Third, the pressure increase inside the endoneural tubes of the graft, resulting from axonal growth within it, hinders the axoplasmic proximodistal flow and, therefore, inhibits the synthesis of neuronal proteins necessary to preserve fiber growth. Although all these reasons are speculative, CCA does actually prevent typical neuroma development, which is precisely the purpose of the operation.

Surgical Technique of Centrocentral Anastomosis

Figure 1 shows a sketch of the CCA technique in a major nerve. The nerve trunk upon which the neuroma is located is exposed through an incision that allows direct access to it. From the trunk, and following a distal direction, the neuroma is dissected and freed of its adherences to neighboring tissues. The neuroma is then excised by sectioning the nerve trunk upon which is located, ensuring that it is sectioned over healthy nerve tissue.

In major nerves, the distal 5–6 cm of the nerve are retracted from the remaining tissues. The nerve is then placed on a tinfoil or gutta-percha plate in order to allow better manipulation. The epineurum of the distal portion of the nerve is then excised in a length proportional to its caliber, after which fascicular dissection can be started. Care should be taken to obtain an even number of fascicular groups. It is desirable that each pair of fascicular groups have similar widths. Having isolated the fascicular groups, their ends are then united by pairs, so that each two fascicular groups form a loop. One of the two fascicular groups of each loop is then sectioned 2 cm above the end-to-end connection. In this manner, an autologous graft interposed between the fascicular groups' ends can be achieved. In our first cases, each fascicular group was anastomosed to the graft with one nylon 8/0 suture stich. However, since the tensile strength between the anastomosed ends is practically nonexistent, at present we only use fibrin glue to unite them, which is sufficient to maintain the apposition. In that way we avoid leaving foreign bodies which could promote fibrous reactions and hinder axonal regeneration towards the graft. At the end of the operation, the terminal end of the sectioned nerve is formed by several closed fascicular loops (Fig. 2). The whole assembly is then placed carefully on a healthy tissue area. The operated limb is protected with a slight compressive and immobilizing bandage, which is maintained for 3 weeks.

In the case of finger amputation, CCA is carried out between the two digital nerves, anterior and posterior, of the same side.

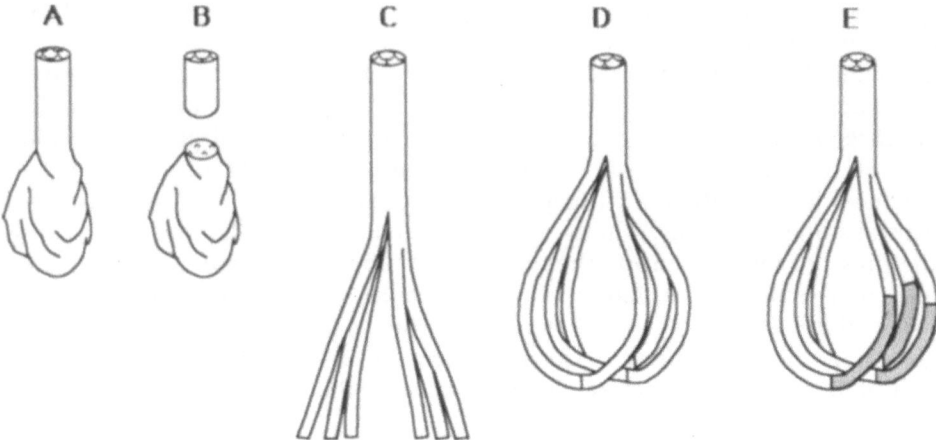

Fig. 1A–E. Surgical steps of the centrocentral anastomosis (CCA) in a major nerve. **A** Neuroma dissection. **B** Neuroma excision through normal nerve tissue. **C** Dissection of a paired number of fascicular groups. **D** First end-to-end union. **E** Proximal section of one fascicular group of each pair and second end-to-end connection. Thus an autologous nerve graft remains interposed between each pair of central fascicular groups

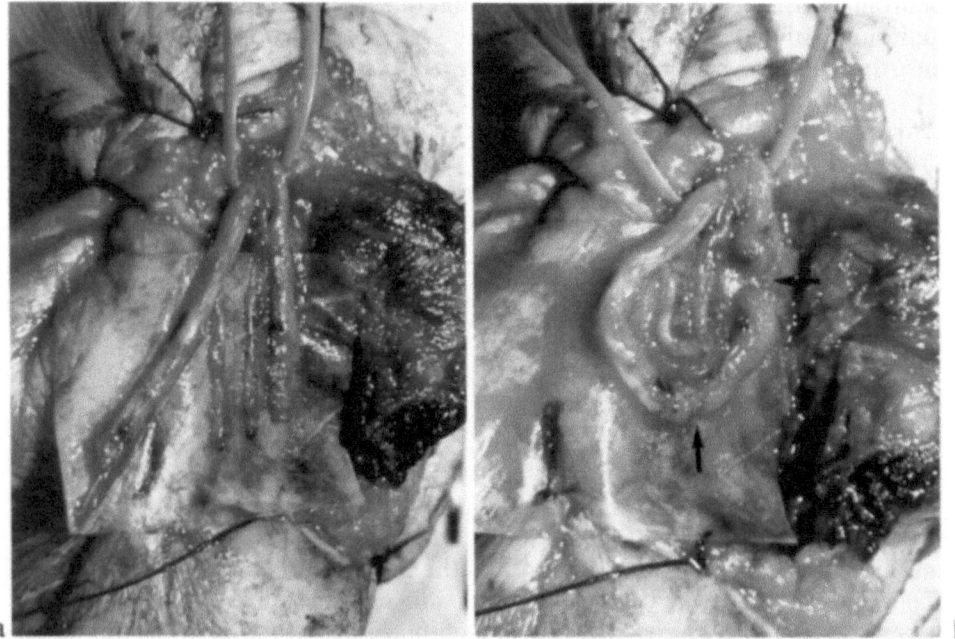

Fig. 2a, b. Operative photographs. **a** Dissection of four fascicular groups in the branches of a peroneal nerve harboring a painful neuroma. **b** Reconstruction of two terminal loops with an interposed nerve graft (*arrows* on the end-to-end connections)

Clinical Material and Results

A total of 43 patients were operated on in a 5-year period, 37 of whom presented with a lower limb painful amputation neuroma (sciatic nerve in 31 cases, cutaneous branches of the femoral nerve in one case, peroneal nerve in two cases, and digital nerves at the tarsus in three cases) and the other six with an upper limb painful amputation neuroma (all six in digital nerves: two cases at hand level and four cases at finger level). The number of painful neuromas of the sciatic nerve is very high, but this can be explained by the fact that one of the hospitals which sent patients to our department is a reference point for the rehabilitation of amputated patients because of vascular disease.

All patients showed the typical clinical symptoms and signs of painful neuroma and were refractory to conservative treatment.

In all cases CCA was the first operation done in order to manage neuroma pain. Results of CCA in 22 selected patients who presented with painful amputation neuromas of major nerves and at least a 1-year clinical follow-up are to be published elsewhere.

The average follow-up period of the total number of cases was 5 months (ranging from 3 to 24 months). Total and immediate suppression of pain was achieved in 90 % of cases. Two patients had to undergo further surgery, as typical pain recurred after a short period of time. In one of them, with a sciatic nerve neuroma, a deep infection of the surgical wound had released the suture. The other case, a digital nerve neuroma, presented with a spontaneous suture dehiscence. Pain was alleviated in both cases after reoperation. In one patient with digital neuroma and another one with tarsus neuroma, symptoms did not improve and the patients refused further surgery. Persistent local discomfort at the stump of the limb was felt by six patients with thigh amputation due to vascular disorders. Such discomfort prevented the continuous use of the prosthesis and we attributed it to a deficiently irrigated limb stump.

In no case of major nerve surgery did phantom pain appear postoperatively.

Discussion

The success of surgery for painful amputation neuroma depends on two kinds of factors. First, it depends on the neuroma environment alterations produced with the purpose of avoiding any external factors, mainly of a mechanic and ischemic nature, which cause pain. Clinical experience shows that in many cases the simple relocation of the nerve end or a simple neurectomy with neuroma excision [5, 12] gives a high percentage of disappearance of pain.

Secondly surgery success depends on the ability to prevent the formation of a new neuroma. End-to-end sutures are, without doubt, the best alternative in the management of pain resulting from nerve section, since they allow physiological regeneration to occur, thus avoiding recurrence of painful neuroma. CCA allows the same physiological approach for cases where the distal end of the sectioned nerve is not accessible due to the amputation.

The mere relocation of the nerve end, it could be argued, might explain the good results of CCA, especially in cases of major nerve neuromas; however, against that, and supporting the elegant conception of CCA, are the experimental findings of no new neuroma formation after this operation, the histological normality of the regenerated fibers inside the graft, and the spontaneous arrest of axonal growth near the second suture [3, 10, 16]. These facts are indisputable and could also be the reason behind the high cure rate of painful neuroma using CCA [10, 13, 15, 16]. Given these good results and considering the simplicity of the technique, we would recommend CCA as the first-choice attempt in surgical treatment for the refractory amputation neuroma pain.

References

1. Ashley L, Stallings J (1988) End-to-side nerve flap for treatment of painful neuroma: 15 year follow-up. J Am Osteopath Assoc 88: 621–624
2. Barberá J, Gonzalez J, Broseta J (1984) Evaluation of centrocentral anastomosis in autotomy following sciatic transection in rats. Pein [Suppl] 2: 444
3. Barberá J, Gonzalez J, Gil JL, Sanjuán A, García F, Lopez A (1988) The quality and extension of nerve fiber regeneration in the centrocentral anastomosis of the peripheral nerve. Acta Neurochir (Wien) [Suppl] 43: 205–209
4. Burchiel KJ, Ochoa JL (1991a) Pathophysiology of injured axons. Neurosurg Clin North Am 2: 105–116
5. Burchiel KJ, Ochoa JL (1991b) Surgical management of posttraumatic neuropathic pain. Neurosurg Clin North Am 2: 117–126
6. Burchiel KJ, Russell LC (1985) Spontaneous activity of ventral roots axons following peripheral nerve injury. J Neurosurg 62: 246–249
7. Devor M (1984) The pathophysiology and anatomy of damaged nerve. In: Wall PD, Melzack R (eds) Textbook of pain. Churchill Livingstone, New York, p 49
8. Devor M, Wall PD (1981) Plasticity in the spinal cord sensory map following peripheral nerve injuries in rats. J Neurosci 1: 679–684
9. Gonzalez-Darder J, Barberá J, Abellán MJ, Mora A (1985) Centrocentral anastomosis in the prevention and treatment of painful terminal neuroma. An experimental study in rats. J Neurosurg 63: 754–758
10. Gorkisch K, Boese-Landgraf J, Vaubel E (1984) Treatment and prevention of amputation neuromas in hand surgery. Plast Reconstr Surg 73: 293–296
11. Govrin-Lippmann R, Devor M (1978) Ongoing activity in severed nerves: source and variations with time. Brain Res 159: 406–410
12. Herndon JH, Hess AV (1991) Neuromas. In: Gelberman RH (ed) Operative nerve repair and reconstruction. Lippincott, Philadelphia, p 1525
13. Kon M, Bloem J (1987) The treatment of amputation neuromas in fingers with a centrocentral nerve union. Ann Plast Surg 18: 506–510
14. Koremann EM, Devor M (1981) Ectopic adrenergic sensitivity in damaged peripheral nerve axons in the rat. Exp Neurol 85: 63–81
15. Lagarrigue J, Chavoin JP, Belahouart L, Scavazza R (1982) Traitement des nevromes douloureux par anastomose nerveuse en anse "piege à neurone". Neurochirurgie 28: 91–92
16. Samii M (1981) Centrocentral anastomosis of peripheral nerves: a neurosurgical treatment of amputation neuromas. In: Siegfried J, Zimmermann M (eds) Phantom and stump pain. Springer, Berlin Heidelberg New York, p 123
17. Scadding JW (1981) The development of ongoing activity, mechanosensitivity and adrenaline sensitivity in severed peripheral nerve axons. Exp Neurol 73: 345–364

18. Seckel BR (1984) Discussion to "Treatment and prevention of amputation neuro-mas in hand surgery". Plast Reconst Surg 73: 297–299
19. Snyder CC, Knowles RP (1965) Traumatic neuromas. J Bone Joint Surg 47A: 641–648
20. Sunderland D (1985) Nervios periféricos y sus lesiones (translation of the second British edition of "Nerves and nerve injures"). Salvat, Barcelona, p 108
21. Wall PD, Devor M (1983) Sensory afferent impulses originate from dorsal root ganglia as well as from the periphery in normal and nerve-injured rats. Pain 17: 321–339
22. Wall PD, Gutnick M (1974) Properties of afferent nerve impulses originating from a neuroma. Nature 248: 740–743
23. Wall PD, Sccading JW, Tomkiewickz MM (1979) The production and prevention of experimental anesthesia dolorosa. Pain 6: 175–182
24. Whipple RR, Unsell RS (1988) Treatment of painful neuromas. Orthop Clin North Am 19: 175–185
25. Wood VE, Mudge MK (1987) Treatment of neuromas about a major amputation stump. J Hand Surg 12A: 302–306
26. Woolf CJ (1983) Evidence for central component of post-injury pain hypersensitivity. Nature 306: 686–688

II. Ophthalmic Surgery

Fibrin Sealant in Ophthalmic Plastic and Reconstructive Surgery

F. J. STEINKOGLER and A. KUCHAR

Abstract

The fibrin sealing technique has been used with good success in eyelid, orbital, and lacrimal surgery for more than 10 years.

In eyelid surgery, the fixation of free autologous skin transplants for covering skin defects after tumor excision has proved advantageous, as early fibrovascular ingrowth into the transplant is stimulated. Sutures for transplant fixation are only necessary in the margin area, because the transplant can be tightly attached to the underlying tissue by fibrin glue. The application of compression bandages for several days can be avoided. The treatment of severe upper eyelid entropion represents a special indication for fibrin sealing. The autologous transplant covering the free anterior tarsal surface is fixed exclusively by fibrin sealant, thus preventing sutures from endangering the cornea.

In orbital surgery, the treatment of postenucleation syndrome, mainly based on orbital volume deficit, can be improved by the use of fibrin sealant for the fixation of the secondary orbital implant. The new fixation technique for the sclera silicone implant in the orbital cavity leads to a strong connection between sclera and orbital tissue, which markedly improves the mobility of the artificial eye.

In lacrimal surgery, there are several indications for the use of fibrin sealant. For reconstructing lacerated canaliculi lacrimales under the microscope, fibrin sealing of the microanastomosis can be utilized. Thus, microsutures adapting the torn ends of the canaliculus are not necessary any more. The glued canaliculus anastomosis has to be stabilized by a silicone tube and by the reconstructed lid.

In canaliculocystostomy, dacryocystorhinostomy, and canaliculodacryocystorhinostomy, the microanastomosis between canaliculi and lacrimal sac and the adaption of the lacrimal and nasal mucosal flaps can be performed by means of fibrin seal fixation. Microsutures, which are particularly difficult to perform at the posterior mucosal flaps, are not needed. In all of these cases a silicone intubation is advantageous and improves the prognosis of these operations.

The different operation techniques are demonstrated and the results are reported.

Introduction

The fibrin sealing technique has developed into a standard method in different surgical fields [24], and its advantages have also been put to use in ophthalmic surgery [1]. There are many fields in ophthalmic plastic and reconstructive surgery in which fibrin sealant can be utilized [1, 17, 24].

In eyelid surgery, the fixation of free autologous skin transplants for covering skin defects after tumor excision has proved advantageous, as early fibrovascular ingrowth into the transplant is stimulated [17]. Severe upper eyelid entropion and particular cases of trichiasis of the lower eyelid are further indications for the use of the fibrin sealing technique [18]. In orbital surgery, the surgical management of postenucleation socket syndrome, consisting in orbital volume deficit, can be improved by utilizing fibrin sealant fixation of the secondary orbital implant [19].

In lacrimal surgery, there are several indications for using fibrin sealant. For reconstructing lacerated canaliculi lacrimales under the microscope, fibrin sealing of the microanastomosis can be utilized [17, 20]. In canaliculocystostomy [20], dacryocystorhinostomy, and canaliculodacryocystorhinostomy, the microanastomosis between canaliculi and the lacrimal sac and the adaption of the lacrimal and the nasal mucosal flaps can be performed by means of fibrin sealing fixation.

Method of Fibrin Sealing

The fibrin sealant Tissucol (Immuno, Vienna) has two components. The first consists of human fibrinogen, factor XIII, and aprotinin, a fibrinolysis inhibitor. The second component contains thrombin and calcium chloride. These components can be mixed easily by means of an application set, provided by the manufacturer. When the two components are mixed, the sealant solidifies, i.e., the thrombin causes the fibrinogen to transform into fibrin, similar to the physiological coagulation process. The rate at which this process takes place depends on the concentration of thrombin used. Thrombin also activates factor XIII, which in turn causes a cross-linking of fibrin chains in the presence of calcium ions. To achieve quick primary agglutination (10–15 s), a thin layer of sealing substance containing 500 IU thrombin is applied to the wound area.

Eyelid Surgery

Fixation of Free Skin Transplants

In tumor surgery of the eyelid area, skin defects normally arise after excision of the tumor (Fig. 1). They can be closed by means of free, full-thickness transplants fixed mainly with fibrin sealant [22]. Skin transplants from the upper lid or from the retroauricular region are used for closing the defects. The excised skin is freed of subcutaneous tissue and prepared for grafting into the defect. For

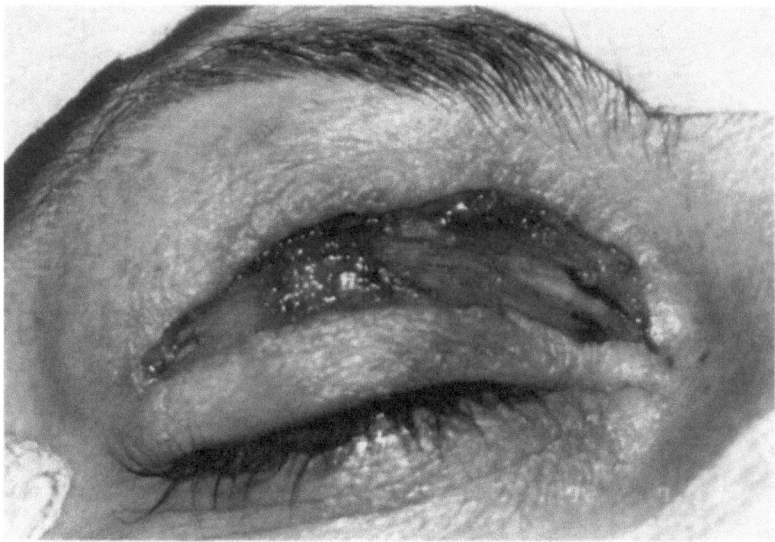

Fig. 1. A 46-year-old woman with recurrent xanthelasma of both upper eyelids combined with dermatochalasis: skin defect after tumor and skin excision of the right upper eyelid

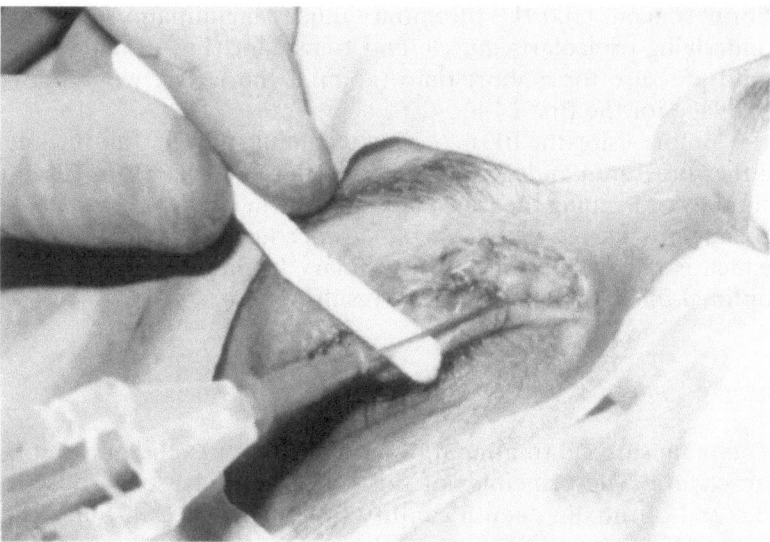

Fig. 2. Same patient as Fig. 1. Only a few sutures fix the free, full-thickness autologous skin transplant to the underlying orbicularis muscle and the skin: the already mixed fibrin sealant is injected under the skin transplant using the application set

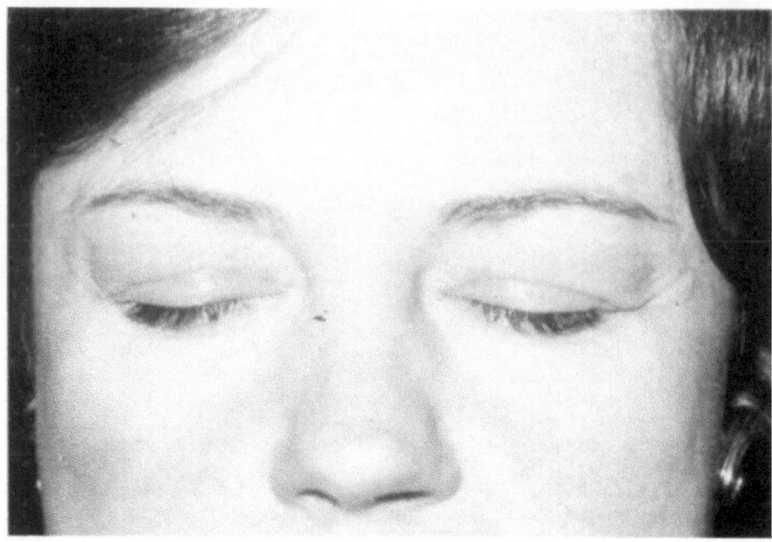

Fig. 3. Same patient as in Figs. 1 and 2; normal lid closure, smooth scars, and symmetric upper lid creases 3 months postoperatively

the fixation of the transplant, fibrin sealant is used after the exact adaption of the transplant into the defect by a few single-stitch sutures. The already mixed fibrin sealant (500 IU thrombin, quick agglutination) is injected between underlying orbicularis muscle and transplant (Fig. 2) and is fixed on it under mild pressure for a short time (about 2 min). The wound is covered with a bandage for the first 24 h.

Before using the fibrin sealing technique of free, full-thickness transplants, either pressure bandages on the free transplant had to be used [16] or special sutures for keeping the transplant in the skin defect had to be made [14]. Fibrin sealing provides us with a one-step procedure for the fixation of the transplant which is easy to perform. The primary healing of the transplant leads to an optimal functional and cosmetic result (Fig. 3).

Severe Upper Eyelid Entropion

The main surgical treatment of a severe upper eyelid entropion is the lid-split procedure. The principles of this procedure have been described ever since the end of the nineteenth century [6, 10, 12, 25, 26]. Since then, there have been different modifications of this procedure. The basic method is the Waldhauer technique [25], which consists of a lid-split procedure combined with a free skin transplantation. It was modified and extended by the fibrin sealing method.

A severe total upper eyelid entropion, with the eyelashes rubbing on the cornea and causing corneal alteration as well as conjunctival irritation, is the indication for this type of operation.

Using local anesthesia, a typical lid-split procedure is performed. After closure of the skin wound, the excised upper lid skin is used as a free, full-thickness skin graft for covering the raw anterior tarsal surface. The fixation of the autologous transplant can be done successfully by using the fibrin sealant. The transplant and the lid wound are covered with an antibiotic ointment and a bandage for 1 day. In the following few days, the operated lid is left without bandage, and only antibiotic ointment and ice packs are applied.

Since severe entropion of the upper eyelid can cause damage of the cornea and even loss of vision, its adequate repair is necessary. This technique provides skin for transplant and therefore no mucosal transplant is necessary, thus avoiding a second wound area.

Using the fibrin sealant technique, quick primary healing of the free skin transplant can be observed without using pressure bandages or cotton rolls, which have to be fixed in the tarsus by sutures.

Trichiasis of the Lower Eyelid

In particular forms of lower eyelid trichiasis (Figs. 4, 5), the same technique can be used for fixation of free autologous conjunctival transplants from the upper fornix after separation of the lashes from the posterior lamella with a lid-split technique.

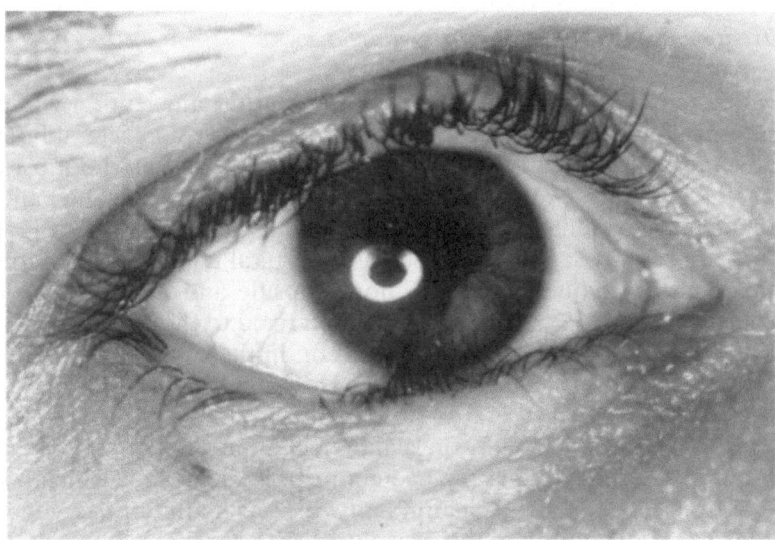

Fig. 4. A 23-year-old man with lower eyelid trichiasis of the right eye after chemical burn

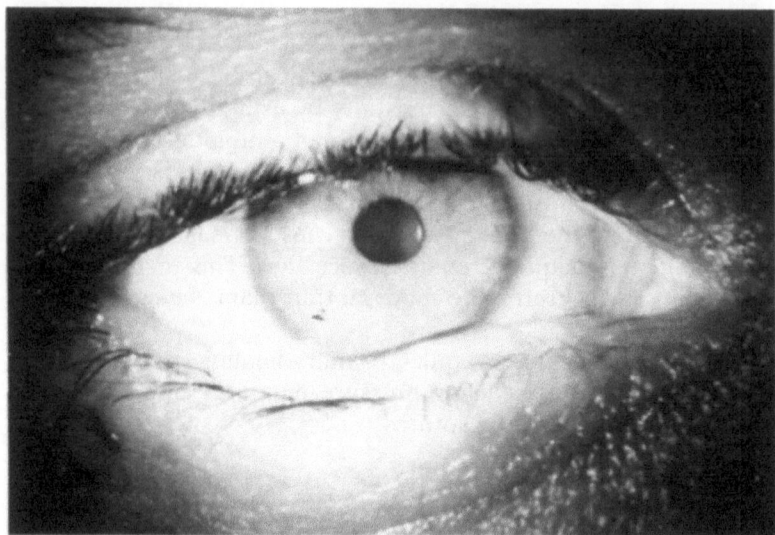

Fig. 5. Same patient after treatment of the right lower lid by means of lid-split procedure and fibrin sealant fixation of a free autologous conjunctival transplant

Orbital Surgery

Treatment of Postenucleation Syndrome

Marked enophthalmus frequently occurs after enucleation without the use of intraorbital implants [9]. Silicone implants encased in scleral homografts [4] or covered with polytetrafluoroethylene are regarded as the most advantageous orbital implants, even in secondary implantation. A silicone ball, 16–20 mm in diameter, covered by alcohol-preserved, homologous sclera [21] or by 1 mm Gore-tex soft tissue patch is used as an orbital implant. A horizontal incision is made in the conjunctiva and Tenon's capsule and the muscle cone opened by sharp dissection [7]. The implant is then fixed to the extraocular muscles either by 4/0 Vicryl (polyglactin 9/0) sutures or, in the case of complete atrophic muscles, by the fibrin sealing technique. The orbital cavity is prepared far back and the attachment of the orbital implant to the orbital connective tissue is achieved by means of a fibrin sealing technique [13, 21, 24]. By using this technique, adequate volume replacement can be achieved, which is especially visible from the side view. The implant works as a kind of new globe and imparts considerable mobility to the prosthesis. At least slight movement of the orbital contents can be transferred to the prosthesis, even if the muscles are atrophic and cannot be identified.

Lacrimal Surgery

Fibrin sealing can be performed in the following lacrimal operation techniques:

Reconstruction of Canaliculi Lacrimales

In patients with traumatic lower lid injuries and laceration of the inferior cana-liculus, bicanalicular silicone ring intubation [15] is used for repairing the lacer-ated canaliculus. Retrograde probing of the canaliculus system under the microscope [3] is followed by readaptation of the torn canaliculi lacrimales by means of fibrin sealant. The freshly prepared gluing substance is applied to the whole circumference of the end-to-end anastomosis. The glued canaliculus anastomosis is stabilized by the silicone tube in its lumen and by the recon-structed lid structures.

The fibrin sealing technique makes the anastomosing procedure easier and quicker. No microsutures are necessary in the actual anastomosis area and therefore less trauma of the canaliculus tissue occurs. The fibrin substance always has a marked hemostyptic effect and is always well compatible, yielding excellent results.

Repair of Canaliculus Communis Stenosis

Stenosis of the common canaliculus is mainly caused by chronic inflammations. It has to be repaired microsurgically. The canaliculus communis is prepared carefully, the scar is resected, and the open canaliculus parts are end-to-end anastomosed [2]. A silicone intubation with the Jünemann probe [11] is done prior to the fixation of the anastomosis by means of fibrin sealant [20] (Fig. 6). The refixation of the lid tendon is followed by conventional wound closure (Fig. 7).

Dacryocystorhinostomy

Postsaccal dacryostenosis is the main indication for the so-called Toti operation [23]. The operation is performed under general anesthesia in the conventional way [8]. After trepanation of the bone and preparation of anterior and poste-rior flaps of nasal and lacrimal sac mucosa, the posterior flaps are adapted using fibrin sealant (Fig. 8). The gluing substance is injected below the mucosa flaps, which are then fixed briefly with mild pressure. The hemostatic effect stops the bleeding of the mucosa. The final steps of the operation are done in the typical way [8]. The advantages of the fibrin sealing technique are espe-cially obvious in this indication. The deep sutures of the posterior mucosa flaps are replaced by fibrin sealing fixation. Diffuse bleeding of the mucosa is stopped due to the hemostatic effect, thus preventing hematoma in the wound area from delaying the healing process.

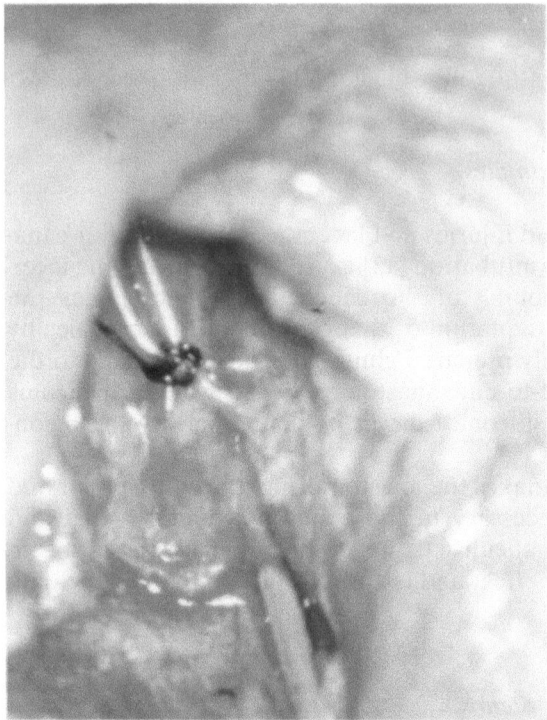

Fig. 6. A 62-year-old woman with canaliculus communis stenosis on the right side. Operation site: fixation of the cranial part of the posterior mucosal anastomosis with fibrin sealant (canaliculi are intubated with silicone tube)

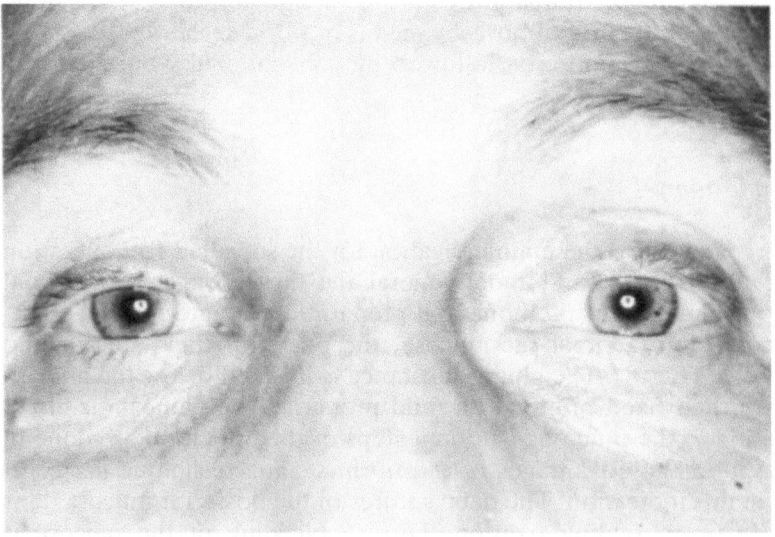

Fig. 7. Same patient as in Fig. 6 showing a normal medial canthus configuration 6 months postoperatively

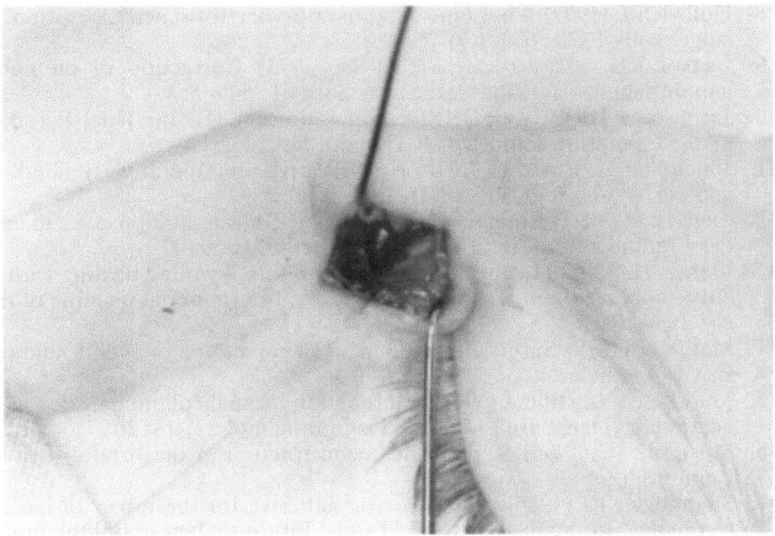

Fig. 8. A 13-year-old boy; operation site. The fibrin sealing technique is used for gluing the posterior mucosal flaps in dacryocystorhinostomy

Canaliculodacryocystorhinostomy

A stenosis of the common canaliculus combined with a postsaccal lacrimal stenosis is the indication for utilizing this combined microsurgical and fibrin sealant procedure. A microscopic canaliculus communis reconstruction combined with dacryocystorhinostomy [5] is performed. Silicone intubation [11] is used to keep the lacrimal passages open. The fibrin sealing technique is used for gluing the anastomosis areas: the common canaliculus anastomosis with the temporal sac is completely covered with sealant; the posterior flaps of the sac and nasal mucosa are glued as in the dacryocystorhinostomy procedure.

References

1. Buschmann W (1982) Wiederherstellung einer weitgehend klaren Linse nach perforierender Verletzung. Klin Monatsbl Augenheilkd 181: 487–489
2. Busse H, Hollwich F (1978) Erkrankungen der ableitenden Tränenwege und ihre Behandlung. Enke, Stuttgart (Bücherei des Augenarztes, vol 74)
3. Busse H, Steinkogler FJ, Friess J (1985) Ring intubation of lacerated canaliculi lacrimales. Orbit 4: 73–75
4. Colin JR (1983) A manual of systematic eyelid surgery. Churchill Livingstone, London, p 96
5. Doucet TW, Hurwitz JJ (1982) Canaliculodacryocystorhinostomy in the treatment of canalicular obstruction. Arch Ophthalmol 100: 306–309
6. Gayet A (1881) Sur un procede nouveau d'autoplastique des paupiers applicable aux entropions graves. Cong. period. internat. sc. med. CR (Amsterdam) 6: 265
7. Härting F, Koorneef HJ, Peeters J, Gillissen P (1985) Complications in orbital implant surgery – worthy of mention? Orbit 4: 105–109

8. Hollwich F (1977) Über eine Modifikation der Totischen Operation. Klin Monatsbl Augenheilkd 170: 633–636
9. Iverson RE, Vistnes LM, Siegel RJ (1973) Correction of enophthalmus in the anophthalmic orbit. Plast Reconstr Surg 51: 545–554
10. Jacobson J (1942) Eine Trichiasisoperation (1887). In: Thiel R (ed) Ophthalmologische Operationslehre, vol I. Thieme, Leipzig, p 49
11. Jünemann G, Busse H (1977) Konservative und operative Behandlung der Störungen der Tränenwege. EFA XII, Essen
12. Machek E (1897) Ein neues Verfahren zur Transplantation des Zilienbodens. Plastik des Lidrandes. Centralbl Prakt Augenheilk 21: 39–47
13. Matras H (1982) Haemostasis and promotion of wound healing with fibrin clot sealants – application in maxillofacial surgery. International meeting of the Joseph Society, 1980. Escher, Salzburg
14. Metha H (1979) Surgical management of carcinoma of eyelids and periorbital skin. Brit J Ophthalmol 63: 578–585
15. Murube del Castillo J (1973) L'intubation bicanaliculaire dans les sections des canalicules lacrymaux. Bull Mm Soc Fr Ophthalmol 22: 18–20
16. Mustarde JC (1966) Repair and reconstruction in the orbital region. Livingstone, Edinburgh, pp 39–43
17. Steinkogler FJ (1986a) Fibrin tissue adhesive for the repair of lacerated canaliculi lacrimales. In: Schlag G, Redl H (eds) Fibrin sealant in ophthalmology and neurosurgery, vol 2. Springer, Berlin Heidelberg New York, pp 92–97
18. Steinkogler FJ (1986b) Lid split surgery and fibrin sealing of free skin transplants. Ophthal Plast Reconstr Surg 2 (4): 183–187
19. Steinkogler FJ (1987) The treatment of the postenucleation socket syndrome. J Cranio Max Fac Surg 15: 31–33
20. Steinkogler FJ (1992) Canaliculocystostomy: combining microsurgery and fibrin sealing of the anastomosis. Ophthalmic Surg 23: 7
21. Steinkogler FJ, Hauff W (1985) Skleraschalen-Silikon Implantate der Orbita nach Enukleation. Klin Monatsbl Augenheilkd 187: 351–352
22. Toledo LS (1983) Blepharoplasty with fibrin seal. Trans Int Congr Plast Surg Montreal, pp 478–479
23. Toti A (1904) Dacryocistorhinostomia. La Clinica Moderna 10: 33–34
24. Tscheliessnigg KH, Hermann W, Dacar E, Stenzl W, Höllerel G (1981) Fibrinklebung – eine Übersicht über Entwicklung, Technik und derzeitigen Stand. Scient Workshop Graz 5–10
25. Waldhauer C (1898) Zur Operation der Trichiasis des oberen Lides. Klin Monatsbl Augenheilkd 36: 47–54
26. Watson TS (1874) On the treatment of trichiasis and distichiasis by a plastic operation. Med Times Gaz 2: 546

Progress in Fibrin Sealing of Eye Lens and Conjunctiva

W. Buschmann

Abstract

Spontaneous healing of lens capsule perforations results in a localized capsule scar on an otherwise clear lens. This course is rare in man.

A retrospective analysis revealed that the post-traumatic protein (fibrinogen) content of the aqueous humor determined the outcome. Usually it is too low in patients. Extended animal experiments supported this concept. It was proven that lack of fibrinogen could be compensated for by fibrinogen-based microsurgical sealing of capsule defects. Application in patients was successful in seven out of 12 anterior capsule perforations (long-term result: visual acuity, 1.0–0.3). Through-and-through perforations of the lens were more difficult to seal: the translental approach to the posterior capsule defect proved best. Conjunctival fistulas were also successfully sealed using fibrinogen. In contrast to lens capsule sealing, however, postoperative topical application of proteinase blockers proved necessary to prevent early clot destruction by tear fluid proteinases.

Introduction

Up until now surgeons have been unable to seal perforating injuries of the lens capsule. Watertight sutures are not possible in this thin capsule, as each stitch would be an additional capsule perforation. Thus, traumatic cataract developed (Fig. 1). Treatment was restricted to removal of the opaque lens and replacement by thick spectacle glasses, corneal contact lenses, or artificial implant lenses. It would be advantageous to save the patient's eye lens in a sufficiently clear condition, because all of the above-mentioned optic aids do have certain disadvantages, especially in view of accommodation and binocular vision. In addition, most of these patients are young people.

Retrospective Analysis

A total of 83 consecutive patients with perforating injuries of the lens capsule, seen at our hospital before fibrinogen-based microsurgery was available, were

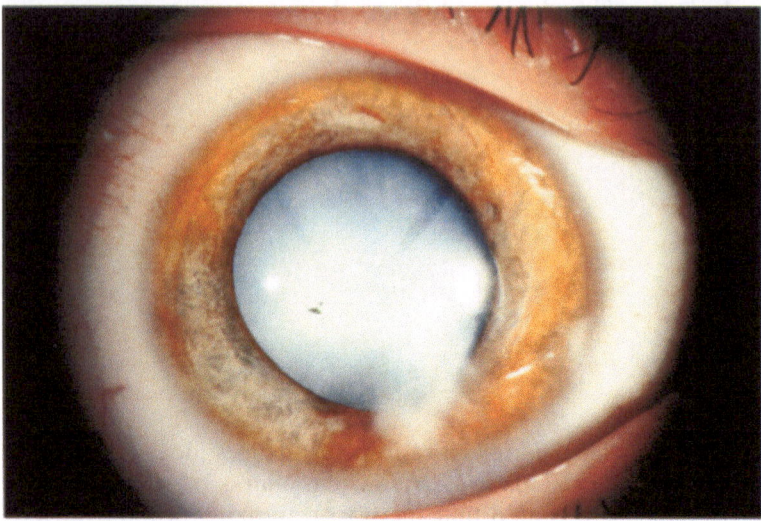

Fig. 1. Traumatic cataract; the regular result of perforating injuries of the lens capsule up to now

analyzed in view of their further course [3]; 96% developed traumatic cataracts, but in 4% spontaneous healing of the capsule rupture was observed. This resulted in a small capsule scar, an otherwise clear lens, and good visual acuity. The question arose as to what was responsible for the favorable course in these few cases.

It appeared to us that the post-traumatic fibrinogen (protein) content of the aqueous humor might be the decisive factor. Posterior synechiae of the iris might or might not have developed – they were not necessary for the healing of the capsule wound and sometimes even disturbed it.

Patients with needle-stitch perforations of cornea and lens capsule whose eye looked as if nothing had happened in the first few days after the accident regularly ended up with traumatic cataracts. These eyes had especially low protein levels in the aqueous humor and a faint Tyndall phenomenon.

In contrast, eyes with marked iris trauma (especially iris contusion), leaking blood/aqueous barrier, and high protein level of the aqueous humor had a comparatively good chance of spontaneous healing of the lens capsule defect.

Animal Experiments

Mongrel dogs and rabbits were used in pilot studies. It was proven that traumatic cataracts developed fairly rarely after lens capsule perforations. Usually they end up with a favorable result: a circumscribed scar only in an otherwise clear lens. The reason for their better prognosis was not very clear in the past. We have seen that the post-traumatic protein level of the aqueous humor was much higher than in our patients. If this makes the difference in the spontaneous healing rate, we wondered whether it could be substituted by a fibrinogen-based tissue adhesive.

In further experiments, white Wistar albino rats after perforating injuries showed a poor protein level of the aqueous and a high incidence of traumatic cataracts, just as in man. Extended experimental series [2, 5] revealed that traumatic cataracts could be prevented and that localized scars formed if the lens capsule defects were sealed by means of fibrinogen-based microsurgery.

Surgical Technique

Treatment of patients was started in 1982. Damaged lens matter was removed from the lesion site by suction, using a blunt needle. The defect of lens cortex and capsule was then filled and sealed by application of fibrinogen and thrombin solution (Tissucol; Immuno, Vienna). The Duploject (Immuno, Vienna) system could not be used. It was not accurate enough for the very small amounts of fibrinogen and thrombin solution we needed (0.002 ml each), and it was possible that only one of the two components appeared at the needle tip. Thus we had to apply the two components successively.

Primarily, we treated the anterior capsule defect only in through-and-through perforations of the lens. Later on we tried to reach the posterior capsule defect around the equator through a basal iridectomy. We avoided the pars plana entrance, because we were worried about dealing with the persisting vitreous layers at the tip of our blunt needle and about subsequent fibrinogen leakage into the vitreous cavity. A sharp needle would also be dangerous as it might cause additional posterior lens capsule defects.

Finally, we applied fibrinogen to the posterior capsule defect by the trans-lental route, using the perforation channel. The blunt needle tip was kept at the anterior capsule lesion at the level of the lens cortex. Thus damaged lens matter was pushed out of the posterior lens defect into the space between the lens and vitreous, where it was absorbed. The defect within the lens was then completely filled by fibrinogen. Thrombin solution was injected into the aqueous humor only, in front of and behind the lens.

Indications

We did not apply fibrinogen in every perforating injury of the lens. Instead, we attempted to differentiate between cases with a good chance of spontaneous healing and those with a poor one. The latter only underwent fibrinogen-based microsurgery. The criteria for selection were derived from our retrospective analysis and from the animal experiments. Patients showing high post-traumatic protein levels in the aqueous humor were not treated by this method, but were carefully followed. Fibrinogen microsurgery proved unnecessary if they developed a strong greyish membrane covering the lesion site. Post-traumatic rosettes and vacuoles then decreased in size and number, and lens astigmatism decreased as well.

Table 1. Results of fibrinogen-based microsurgical capsule wound sealing in relation to time interval between injury and microsurgery

Time interval	Visual acuity reached 0.3–1.2 (n)	Progressive traumatic cataract (n)
5–24 h	8	12
1–3 day	3	3
> 3 days	2	3

Patients with low post-traumatic protein levels of the aqueous humor were, however, considered to be at high risk for cataract development and were treated by fibrinogen-based sealing. They usually had no or only small iris traumas. Fibrinogen sealing was started at once in the case of gaping capsule defects with somewhat protruding lens cortex and lack of a covering grey membrane at the lesion site.

Many patients, however, had a moderate protein level of the aqueous and a thin covering membrane at the capsule defect. In these patients, the outcome of the spontaneous course was open. We dilated the pupil and reexamined these patients using a slit-lamp microscope at intervals of a few hours. Increase in the membrane bulging and in the defect size as well as in the size and number of rosettes and vacuoles revealed a poor spontaneous course and thus fibrinogen surgery was started. Size and number of equatorial vacuoles and extent of lens astigmatism are valuable indicators as well. Thus fibrinogen microsurgery was used many hours or even several days after trauma and primary surgical care.

The above-mentioned thin membranes are insufficient in view of permanent sealing of the capsule wound, but they protect the lens for several hours or even days from fast destruction. Thus we were able to succeed in some cases even if microsurgical sealing was performed rather late after injury (Table 1).

Results

The rate of spontaneous healing of lens capsule defects was 4 %–10 % in our patients in the period before we started the fibrinogen sealing technique (in 1981), as was shown by our retrospective analysis (see above). It remained nearly unchanged afterwards. Thus we succeeded in selecting the patients who did not need fibrinogen sealing and treated only those who otherwise would have developed traumatic cataracts.

The total rate of favorable courses (localized capsule scar, visual acuity of 1.0–0.3) then increased to 25 %. The results of early treatment were, of course, better, but we were successful even in a number of patients treated rather late (Table 1) or repeatedly (in the case of insufficient first approach).

Our first series included 31 consecutive patients treated from 1982 to 1984, among which there were 12 anterior capsule lesions. We were able to save

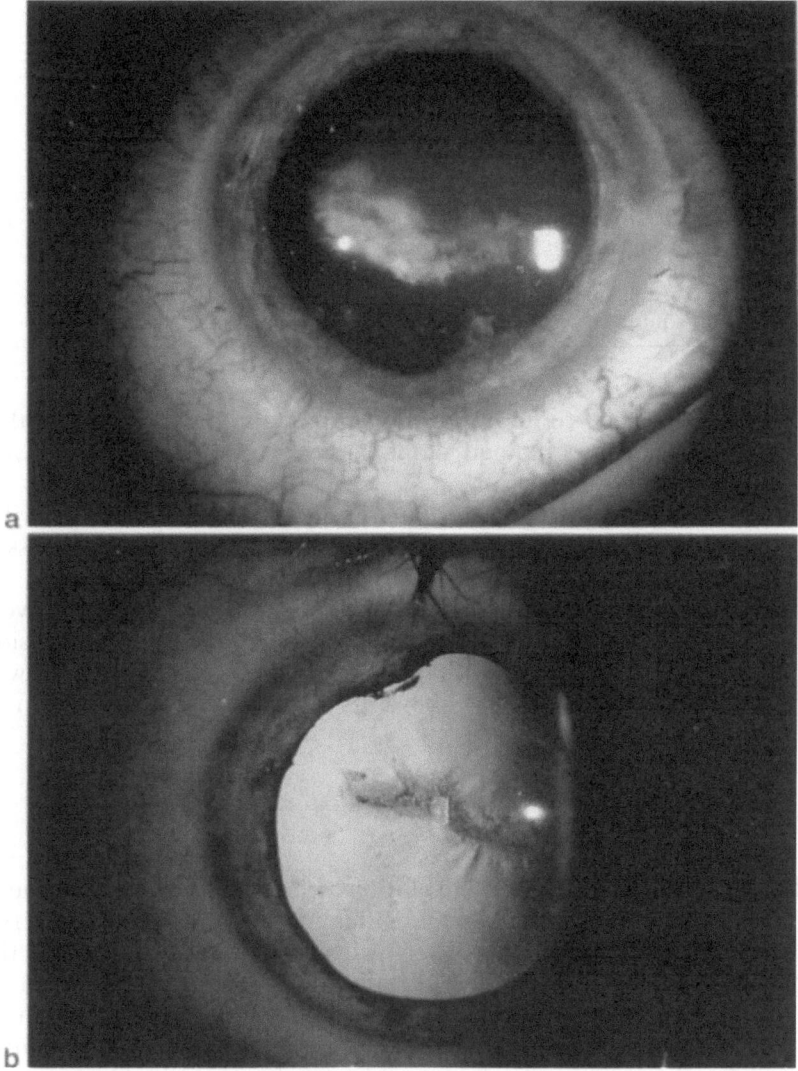

Fig. 2a, b. Extended rupture of the anterior capsule of the lens (caused by a wire), sealed with fibrinogen. **a** 15th postoperative day. **b** Ten weeks postoperatively. Localized scar at the anterior capsule, which does not prevent fairly good visual acuity (0.5), lens otherwise clear. Follow-up now 7 years with no change

seven out of the 12 injured lenses (Fig. 2; visual acuity reached 0.3–1.0). In five cases the course was unfavorable and traumatic cataracts developed. Through-and-through perforations of the lens are naturally more difficult to seal (Table 2). Primarily, we had no technique for the posterior capsule defect and treated the anterior capsule lesion only. Our results – one success in 11 cases – were not very good.

Table 2. Results of fibrinogen sealing in through-and-through perforations of the eye lens (anterior and posterior capsule defect)

Microsurgical technique	Visual acuity reached 0.3–1 (n)	Traumatic cataract (n)	Total (n)
Sealing of anterior capsule only	1	10	11
Posterior capsule sealing attempted past lens equator	1	3	4
Posterior capsule sealing attempted by translental route	4	0	4

Thus we tried to apply fibrinogen past the lens equator to the posterior defect. The results obtained – one success out of four cases – were still not satisfying.

Then we decided to use the translental route I have described before, which proved successful. All four lenses in this group were successfully sealed (Fig. 3). Other examples have been published before (e.g., [1]).

The patients have been followed for 4–10 years postoperatively. Failures of capsule sealing or too late treatment resulted in cataract and vision decrease within weeks or months. No patient has been observed up to now in whom a favorable 1-year result was followed by cataract development in the further course.

Complications

The fibrinogen and thrombin solutions were surprisingly well tolerated, even after repeated application, and no inflammatory reaction was observed. Proper limitation of the amount applied proved difficult, especially if the anterior chamber was filled with aqueous humor instead of air. One could scarcely see the applied fibrinogen until clotting began to stain it greyish. Therefore, surplus fibrinogen was observed in some cases. It caused a transient increase of the intraocular pressure, which could easily be controlled by systemic carboanhydrase blockers. These, however, delayed to some extent the absorption of the surplus fibrin. A fibrin blockade of the chamber angle must be avoided and did not occur. Parts of the iris and pupil margin were sometimes reached by the fibrin clot (forming transient posterior synechiae). No problem evolved if part of the pupil remained free and the aqueous humor circulation was not blocked. All of these artificial synechiae disappeared spontaneously, leaving the pupil free, within a few days if no attempt was made to free the iris mechanically at the end of the operation (such attempts would result in permanent synechiae due to iris trauma). A basal iridectomy was performed if we were in doubt regarding aqueous humor circulation.

Application of fibrinogen into the vitreous would cause shrinking and traction to the retina. This has to be avoided, and therefore proper limitation of the

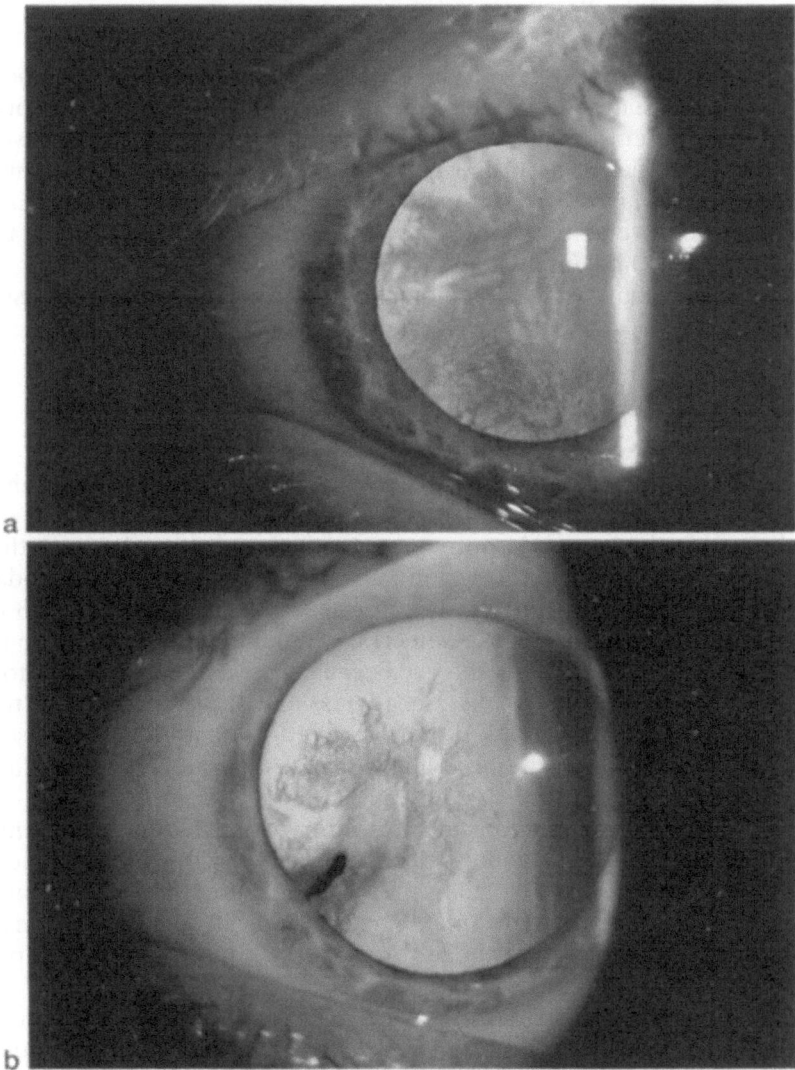

Fig. 3a. Through-and-through perforation of the lens (by foreign body). Large traumatic rosette. **b** Reduction of rosette size and density, 60th day after fibrinogen sealing of anterior and posterior capsule defects (translental approach). Increase in visual acuity

amount applied is especially important in through-and-through perforations of the lens. We had no vitreous or retina problems in our patients, but automatic dose limitation would nevertheless be safer (see below).

Insufficient Sealing

Patients treated also have to be reexamined, as was described above ("Indications"). Repeated fibrinogen surgery, including removal of degenerated, swollen lens matter from the lesion site, was performed if the capsule wound sealing proved insufficient according to the criteria described above. This was necessary in four of our patients, mainly due to our lack of experience in the first few years. No adverse reactions were observed after second or even third fibrinogen surgery, and finally we succeeded. However, the resulting scar area or rosette remnants were larger than in the other patients. The visual outcome was 0.8–0.4.

Postoperative Care

Antibiotics are given just as in other patients after perforating injuries. Cycloplegia has to be continued for 3–4 months. This allows us to evaluate the changes in the lens and, more importantly, is necessary because the fibrin clot and the early scar at the lesion site cannot take the accommodation forces before new capsule material is formed, which takes about 3 months [6], depending on the size of the defect. We discontinued the atropine treatment in one patient 6 weeks after surgery because he wanted to go back to work (scaffold worker). After 3 weeks, the regressing subcapsular rosette turned into a growing one (big vacuoles at the rosette edges) and the capsule scar was leaking, so we had to repeat fibrinogen surgery. Again, regression of the rosette was observed.

Careful reexaminations at short intervals, including retroillumination and photos, enable the surgeon to recognize very early whether or not the course will be favorable. In particular, the size of rosettes and of their marginal vacuoles has to be compared. Small vacuoles indicate a good prognosis. Size and number of vacuoles near the lesion or at the equator are also important, as in preoperative evaluation.

To avoid any possible risk of permanent cycloplegia, we aim at full cycloplegia only during the first 2–3 weeks. Then the atropine applications are reduced (e.g., every second night only) so that small reactions of the pupil to light become visible. All patients regained their age-related accommodation in the long run after withdrawal of the atropine drops.

Progress and Further Development

Proper volume limitation was somewhat difficult when applying the fibrinogen. It is nearly invisible within the aqueous humor of the eye unless clotting has started. Therefore, we tried to facilitate volume determination in two ways.

First, staining of the fibrinogen was attempted using fluorescein, which is known to be well tolerated by the eye. Clotting was not disturbed by the fluorescein in experimental adhesion tests. The visibility of the fibrinogen was markedly improved, especially if a corresponding blue filter was used in the microscope.

Second, in cooperation with Steinhagen Gerätebau, we developed a microapplicator for simultaneous application of predetermined small volumes of fibrinogen and thrombin solution. The pistons of two 1-cc syringes are moved simultaneously and stepwise, turning a screw by applying finger pressure to a lever.

Volumes of 0.5, 1, 1.5, 2, and 2.5 µl (= mm³) can be predetermined. Repeated finger pressure results in repeated application of the predetermined volume. Experimental adhesion tests have shown that even at the smallest volume both components were properly applied. Tests with colored solutions confirmed this result.

We succeeded in finding a company which made special twin needles of small size for us. Both tissue adhesive components are released next to each other at the blunt twin-needle tip. Thus, the probability of clotting inside the needle is reduced. The above-mentioned advanced techniques still have to be tested clinically, as we have only just got the microapplicator and the twin needles. We would like to cooperate with interested colleagues and would make the microapplicator and twin needles available to them.

The traumatic rosettes increased to some extent during application of the tissue adhesive. It seemed to us that the thrombin–calcium chloride solution is mainly responsible for this effect. We do not yet know whether it would be helpful (and tolerable in view of undisturbed clotting) to reduce the calcium chloride content.

Conjunctival Fistulas

Conjunctival fistulas are another situation which is often very difficult to handle. They are found after cataract or glaucoma surgery, especially in elderly patients with atrophic conjunctiva. Sutures do not hold; new ruptures of the thin conjunctiva might occur if suturing were attempted. The anterior chamber becomes shallow, and a very dangerous situation for the eye develops, so we decided to try fibrinogen sealing.

Surgical Technique

The conjunctival epithelium must be removed around the fistula. Then, all means have to be used to dry the lesion area. The patient receives carboanhydrase blocker preoperatively to reduce the production of aqueous humor. Additionally, some aqueous humor is released from the eye by slight pressure. Efficient swab tips are used to dry the tissue around the fistula. Fibrinogen and thrombin solution are applied successively and repeatedly to form a large, solid clot. The tear fluid contains much more proteolytic enzymes than the aqueous humor. Therefore, the aprotinin content of the fibrinogen solution is not sufficient to prevent early clot destruction, so we developed aprotinin eye drops [4], containing 10.0 cc Trasylol (aprotinin), 5.0 cc Methocel (methylcellulose), and 5.0 cc 0.9 % natrium chloride. The mixture was sterile filtered and filled into four 5-ml bottles for topical application to the eye.

No clot destruction takes place as long as these drops are applied at 1- to 2-h intervals in the daytime and 3- to 4-h intervals at night. The clot may be lost after about 1 week if healing and epithelization of the former fistula region are completed. If not, withdrawal of the aprotinin eye drops after 1 week results in fast clot destruction within 1–2 days.

The conjunctiva is then sealed, but the subconjunctival filtering effect (in the case of former glaucoma surgery) is not blocked, saving the eye from recurrence of increased intraocular pressure.

References

1. Buschmann W (1987) Microsurgical treatment of lens capsule perforations, part II. Ophthalmic Surg 18: 276–282, 731–737
2. Buschmann W, Gehrig O, Raab H (1981) Zur Behandlung von Verletzungen der vorderen Linsenkapsel. Ber Dtsch Opthalmol Ges 78: 533–540
3. Buschmann W, Waller W, Behringer D (1984a) Bisherige Ergebnisse in der Behandlung von Verletzungen der Linsenkapsel. Fortschr Ophthalmol 81: 59–61
4. Buschmann W, Stemberger A, Blümel G, Leydhecker W (1984b) Fibrinklebung und antifibrinolytische Nachbehandlung von Bindehautwunden. Klin Monatsbl Augenheilkd 184: 185–188
5. Buschmann W, Gehrig O, Vogt E, Raab H, Römer M (1987) Microsurgical treatment of lens capsule perforations, part I (see [1])
6. Schirmer O (1889) Histologische und histochemische Untersuchungen über Kapselnarbe und Kapselkatarakt nebst Bemerkungen über das physiologische Wachstum und die Struktur der vorderen Linsenkapsel. Graefes Arch Ophthalmol 35: 220–270

Morphological Reactions Following Fibrin Retinopexy in Rabbit Eyes

K.-H. EMMERICH, F. J. STEINKOGLER, and G. EDEL

Abstract

The authors report on the transvitreal application of commonly available fibrin sealant in experimental retinal detachment surgery. The feasibility of transvitreal fibrin sealing was investigated in 50 rabbit eyes. Operation model, methods of application, and results are shown. Ophthalmoscopic and histologic findings in the chosen model demonstrate fibrin retinopexy as a well-tolerated procedure. Fibrin retinopexy does not induce proliferative reactions of intraocular structures.

Introduction

In a rabbit study, possibilities and reactions following subretinal fibrin application were investigated. Stimulated by the introduction of cyanoacrylate sealants in vitreoretinal surgery [4, 6, 7, 13] and first experiences with subretinal fibrin application with homologous fibrin in rabbit eyes [9], the aim of our study was the investigation of morphological changes and proliferative reactions on the application of commercially prepared fibrin sealant that was heterologous for the animals.

Material and Methods

For subretinal fibrin application, a two-component fibrin sealant (Tissucol; Immuno, Heidelberg) was used. The use of a two-syringe application system (Duploject; Immuno, Vienna) ensures the automatic mixture of the two sealant solutions, resulting in reactions identical to the ones that take place in the final stage of blood coagulation [1, 8]:

1. Conversion of highly concentrated fibrinogen into fibrin
2. Activation of factor XIII
3. Cross-linkage of fibrin

To ensure these reactions, it is necessary that the sealants are optimally mixed. By using a Duploject system, the liquid sealant passes through the application needle at a flow rate which is high enough to prevent clogging of the needle [10–12]. For the investigations, commercially available frozen human fibrin sealant was used. After defrosting within approximately 30 min, a second sealant solution was prepared by dissolving thrombin in aprotinin–CaCl$_2$ solution. Aprotinin prevents premature fibrinolysis; calcium ions are an essential coenzyme of blood coagulation. Mixing ratio of the solutions was chosen with an expected setting time of 16 s.

We investigated the feasibility of transvitreal fibrin sealing in 50 rabbit eyes. At least 1 week prior to the scheduled vitrectomy, a transscleral cryocoagulation in the region of the vitrectomy entrance 4.5 mm from the limbus corneae was performed.

After extensive posterior vitrectomy (Fig. 1), a retinal hole was made with the blunt head of the ocutome. After ballooning-up the retina through the hole, the needle of the Duploject system was introduced in the middle of the hole in such a way that the sealant could be injected between retina and pigment epithelium (Fig. 2). The amount of fibrin sealant injected was between 0.05 and 0.2 ml.

The animals were included in our experimental series on the basis of safe subretinal fibrin sealing. The test animals were consecutively numbered, and the observation period and the time of enucleation were determined in advance by randomization between 3 and 84 days. For further investigations the enucleated rabbit eyes were fixed in a 4 % formalin solution for at least 1 week. Then the eyes were opened at the equator and macroscopically examined. Hereafter, histologic examinations were performed in the Gerhard Domagk Institute for Pathology at the Westphalian Wilhelms University in Münster.

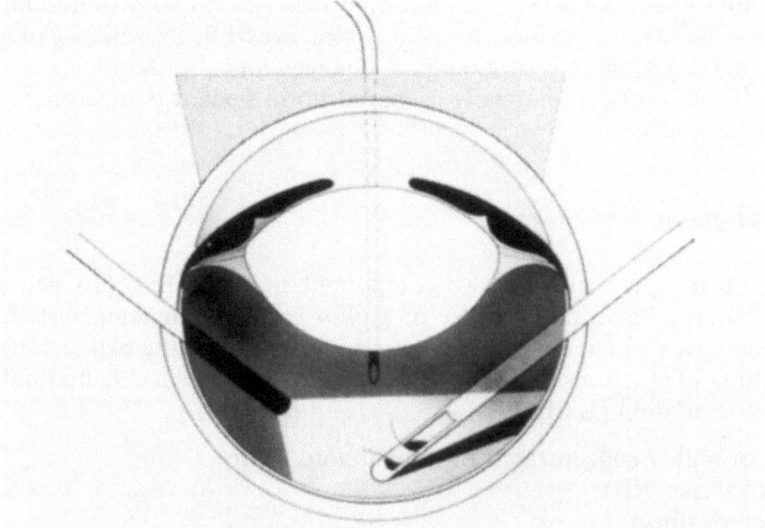

Fig. 1. Vitrectomy in the rabbit's eye

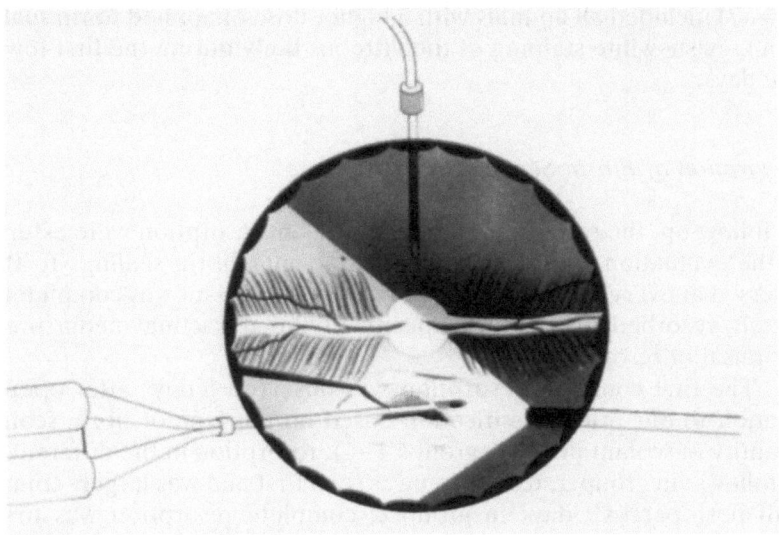

Fig. 2. Subretinal fibrin sealing

Results

Operative Results

Depending on the quantity of fibrin sealant used, the operated animals were divided postoperatively into four groups (Fig.3). In the animals in group 1 ($n = 12$) fibrin sealant was only found subretinally. Postoperatively, in group 2 ($n = 22$) fibrin sealant was not only seen subretinally, but also preretinally, and the edges of the lesion were clearly visible. If the edges of the hole could be vaguely discerned, the animals were classed as group 3 ($n = 9$). Group 4

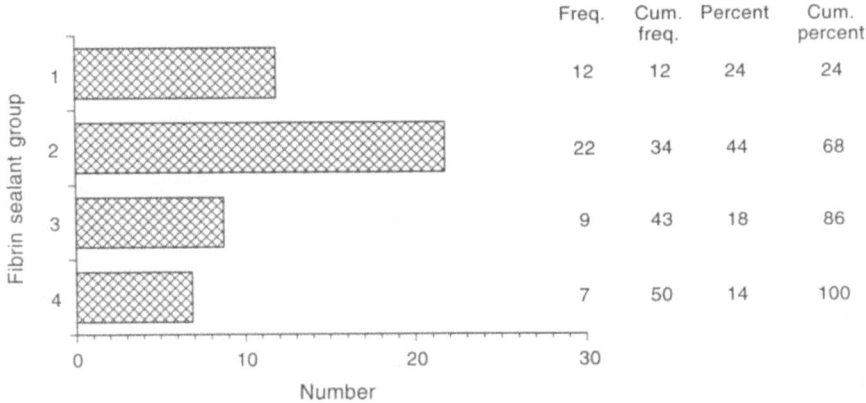

Fibrin sealant group	Freq.	Cum. freq.	Percent	Cum. percent
1	12	12	24	24
2	22	34	44	68
3	9	43	18	86
4	7	50	14	100

Fig. 3. Distribution of test animals in groups 1–4

($n = 7$) included all animals with a higher dose of applied fibrin sealant leading to a greyish–white staining of the vitreous body during the first few postoperative days.

Absorption of Fibrin Sealant

At follow-up, the progress and time of sealant resorption were essential criteria in the evaluation of the success of intraocular fibrin sealing. To this end, we assessed at every follow-up whether the fibrin sealant was completely or incompletely resorbed or whether opacity of the refracting media prevented the appraisal of resorption.

The first complete resorption was observed 5 days after operation. With relation to our prior classification based on the type of fibrin sealing and the quantity of sealant present (groups 1–4), resorption in the different groups was as follows: in group 1, resorption was seen first and was largely complete by the 14th postoperative day; in group 2, complete resorption was first observed 7 days after operation and, with one exception, was complete by the 14th day; in group 3, the sealant was found to be completely resorbed in one test animal

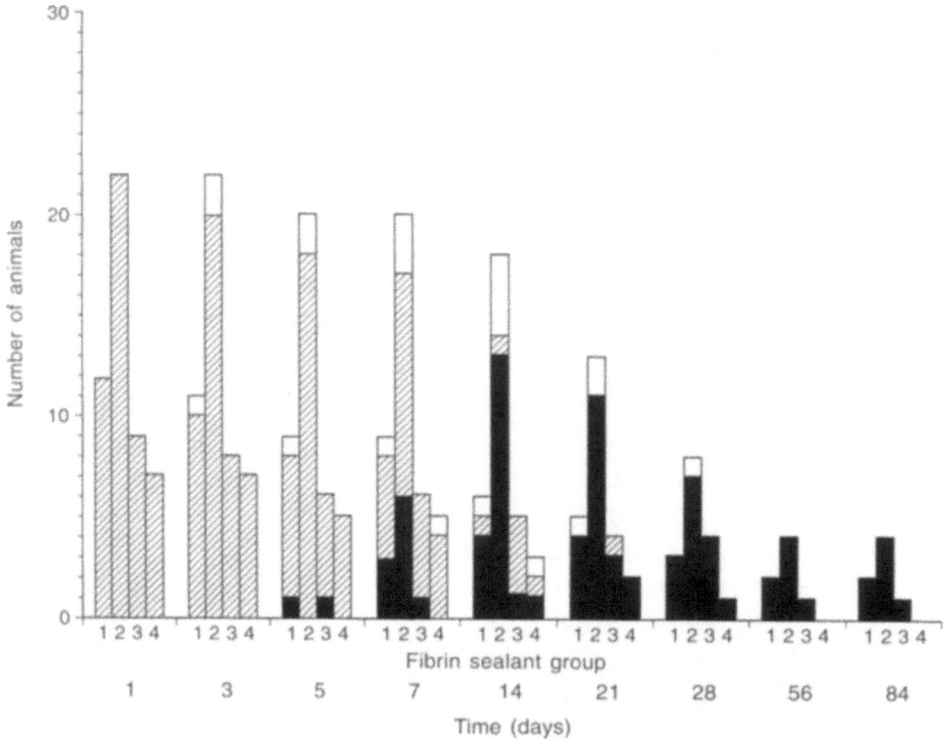

Fig. 4. Postoperative fibrin resorption in groups 1–4. *Black bars*, complete resorption; *shaded bars*, incomplete resorption; *white bars*, could not be determined

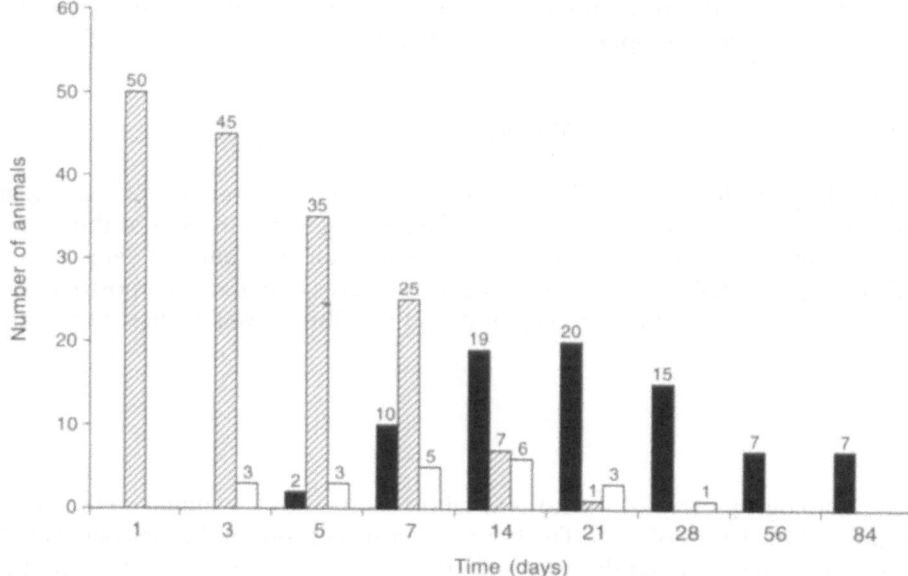

Fig. 5. Postoperative fibrin resorption; absolute distribution at different follow-up periods. Numbers beneath the three-dimensional columns indicate number of test animals. *1*, complete resorption; *2*, incomplete resorption; *9*, could not be determined

on day 7, but in the rest of the animals not until days 21 and 28; in group 4, the first complete resorption was seen as late as day 14 after operation. Figures 4 and 5 show the postoperative resorption of fibrin sealant in each of the four groups of test animals.

Macroscopical Findings after Enucleation

Development of a Retinal Detachment

In 47 out of 50 eyes in our series, the retina could be judged at the time of enucleation. Three eyes had developed a panophthalmia with diffuse infiltration of the vitreous body.

In 39 eyes the retina was attached, and in eight eyes the retina was detached at the time of enucleation. Detached retinas could be seen both at the first enucleation dates on days 3 and 7 and at the last dates on days 42 and 84 without any tendency to a longer-lasting postoperative follow-up period. The distribution of the operated eyes with detached retina between groups 1–4 shows a different pattern; the probability of a retinal detachment was lowest in group 1 and highest in group 4: in group 1, we did not see an amotio retinae at any enucleation date; in group 2, four of 20 operated eyes had developed a retinal detachment; and in group 4, the highest incidence of an amotio retinae

112   K.-H. Emmerich et al.

was observed. Groups 3 and 4 together, both with a higher quantity of fibrin sealant at the time of operation, showed an amotio retinae in four of 16 eyes.

Development of Preretinal Fibrosis

In the later postoperative follow-up period, in some operated eyes a preretinal fibrosis was seen ophthalmoscopically. Macroscopically, in nine of the 39 eyes with attached retina, a preretinal fibrosis was seen. The earliest date of recognizing a preretinal fibrosis in the enucleated eyes was the 14th postoperative day. The frequency of occurrence of preretinal fibrosis was highest in groups 3 and 4.

Histologic Findings

The histologic pattern of the normal rabbit retina shows – similar to the human retina – three layers of cells. The fuzzy structures of rods and cones between the pigment epithelium and the outer plexiform layer can frequently be seen if the retina is artificially detached in the microscopical slide preparation.

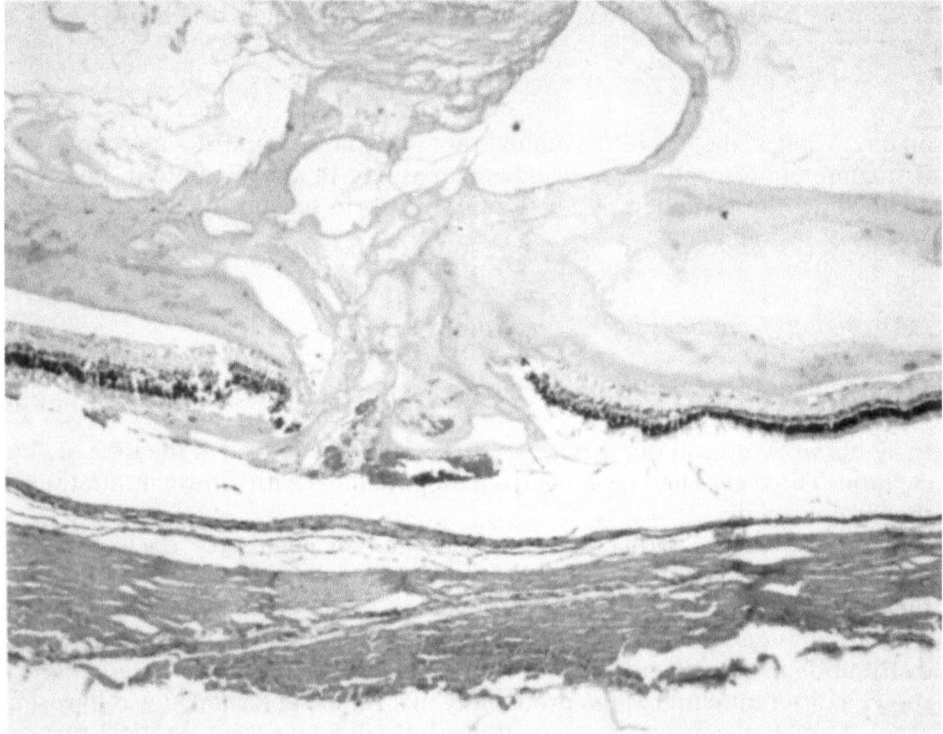

Fig. 6. Second postoperative day; retinal hole, partially preretinal, partially subretinal fibrin (H & E, × 100)

Histologic examination of the eyes on the second postoperative day revealed signs of a fresh traumatic injury of the retina and partial preretinal eosin red-colored fibrin sealant. The layer of the retina was preserved, and in some parts intraretinal hemorrhages could be seen (Fig. 6).

The histologic findings on the third postoperative day showed a different strength of inflammatory reaction of the retina.

Histologic examinations on the seventh postoperative day showed first signs of fibrin resorption. At the margins of the fibrin clot, fresh granulative tissue could be recognized.

On the 14th postoperative day, the quantity and activity of granulative tissue showed great differences depending on the quantity of fibrin sealant. At this point in time the first signs of a tender preretinal membrane – consisting of one cell layer – were observed. In the fibrin clot, active resorption signs with development of a granulative tissue were seen.

The proliferative activity of the granulative tissue decreased on the 21st day. Only rests of fibrin could be found, and the preretinal membrane could be seen better, still consisting of one cell layer. A proliferative tendency of the membrane was not observed.

Histologic examinations on the 42nd postoperative day showed a glial scar where the former retinal hole was situated. Around the former hole, small cystoid-degenerative tissue reactions were seen. The inflammatory reaction further decreased. Only residues of capillaries could be recognized as rests of the granulative tissue. Degenerative reactions were strictly localized on the area of the retinal hole, the glial scar, or the direct neighborhood (Fig. 7). On the 84th postoperative day, no more inflammatory reactions were seen; in particular, no proliferative activity was observed. The tender preretinal membrane showed no increase in thickness.

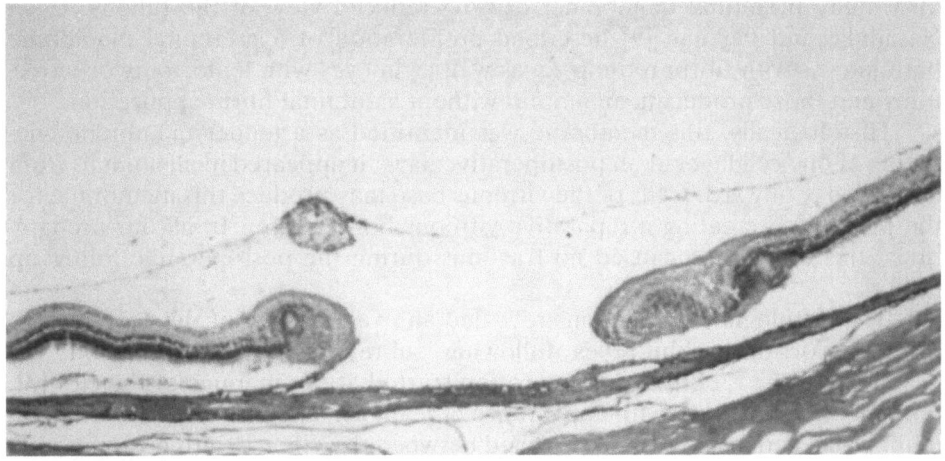

Fig. 7. The 42nd postoperative day; rolled edges of the retinal hole; preretinal membrane, attached retina (H & E, × 100)

Discussion

The traditional methods of inducing chorioretinal adhesions by thermic lesions take some time to attain maximal strength. Chorioretinal adhesions induced by synthetic tissue sealants attain the maximal strength more rapidly, but they lead to local toxicity. The principle of fibrin adhesion harnesses the physiological process of the final phase of blood coagulation. Owing to its nontoxicity, the sealant can be used in neurosurgical interventions, for example [5]. After the first results of retinopexy with autologous fibrin sealant were obtained by Nasaduke and Peyman [9], our group was able to demonstrate the subretinal fibrin application of heterologous, commonly available fibrin sealant [2].

Morphological reactions after fibrin retinopexy are characterized by the time of fibrin resorption. Progress and time of sealant resorption depend on the quantity of applied sealant and show a good correlation to a classification into four groups. Ophthalmoscopically, the most rapid resorption was observed within 5 days, and in all animals except one, the resorption was complete by the 21st postoperative day.

Eight of 47 eyes developed an amotio retinae postoperatively. The incidence of developing a retinal detachment showed no correlation to longer follow-up periods. The incidence of developing an amotio retinae was higher in groups 3 and 4 with greater quantity of applied sealant, corresponding to the operative trauma. Tractive processes causing retinal detachment were not seen during the follow-up period.

Nasaduke and Peyman [9] reported the appearance of golden or white synchisis scintillans-like particles in the vitreous body following fibrin retinopexy. We did not obtain similar findings in our larger collective in a later follow-up period.

One morphological reaction in our examination group was the appearance of a milky preretinal membrane, causing reduced view of the fundus. Even Nasaduke and Peyman [9] described proliferation of a preretinal membrane both in eyes with fibrin retinopexy as well as in eyes with lentectomy or vitrectomy and those producing an amotio without subretinal fibrin application.

Histologically, this membrane was identified as a tender membrane consisting of one cell layer at all postoperative days; it appeared in all animals from the 14th day onward. Cells of the vitreous base may produce this membrane for the purpose of creating a reparative vitreous border layer. In all our preparations, this membrane caused no tractions during the postoperative follow-up period.

The histologic examinations revealed an exact picture of the proliferative reactions of the rabbit eyes following subretinal fibrin application. As described in the rabbit's skin, resorption started at the margins of the clot [3]. Foreign body reactions with appearance of giant cells were not observed. Maximum proliferative activity was reached between the 7th and 14th postoperative day, and inflammatory and reparative activity decreased during the postoperative course. Intensity and quantity of granulative tissue mainly depended on the amount of applied sealant and operative trauma.

Even the histologic findings demonstrate fibrin retinopexy in the chosen experimental model to be a well-tolerated procedure. Fibrin retinopexy does not induce proliferative reactions of intraocular structures, which would not suggest a possible clinical application. We noticed the appearance of a preretinal membrane, consisting of one cell layer from the 14th postoperative day onward. This membrane caused no tractions or proliferative activity.

At least in the rabbit eye, the subretinal application of heterologous, commonly available fibrin sealant with a temporary tamponade of the retinal hole is possible. After further improvement of the armamentarium to suit the requirements of vitreoretinal surgery, an additional method for the surgical treatment of some kinds of complicated retinal detachment should be available in the future.

References

1. Bloom AL (1981) Inherited disorders of blood coagulation. In: Bloom AL, Thomas PD (eds) Hemostasis and thrombosis. Churchill Livingstone, Edinburgh, pp 321–370
2. Emmerich KH, Busse H, Slezak H, Steinkogler FJ (1989) Experimentelle transvitreale Fibrinklebung der Netzhaut. Klin Monatsbl Augenheilkd 194: 42–47
3. Heine WD, Edinger D, Braun A (1982) Wundheilung nach Fibrinklebung – histopathologische Untersuchungen. In: Cotta H, Braun A (eds) Fibrinkleber in Orthopädie und Traumatologie. Thieme, Stuttgart, pp 27–34
4. Hida T, Sheta SM, Proia AD, McCuen BW II (1987) Experimental transvitreal cyanoacrylate retinopexy in a primate model. Am J Ophthalmol 103: 782
5. Kletter G (1986) The use of fibrin adhesive in neurotraumatology. In: Schlag G, Redl H (eds) Fibrin adhesive in operative medicine. Ophthalmology-Neurosurgery, vol 2. Springer, Berlin Heidelberg New York, pp 116–122
6. McCuen BW II, Hida T, Sheta SM, Isbey EK, Hahn DK, Hickingbotham D (1986) Experimental transvitreal cyanoacrylate retinopexy. Am J Opthalmol 102: 199
7. McCuen BW II, Hida T, Sheta SM (1987) Transvitreal cyanoacrylate retinopexy in the management of complicated retinal detachment. Am J Ophthalmol 104: 127
8. Murano G (1980) Plasma protein function in hemostasis. In: Murano G, Bick RL (eds) Basis conceptions of hemostasis and thrombosis. CRC Press, Boca Raton, Florida
9. Nasaduke I, Peyman GA (1986) The use of autogenous rabbit fibrin sealant to plug retinal holes in experimental detachments. Ann Ophthalmol 18: 324
10. Redl H, Schlag G, Baucher E (1982) Grundlagen der Fibrinklebung. In: Cotta H, Braun A (eds) Fibrinkleber in der Orthopädie und Traumatologie. Thieme, Stuttgart, pp 18–21
11. Redl H, Schlag G (1986) Fibrin sealant and its modes of application. In: Schlag G, Redl H (eds) Fibrin sealant in operative medicine. Ophthalmology-neurosurgery, vol 2. Springer, Berlin Heidelberg New York, pp 13–26
12. Seelich T, Redl H (1984) Applikationstechniken. In: Scheele J (ed) Fibrinklebung. Springer, Berlin Heidelberg New York, pp 11–16
13. Sheta SM, Hida T, McCuen BW II (1986) Experimental cyanoacrylate retinopexy through silicone oil. Am J Ophthalmol 102: 717

Fibrin Adhesive for Wound Closure in Small-Incision Cataract Surgery

M. RAUBER, U. MESTER, and M. ZUCHE

Abstract

The scleral pocket technique has dramatically changed wound closure after phacoemulsification with posterior chamber lenses (PCL). The use of the single-stitch technique as well as wound closure using fibrin adhesive became possible.

The application of this biological substance is rapid, easy, and nonirritating, resulting in a very firm wound adaptation. This prevents the inferior edge of the scleral incision sagging away from the superior edge, thus reducing the potential for against-the-rule astigmatism.

A comparative study of 385 consecutive patients was conducted: 167 patients received only fibrin glue for wound closure, and 218 patients were operated on using the single-stitch procedure. No complications were observed in either group. Surgically induced astigmatism was smaller in the fibrin group (vector analysis, 0.8 D) than in the single-stitch group (vector analysis, 0.99 D). There was only a minimal, statistically insignificantly different against-the-rule astigmatism development: single-stitch group, 0.07 D (Cravy) and −0.09 D (Naeser); fibrin adhesive group, −0.13 D (Cravy) and −0.17 D (Naeser). These results suggest that postoperative against-the-rule astigmatism can be prevented with fibrin glue. We therefore continue to use fibrin adhesive for routine wound closure in small-incision cataract surgery.

Introduction

The scleral pocket technique in small-incision cataract surgery has dramatically changed wound closure after phacoemulsification with PCL implantation. Many surgeons have switched to single- or no-stitch techniques with excellent postoperative results. One benefit of this innovation is the reduction of postoperative astigmatism. In practice, however, some surgeons have observed a postoperative increase in against-the-rule astigmatism [13, 17, 22, 23]. To avoid this complication, several modifications of wound construction and wound closure have been developed. Shepherd [20] described the one-stitch horizontal wound closure to minimize postoperative astigmatism. Other surgeons have developed different configurations of cataract incision to avoid postoperative

astigmatism [4–6, 10, 15, 16, 21, 22]. An alternative technique to prevent astigmatism consists in the reinforcement of the scleral incision with fibrin adhesive.

Materials and Methods

Fibrin glue is a biological, nonirritating substance which is absorbed within a
few days, inducing collagen formation and cross-linking, thus promoting natural wound healing [19]. This fibrin sealant (Tissucol; Immuno, Heidelberg)
consists of two components: sealer protein–aprotinin and thrombin–$CaCl_2$
solution. It is available as a kit containing freeze-dried powder, freeze-dried
thrombin, calcium chloride, and aprotinin solution. As the two components
combine during application, fibrin sealant consolidates and adheres to the site
of application. The tensile strength of a clot formed with fibrin sealant was
found to be approximately 200 g/cm^2 (17 kPA) [18]. The clotting procedure is
very fast, leading to firm adhesion after a few seconds. Fibrin glue can also be
used on wet tissue surfaces.

The application of fibrin glue is performed using a double syringe (Tissucol
Duo S; Immuno, Heidelberg) which allows thorough mixing of the two sealant
components by single-handed operation immediately prior to wound closure
(Fig. 1). For optimal mixing it is important to apply the glue at 36 °C.

We evaluated the effect of fibrin glue for wound closure on postoperative
astigmatism in a comparative study with 385 consecutive patients.

In all cases phacoemulsification with PCL implantation was performed
using the small-incision technique. The straight scleral incision was started
2.5 mm posterior to the limbus, followed by a half-thickness scleral dissection
entering the anterior chamber 0.5 mm anterior to the vascular arcade at the
limbus. After capsulorhexis and phacoemulsification, the incision was enlarged

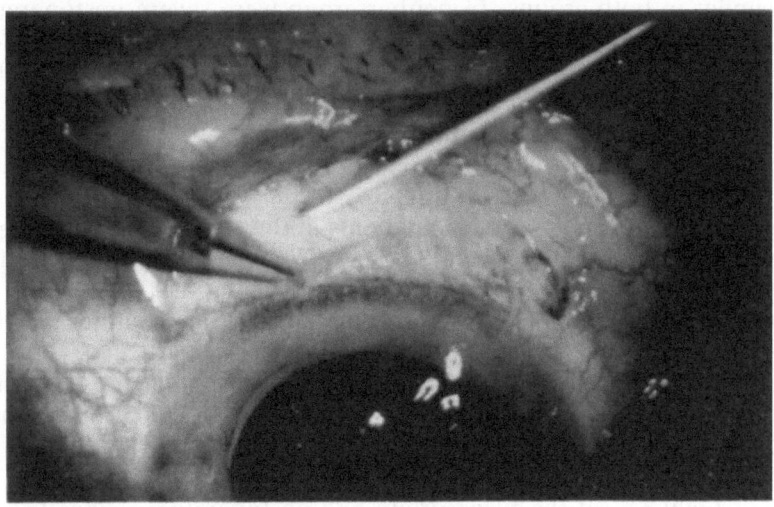

Fig. 1. Application of fibrin glue using a double syringe

to a length of 5.5 to 6.0 mm, allowing the implantation of biconvex PCL with a diameter of 6.0 and 6.5 mm.

Wound closure was carried out by two alternative methods: 167 patients received fibrin glue, and 218 were operated on using the single-stitch procedure and a horizontal mattress suture (Nylon 10/0) according to the technique described by Shepherd [20]. The patients were distributed to each group at random.

Wound closure with fibrin adhesive was performed with a double syringe. A thin film of glue was applied to the posterior part of the scleral pocket. The conjunctiva was finally fixed onto the sclera with several drops of fibrin. After application of the glue, fibrin consolidates within a few seconds. The wound should be as dry as possible, thus enhancing the adhesive strength of fibrin.

Evaluations were made preoperatively and postoperatively at 1 day, 1 week, and 6 months. Analysis of astigmatism was restricted to keratometric readings (Haag-Streit keratometer).

Surgically induced keratometric astigmatism was examined in three ways:

1. The vector analysis method of determining the magnitude of the surgically induced astigmatic vector, described by Jaffe and Clayman [9]
2. The method described by Cravy [3]
3. The polar value method of Naeser [14] for determining with-the-rule or against-the-rule change

The obtained data were tested statistically using the U test (Wilcoxon, Mann, and Whitney), the chi-squared test, the unpaired two-tailed t test, and the Wilcoxon rank test.

Results

Preoperative ocular findings, visual acuity, and astigmatism were statistically similar in both groups. In neither group were severe postoperative complications observed. Postoperative inflammation was minimal in all eyes, without any difference between those eyes in which glue was used and those in which sutures were used. Transient hyphema was found in seven eyes in the single-stitch group and one in the fibrin adhesive group. Prolonged mild corneal decompensation occurred in one eye in each group. Visual acuity increased postoperatively in both groups: 3% of the patients in the single-stitch wound closure group and 4% of the patients in the fibrin adhesive group had a visual acuity of 0.5 or more preoperatively. This percentage increased to 19% and 24%, respectively, on the first postoperative day and to 74% and 81%, respectively, after 6 months. These functional results do not differ significantly in the two groups.

Focusing our interest on keratometric astigmatism 6 months postoperatively, we were able to make several observations; the total amount of astigmatism was small in most cases: 1.12 D in the single-stitch group and 0.89 D in the fibrin group (U Test, $p < 0.05$; Table 1).

Only 3% of the fibrin group had postoperative astigmatism greater than 1.75 D, compared to 11.9% of the single-stitch group. In 37% of cases,

Table 1. Mean pre- and postoperative astigmatism in diopters ($\pm$ standard deviation) Mean postoperative astigmatism was significantly less for the fibrin group at 6 months (p <0.05).

	Single-stitch group	Fibrin group	Total
Preoperative astigmatism	0.65 $\pm$ 0.89	0.66 $\pm$ 0.86	0.65 $\pm$ 0.88
Astigmatism 1 day postoperatively	0.37 $\pm$ 0.54	0.40 $\pm$ 0.57	0.38 $\pm$ 0.55
Astigmatism 1 week postoperatively	0.56 $\pm$ 0.57	0.58 $\pm$ 0.78	0.58 $\pm$ 0.70
Astigmatism 6 months postoperatively	1.12 $\pm$ 1.01	0.89 $\pm$ 0.81	1.02 $\pm$ 0.94

the postoperative astigmatism was smaller than preoperatively in the single-stitch group, compared to 49 % in the fibrin group (significantly different, chi-squared test, p <0.05). Astigmatic change was significantly smaller in the fibrin group, evaluated by vector analysis (0.84 D compared to 0.99 D; U test, <0.05). On the other hand, calculation methods evaluating astigmatic change with/against-the-rule resulted in similarly small values: the astigmatic swing was –0.07 D against-the-rule in the single-stitch group using the Cravy method [3] and –0.09 D by Naeser's method, compared to –0.13 D and –0.17 D, respectively, in the fibrin group (Table 2). Also, the distribution of the axis of the corrective cylinder required to eliminate the astigmatic error [9] did not show any significant difference.

Table 2. Mean induced astigmatism for single-stitch and fibrin wound closure, 6 months postoperatively; calculation with three different methods

	Single-stitch group	Fibrin group	Total
Vector analysis of astigmatic change by [9]	0.99** $\pm$ 0.68	0.84** $\pm$ 0.63	0.92 $\pm$ 0.67
With/against-the-rule change [3]	–0.07 $\pm$ 1.07	–0.13 $\pm$ 0.97	–0.10 $\pm$ 1.03
With/against-the-rule change [14]	–0.09 $\pm$ 1.14	–0.17 $\pm$ 1.00	–0.13 $\pm$ 1.08

Results expressed as mean change ($\pm$ standard deviation) in diopters.
** Statistically different (p <0.05).

Table 3. Synopsis of recently published data concerning surgically induced astigmatism in cataract surgery

Author	Year	No. of patients	Surgical procedure	Follow-up	Induced astig-matism[a]	With/against-the-rule astig-matism
Buzard and Shearing [2]	1991	43	5-mm incision, no stitch	6.9 weeks	0.74	
		88	5-mm incision, one stitch	6.9 weeks	0.86	
		42	6-mm incision, one stitch	6.9 weeks	0.85	
		12	6.5-mm incision, one stitch	6.9 weeks	0.6	
Fine [4]	1991	295	4-mm incision, silicone IOL	5 months		−0.14
Golychev [7]	1990	130	ICCE, step-shaped incision	7 months	1.8	
Masket [13]	1991	20	4-mm incision, no stitch	4 months		−0.27
[13]	1991	50	4-mm incision, anchor suture	4 months		−0.01
Shepherd [20]	1989	99	4-mm incision	3 months		−0.22
Singer [22]	1991	45	6- to 7-mm frown incision	6 months	0.84	−0.69
		32	Scleral pocket (6–7 mm)	6 months	1.15	−1.0
Steinert et al. [23]	1991	65	4-mm incision, silicone IOL	3 months	0.82	−0.21
		65	6-mm incision, PMMA IOL	3 months	1.03	−0.2
Talamo et al. [24]	1991	137	ECCE, four sutures	6 months		−0.29
Our results	1992	167	5.5- to 6.5-mm incision, fibrin	6 months	0.84	−0.13
		218	5.5- to 6.5-mm incision, single stitch	6 months	0.99	−0.07

ICCE, intracapsular cataract extraction; IOL, intraocular lens; PMMA, polymethyl methacrylate; ECCE, extracapsular cataract extraction.
[a] Calculated by vector analysis.

Discussion

In all patients proper wound closure was achieved either by the single-stitch technique or by using fibrin glue. No adverse effects of the applied fibrin glue could be detected. The excellent biocompatibility of this adhesive was expected, since Buschmann [1] had used fibrin intraocularly to close traumatic defects of the lens capsule without any side effects due to the glue. With our technique, the fibrin adhesive is not given intraocularly; only a thin film of glue is applied into the external wound gap and onto the sclera. The self-sealing scleral pocket incision prevents glue penetration into the anterior chamber.

No case demonstrated early or late wound leaks. Postoperative inflammation was minimal in all eyes, without any difference between those eyes in which glue was used and those in which sutures were used. Henrick [8] found that the application of fibrin glue leads to an equal or superior wound closure of scleral incisions compared to suturing, according to his results of experimental studies performed with fibrin adhesive in animals. Discussing his results, Henrick concluded that fibrin glue might be advantageous for reinforcement of scleral cataract incisions in humans. Our main concern in securing the scleral pocket incision after phacoemulsification with in-the-bag implantation of an intraocular lens was to prevent the development of postoperative against-the-rule astigmatism. There are numerous reports confirming the self-sealing properties of scleral pocket incisions in cataract surgery without suture; however, some of them report the development of postoperative against-the-rule astigmatism [13, 17, 22, 23], which may be due to an intra- or postoperative dehiscence of the scleral wound lips caused by increased intraocular pressure. Particularly after the use of viscoelastic substances during surgery, postoperative increase of intraocular pressure is a common finding, despite irrigation procedures at the end of surgery [11].

To avoid the development of postoperative against-the-rule astigmatism, some surgeons advocate sophisticated incision techniques [6, 12, 16, 21, 22] or suturing of the scleral wound [13, 15, 20]. Other authors prefer foldable intraocular lenses, allowing the reduction of the incision length to 3.5–4.0 mm [4, 23]

The idea of wound closure with fibrin adhesive was to reinforce the scleral wound in small-incision cataract surgery in order to prevent postoperative development of astigmatism. This technique allows the implantation of intraocular lenses of proven material (polymethyl methacrylate, PMMA) and size without performing time-consuming scleral incisions of sophisticated geometry or suturing. Our results with fibrin sealant and wound closure with a horizontal suture demonstrate that postoperative against-the-rule astigmatism is minimal in both groups (0.13 versus 0.07 D). Compared to data gained with different surgical techniques (Table 3), our results are promising.

Regarding the additional effects of wound reinforcement and facilitation of the surgical procedure, we conclude that wound closure with fibrin adhesive is likely to be a beneficial improvement in small-incision surgery.

References

1. Buschmann W (1982) Wiederherstellung einer weitgehend klaren Linse nach perforierender Verletzung. Klin Monatsbl Augenheilkd 181: 487–489
2. Buzard KA, Shearing SP (1991) Comparison of postoperative astigmatism with incisions of varying length closed with horizontal sutures and with no sutures. J Cataract Refract Surg 17: 734–739

3. Cravy TV (1979) Calculation of the change in corneal astigmatism following cataract extraction. Ophthalmic Surgery 10: 38–48
4. Fine IH (1991) Architecture and construction of a self-sealing incision for cataract surgery. J Cataract Refract Surg 17: 672–676
5. Fish JR (1991) Creation of a no-stitch cataract incision. J Cataract Refract Surg 17: 713–715
6. Freeman JM (1991) Scleral stretch incision for cataract surgery. J Cataract Refract Surg 17: 696–701
7. Golychev VN (1990) The effect of the incision in cataract extraction on corneal astigmatism. Oftalmol Zh 3: 160–161
8. Henrick A, Kalpakian B, Gaster RN, Vanley C (1991) Organic tissue glue in the closure of cataract incision in rabbit eyes. J Cataract Refract Surg 17: 551–555
9. Jaffe NS, Clayman HM (1979) The pathophysiology of corneal astigmatism after cataract extraction. Trans Am Acad Ophthalmol Otolaryngol 79: 615–630
10. Koch PS (1991) Structural analysis of cataract incision construction. J Cataract Refract Surg 17: 661–667
11. Lane SS, Naylor DW, Kullerstrand LJ, Knauth K, Lindstrom RL (1991) Prospective comparison of the effects of Occucoat, Viscoat and Healon on intraocular pressure and endothelial cell loss. J Cataract Refract Surg 17: 21–26
12. Maloney WF, Shapiro DR (1991) Universal small incision for cataract surgery. J Cataract Refract Surg 17: 702–705
13. Masket S (1991) Horizontal anchor suture closure method for small incision cataract surgery. J Cataract Refract Surg 17: 689–695
14. Naeser K (1990) Conversion of keratometer readings to polar values. J Cataract Refract Surg 16: 741–745
15. Pacifico RL, Morrison C (1991) Astigmatically neutral sutured small incision. J Cataract Refract Surg 17: 710–712
16. Pallin LS (1991) Chevron sutureless closure: a preliminary report. J Cataract Refract Surg 17: 706–709
17. Parker WT, Clorfeine GS (1989) Long-term evolution of astigmatism following planned extracapsular cataract extraction. Arch Ophthalmol 107: 353–357
18. Redl H, Schlag G (1986) Fibrin sealant and its modes of application. Springer, Berlin Heidelberg New York (Fibrin sealant in operative medicine, vol 2), pp 13–26
19. Schlag G, Redl H, Turnher M, Dinges HP (1986) The importance of fibrin in wound repair. In: Schlag G, Redl H (eds) Opthalmology – Neurology. Springer, Berlin Heidelberg New York (Fibrin sealant in operative medicine, vol 2)
20. Shepherd JR (1989) Induced astigmatism in small incision cataract surgery. J Cataract Refract Surg 15: 85–88
21. Siepser SB (1991) Sutureless cataract surgery with radial transverse incision. J Cataract Refract Surg 17: 716–718
22. Singer JA (1991) Frown incision for minimizing induced astigmatism after small incision cataract surgery with rigid optic intraocular lens implantation. J Cataract Refract Surg 17: 677–688
23. Steinert RF, Brint FS, White SM, Fine IH (1991) Astigmatism after small incision cataract surgery. Ophthalmology 98: 417–424
24. Talamo JH, Stark WJ, Gottsch JD, Goodman DF, Pratzer K, Cravy TV, Enger C (1991) Natural history of corneal astigmatism after cataract surgery. J Cataract Refract Surg 17: 313–318

Wound Closure with Fibrin Adhesive in Cataract Surgery

U. MESTER

Abstract

The scleral flap technique has considerably improved wound closure in cataract surgery, allowing a sutureless wound construction. Some remaining problems are postoperatively induced astigmatism, wound leakage with the risk of intraocular infection, and dehiscence of the conjunctiva. The application of fibrin glue can minimize these potential complications by reinforcing the scleral wound and firmly positioning the conjunctiva. Clinical experience in a large number of cataract procedures has confirmed the beneficial effects of fibrin sealant; no side effects have been observed.

Introduction

The current standard procedure in cataract surgery is phacoemulsification using the small incision technique, i. e., entry into the anterior chamber of the eye via a scleral flap, capsulorhexis in the capsulectomy procedure, and intraocular lens implantation within the capsular bag (Fig. 1). Other techniques are reserved for difficult cases or are still in the experimental stage.

Surgical entry to the lens via a lamellar scleral tunnel has led to significant improvements: a good surgeon can close a sutureless wound by means of its valve construction. The high tensile strength makes it possible to insert rigid polymethyl methacrylate intraocular lenses as the wound can be extended to 6.5 mm [9, 19, 11].

An important aspect of cataract incision and scleral tunnel technique is that postoperative astigmatism is minimized. However some authors have observed a tendency to development of postoperative astigmatism [27], even when the scleral flap was secured with a horizontal suture [34] or when special wound constructions were used [35].

An additional complication that may arise in a sutureless tunnel incision is the impairment of the stability of wound edges, especially after long intraoperative manipulations or in the case of scleral thinning. Although this seldom results in permanent damage and wound healing is merely delayed, a filtration bleb may form in individual cases which could lead to an intraocular infection [24].

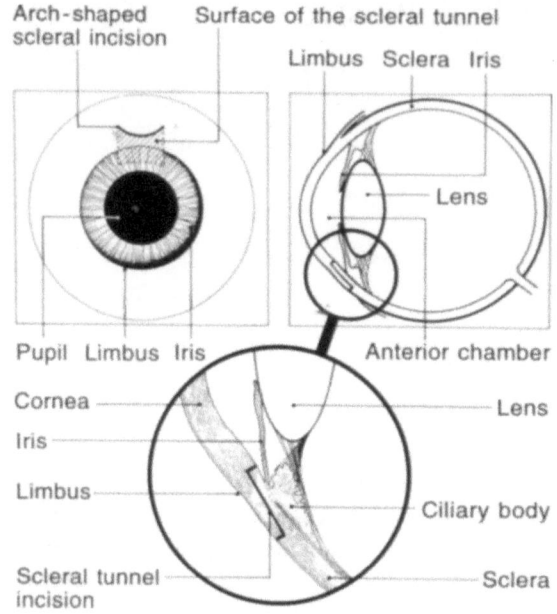

Arch-shaped   Surface of the scleral tunnel
scleral incision

Limbus Sclera Iris

Lens

Pupil Limbus Iris

Anterior chamber

Cornea   Lens

Iris

Limbus   Ciliary body

Scleral tunnel   Sclera
incision

Fig. 1. Small incision technique for cataracts

Conjunctival closure is beneficial in these cases. It is advisable to avoid using a conjunctival suture in sutureless wound closure. Conjunctival positioning with bipolar diathermy forceps, a widespread technique, often does not provide enough stability if the scleral tunnel incision is insufficient. Efforts to optimally close a wound using the scleral flap technique have led to the use of fibrin glue, because such complications are then minimized or avoided altogether.

Materials and Methods

Fibrin Glue

Fibrin glue is a biological, nontoxic product made from human blood. Heat treatment precludes the risk of infection [32]. During the last 20 years numerous papers have been published on the successful application of fibrin glue in all specialist surgical fields. It has been conclusively demonstrated that even large, hemorrhaging wound areas or wounds in inaccessible operating areas can be closed reliably. Not only have the hemostatic effects of fibrin glue proved to be beneficial, but fibrin glue is also suitable for application on a damp wound surface. Redl et al. [30, 31] calculated a strength of 1200 g/cm^2 for a fibrin clot. Rat skin fixed with fibrin glue demonstrated a tensile strength of 200 g/cm^2 after 10 min. Fibrin additionally promotes the natural healing process by stimulating fibroblast growth, promoting wound healing for up to 10 days [33]. Fibrin has been shown to be resorbed by phagocytasing macrophages on the third postoperative day. After 7 days new collagenous fibers appear during simultaneous, continual breakdown of the fibrin [28]. Henrick et al. [14] found fibrin in the wound area after 30 days at histological examination.

Application in Ophthalmology

Unlike other surgical disciplines, the use of fibrin glue in ophthalmology has not yet become generally accepted. Several reports on very interesting potential applications of fibrin glue have been published. There are, however, still too few cases or the procedure is still in the experimental phase. Buschmann [3] reported successful clinical results in the repair of traumatic lesions with fibrin glue after carrying out experimental studies. There have been few cases to date, however.

Härting and Mellin [13] reported on animal experiments with fibrin glue in conjunctival and scleral surgery and Mellin et al. [21] on the anchoring of the ciliary body with fibrin. Animal experiments of fibrin glue in retinal surgery were conducted by Nasaduke and Peyman [26] and Emmerich et al. [8]. Steinkogler [36] used this glue to repair lacerated canaliculi lacrimales, Aichmair [1] in strabismus surgery. There are very early reports on fibrin glue in corneal surgery by Holtmann and Stein [16] and Freyler and Klemen [10].

More recent publications discuss the use of fibrin in mucous membrane transplants grafting in the orbita [37] or the fixation of autologous conjunctival transplants in the surgical treatment of pterygium [5].

These studies are meant to serve as a general guide to the history of fibrin glue in ophthalmology; numerous other publications are available, too. Fibrin glue has not yet found widespread application in ophthalmic surgery; however, the aforementioned complications in the sutureless scleral flap technique used in cataract surgery have led to the conjecture that the routine application of fibrin glue may be beneficial. In September 1991, Henrick et al. published the results of animal experiments using fibrin to position the scleral flap [14]. The authors compared this procedure with wound closure using a continuous 10–0 nylon suture and found the same wound strength. There was no significant difference with regard to postoperative irritation either. The animals treated with fibrin glue had more cells in the anterior chamber on the 30th postoperative day, which appeared to result from the use of human fibrin in rabbits. No toxic or allergic reactions to human fibrin glue in clinical applications in the eye were observed by Buschmann [4].

Fibrin Sealant Technique in Cataract Surgery

The fibrin glue we used (Tissucol Duo S human fibrinogen, human thrombin steam-treated, 0.5 ml, Immuno, Heidelberg) consists of two deep-frozen solutions in syringes. A syringe with 0.5 ml glue protein contains human plasma protein with fibrinogen, factor XIII, fibronectin, plasminogen, and aprotinin. The syringe with 0.5 ml thrombin solution contains $CaCl_2$ (Fig. 2) in addition to

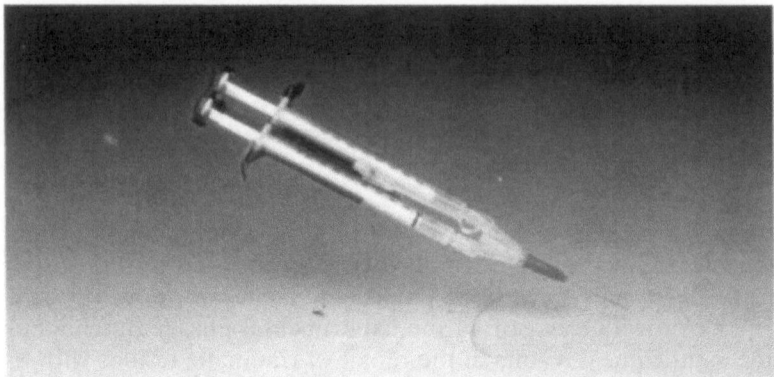

Fig. 2. Tissucol Duo S human fibrinogen, human thrombin, steam-treated 0.5 ml (Immuno, Heidelberg). Sterilized Duploject double syringe with deep-frozen fibrin glue components

thrombin. The high thrombin concentration provides almost instantaneous hardening of the fibrin glue (within a few seconds). Both syringes are thawed and warmed to 36 °C. The two components mix best at body temperature. The use of a double syringe system (Duploject, Immuno, Heidelberg) to apply fibrin glue on the eye has proved to be invaluable. It consists of a holding device for the two syringes and a common plunger which mixes the fibrin and thrombin systems as they are injected through a disposable needle applicator. The optimum mixture (temperature-dependent) of the two components is identifiable by the viscous consistency of the extravasating sealant. The deep-frozen syringes are delivered in sterile packaging together with the double syringe systems and only require warming in a water bath. The double syringe offers the advantage of being able to apply the ready-mixed adhesive with a thin-needle applicator, thus enabling fine dosage. We consider this procedure to be more beneficial than that proposed by Kammann et al. [17] in which the two components are applied in layers. The very thin application of the fibrin glue using the double syringe permits direct positioning of the conjunctiva on the sclera. Four to five fine drops instilled onto the scleral wound are sufficient. They combine to form a thin film (Fig. 3). Thick layers of fibrin are to be avoided: biological breakdown of the fibrin results in a preformed subconjunctival filtration bleb if the scleral wound is not watertight. Injection of glue into the scleral flap is unnecessary. Although there is no risk of complications, an episcleral application is sufficient.

Because of high thrombin concentration, the fibrin hardens within a few seconds. The conjunctiva must therefore be positioned quickly. It is beneficial to hold the conjunctiva with a forceps and to extend it over the exposed sclera while positioning it on the sclera, using slight pressure and the stroke of a second closed anatomic forceps (Fig. 4). If the conjunctiva is positioned too slowly the fibrin glue will have already gelled. In this case it is advisable to remove the fibrin film with forceps and to repeat the procedure. The needle applicator

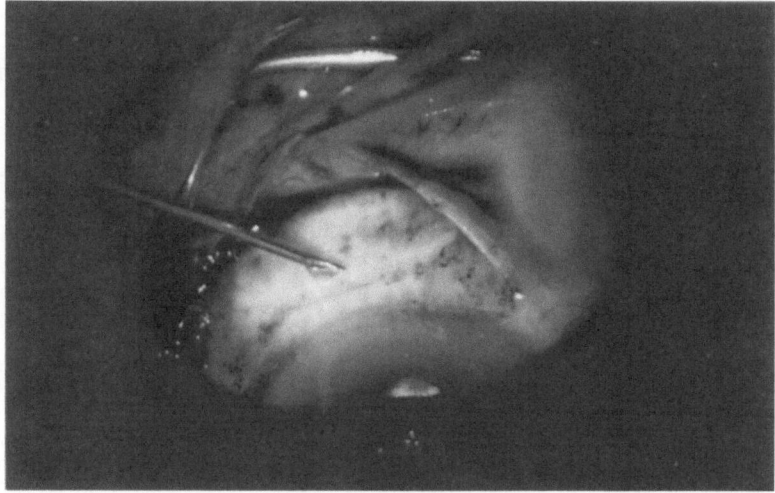

Fig. 3. Application of the ready mixed fibrin glue using the double syringe. Four to five drops are instilled onto the exposed sclera and combine to form a thin fibrin film

must also be replaced as the fibrin will have also gelled to it. The glue is most effective on dry wound surfaces, but can also be used in wet environments. A wet wound delays the hardening of the fibrin somewhat. The anchoring of the conjunctiva, although reliable, is delayed if fluid escapes from the anterior chamber during positioning of the conjunctiva. As optimum hardening of the fibrin after positioning of the conjunctiva has not yet been attained,

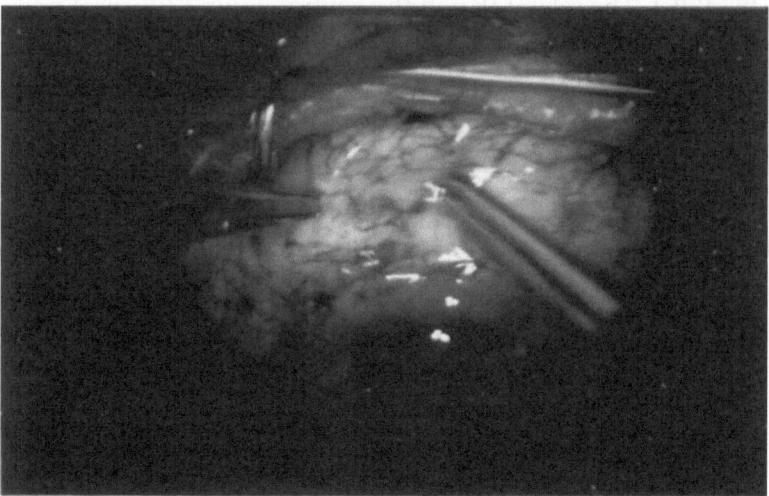

Fig. 4. The conjunctiva is held by forceps and stretched over the wound surface in the original position. Other forceps are used to exert slight pressure to position the conjunctiva on the sclera. The forceps slides over the conjunctival flap and exerts slight pressure so that it is positioned on the sclera within a few seconds

a subsequent subconjunctival injection of antibiotics or steroids should be given at the 6-o'clock position rather than in the wound area. Extensive fixation of the conjunctiva in the operating field obviates the spreading of the fluid applied subconjunctivally.

A maximum of 0.1 ml fibrin glue is required for the repair of a cataract incision. A Tissucol Duo S Packet is, therefore, sufficient for the treatment of 10–15 eyes, of course providing the needle applicator is changed and sterilization is ensured. A smaller packet of glue components is desirable, however.

Clinical Experience and Results

Fibrin Glue in Cataract Surgery

We began using fibrin glue in cataract surgery in April 1991. Our expectations were as follows:

1. Avoidance of the postoperative-induced astigmatism
2. Protection of the scleral tunnel incision from leaks, filtration blebs, and intraocular infections
3. Improvement of conjunctival positioning
4. Simplification of surgical procedures

The first results were disclosed in 1992 [22]. We were particularly interested in postoperative astigmatism. Two groups of patients were compared: 167 eyes were treated with fibrin glue after phacoemulsification with scleral tunnel incision and "in-the-bag" placement of a posterior chamber intraocular lens (PC-IOL). The scleral flap in the control group (218 eyes) was secured with a horizontal 10–0 nylon suture. The other conditions were the same in both groups: a lamellar scleral incision was made beginning 2.5 mm to the surgical limbus and then carried forward in a lamellar plane 0.5 mm into clear cornea. The wound was extended 5.5–6 mm for insertion of the polymethyl

Table 1. Mean induced astigmatism (in diopters) for single-stitch and fibrin wound closure 6 months postoperatively as calculated using three methods

Calculation method	Single-Stitch		Fibrin		Total	
	Mean change	SD	Mean change	SD	Mean change	SD
Vector analysis astigmatic change (Jaffe and Clayman [15])	0.99	0.68	0.84*	0.63	0.92	0.67
With/against-the-rule change (Cravy [6])	−0.07	1.07	−0.13	0.97	−0.10	1.03
With/against-the-rule change (Naeser [25])	−0.09	1.14	−0.17	1.00	−0.13	1.08

* $p < .05$.

methacrylate intraocular lens. The postoperative observation period lasted 6 months. The following picture of postoperative astigmatism was obtained: using Cravy's method of calculation [6] the group with fibrin glue demonstrated induced astigmatism with –0.13 D and the group with a suture with –0.07 D. The same values calculated by Naeser [25] were –0.17 or –0.09. As these are comparatively low values the differences are insignificant [23] (Table 1).

Discussion

The rate of postoperative astigmatism due to an effect of fibrin glue is comparable to that obtained with the use of sutures. The pathogenetic mechanism of postoperative astigmatism in the tunnel incision technique may be influenced by an increase in intraocular pressure resulting from the use of viscoelastic substances. Considerable increases in pressure were observed during the first 24 h after surgery although the material we used (Healon, Pharmacia, Erlangen) can largely be removed at the end of the operation, unlike other viscoelastic substances [2], so that postoperative increases in pressure are less pronounced [20, 12]. The experiments on cadaver eyes conducted by Frieling and Steinert [11] did not demonstrate topographic changes in the cornea resulting from pressure increases after tunnel incision. However, only the short-term effect was measured and a very long, 4-mm scleral tunnel was fashioned. A significant increase in intraocular pressure leads to marked dehiscence of the scleral wound with displacement of the scleral flap lamellae. This is of no real consequence as the wound remains watertight. Sealing the scleral lamellae in this position will lead to weakening of the tissue in the wound area, which causes long-term development of astigmatism. The aforementioned high tensile strength of fibrin glue during the first 3 days after surgery as well as its elasticity [29] counteract the pathogenetic mechanism caused by temporarily increased intraocular pressure. These results and those of other researchers confirm the beneficial effect of fibrin glue on postoperative astigmatism [23, 7]. The use of fibrin glue to close a scleral wound is particularly beneficial in the case of scleral thinning, poor tunnel incision, or loss of tension of the scleral tissue resulting from long intraoperative manipulations [18].

Fibrin glue is not only useful for the avoidance of postoperative induced astigmatism, but also as a prophylactic agent in the treatment of other complications. The author has treated more than 7000 cataract patients with the fibrin sealant technique. Postoperative filtration blebs were only observed at the beginning when no conscious effort was made to apply the fibrin layer thinly to maintain close contact of the sclera and the approximated conjunctiva. The technique of applying fibrin glue is described in more detail below. Conjunctival dehiscence was not observed in any of the cases. The wound was completely watertight in the few eyes in which postoperative intraocular infection (5) was suspected, which means that the microorganisms must have entered the eye intraoperatively.

Clinical experience has confirmed that the use of fibrin glue considerably facilitates cataract operations using the scleral flap technique. This not only applies to the preparation of the scleral tunnel, but also to phacoemulsification. Complicated construction of the scleral flap, preferred by many surgeons, or a very long tunnel incision are unnecessary. A tunnel incision 2 mm in length is sufficient to attain a reliable, watertight wound postoperatively when fibrin glue is used. We fashioned a slightly arched scleral incision; the limbal margin is antidromic. The flap was made 0.5–1.0 mm into the cornea. The advantage of this relatively short and slightly arched incision is that, particularly during phacoemulsification, the cornea is only very slightly strained. As the operating field is easily viewed, intraoperative complications resulting from poor visibility are avoided. The use of fibrin glue not only shortens and facilitates surgical intervention, but also increases the safety factor. This also applies to conjunctival positioning: in one operation fibrin is applied to the sclera prior to the positioning of the conjunctiva over the sclera. The glue is applied and the conjunctiva is positioned and firmly anchored in less than 10 s. A firm, flat covering of the scleral wound by the conjunctiva is attained, which closes the wound more reliably.

References

1. Aichmair H, Lintner F, Aichmair M (1986) Fibrin sealing in surgery of extraocular muscles: experiments in rabbits. In: Schlag G, Redl H (eds) Fibrin sealant in operative medicine, vol 2. Springer, Berlin Heidelberg New York, pp 70–73
2. Assia E, Apple DJ, Lim ES, Morgan RC, Tsai JC (1992) Removal of viscoelastic material after experimental cataract surgery in vitro. J Cataract Refract Surg 18:3–6.
3. Buschmann W (1982) Wiederherstellung einer weitgehend klaren Linse nach perforierender Verletzung. Klin Monatsbl Augenheilkd 181: 487–489
4. Buschmann W (1986) Fibrin sealant in the treatment of perforating injuries of the anterior and posterior lens capsule. In: Schlag G, Redl H (eds) Fibrin sealant in operative medicine, vol 2. Springer, Berlin Heidelberg New York
5. Cohen RA, McDonald MB (1993) Fixation of conjunctival autografts with an organic tissue adhesive. Arch Opthalmol 111: 1167–1168
6. Cravy TV (1979) Calculation of the change in corneal astigmatism following cataract extraction. Ophthalmic Surg 10: 38–49
7. Dietze U (1993) Vergleich von frühpostoperativen Ergebnissen nach Phakoemulsifikation mit fibrinverklebtem und mit nicht verklebtem Tunnelschnitt sowie nach herkömmlicher Schnittechnik. Symposium Fibrinklebung in der Augenheilkunde, Heidelberg, October 1993.
8. Emmerich KH, Edel G, Gerding H (1993) Fibrinklebung der Netzhaut. Symposium Fibrinklebung in der Augenheilkunde, Heidelberg, October 1993
9. Ernest PH, Kiessling LA, Lavery KT (1991) Relative strength of cataract incisions in cadaver eyes. J Cataract Refract Surg 17: 668–671
10. Freyler H, Klemen U (1978) Fibrinklebung in der Hornhautchirurgie. Graefes Arch Clin Exp Ophthalmol 207: 27–39
11. Frieling E, Steinert RF (1993) Intrinsic stability of "self-sealing" unsutured cataract wounds. Arch Ophthalmol 111: 381–383
12. Fry LL (1989) Postoperative intraocular pressure rises: comparison of Healon, Amvisc, and Viscoat. J Cataract Refr Surg 15: 415–420
13. Härting F, Mellin KB (1981) Tierexperimentelle Erfahrungen mit dem Fibrinkleber in der Bindehaut- und Sklerachirurgie. Klin Monatsbl Augenheilkd 179: 23–25
14. Henrick A, Kalpakian B, Gaster RN, Vanley C (1991) Organic tissue glue in the closure of cataract incisions in rabbit eyes. J Cataract Refract Surg 17: 551–555

15. Jaffe NS, Clayman HM (1975) The pathophysiology of corneal astigmatism after cataract extraction. Trans Am Acad Ophthalmol Otolaryngol 79: 615–630
16. Holtmann HW, Stein HJ (1977) Experimentelle Untersuchungen zur Hornhaut-wundklebung mittels hochkonzentriertem Fibrinogen. Ber Dtsch Ophthalmol Ges 77: 220–224
17. Kammann J, Dornbach G, Vollenberg C, Linares I (1993) Technik und Ergebnisse des Wundverschlusses durch Klebetechnik nach Phakoemulsifikation und IOL-Implantation. In: Neuhann I, Hartmann C, Rochels R (eds) Sechster Kongreß der Deutschsprachigen Gesellschaft für Intraokularlinsen Implantation. Springer, Berlin Heidelberg New York
18. Klemen U (1993) Nahtlose Kataraktoperationstechnik – Wundklebung mit Fibrinogen. Symposium Fibrinklebung in der Augenheilkunde, Heidelberg, October 1993
19. Kondrot EC (1991) Rupturing pressure in cadaver eyes with three types of cataract incisions. J Cataract Refract Surg 17: 745–748
20. Lane SS, Naylor DW, Kullerstrand LJ, Knauth K, Lindstrom RL (1991) Prospective comparison of the effects of Occucoat, Viscoat, and Healon on intraocular pressure and endothelial cell loss. J Cataract Refr Surg 17: 21–26
21. Mellin KB, Waubke TN, Härting F (1981) Modifikation des Operationsverfahrens zur Anheftung des Ziliarkörpers nach Mackensen und Corydon. Klin Monatsbl Augenheilkd 178: 68
22. Mester U, Zuche M, Rauber M (1992) Phaco with PCL-small incision technique with fibrin adhesive for wound closure. Second Congress of the American Society of Cataract and Refractive Surgery, San Diego, April 1992
23. Mester U, Zuche M, Rauber M (1993) Astigmatism after phacoemulsification with posterior chamber lens implantation: small incision technique with fibrin adhesive for wound closure. J Cataract Refract Surg 19: 616–619
24. Miller KM, Glasgow BJ (1993) Bacterial endophthalmitis following sutureless cataract surgery. Arch Ophthalmol 111: 377–379
25. Naeser K (1990) Conversion of keratometer readings to polar valucs. J Cataract Refract Surg 16: 741–745
26. Nasaduke I, Peyman GA (1986) Intraocular effects of rabbit fibrin sealant used in experimental retinal holes and detachments. In: Schlag G, Redl H (eds) Fibrin sealant in operative medicine, vol 2. Springer, Berlin Heidelberg New York, pp 74–84
27. Pfleger T, Scholz U, Skorpik C (1993) Postoperativer Astigmatismusverlauf bei Kleinschnittkataraktchirurgie und Nostitch-Wundverschluß. In: Neuhann T, Hartmann C, Rochels R (eds) Sechster Kongreß der Deutschsprachigen Gesellschaft für Intraokularlinsen-Implantation. Springer, Berlin Heidelberg New York
28. Pflüger H (1986) Lysis and absorption of fibrin sealant. In: Schlag G, Redl R (eds) Fibrin sealant in operative medicine, vol 2. Springer, Berlin Heidelberg New York, pp 39–50
29. Redl H, Schlag G (1986) Properties of different tissue sealants with special emphasis on fibrinogen-based preparations. In: Schlag G, Redl H (eds) Fibrin sealant in operative medicine, vol 2. Springer, Berlin Heidelberg New York, pp 27–38
30. Redl H, Stanek G, Hirschl A, Schlag G (1982) Fibrinkleber-Antibiotika-Gemische – Festigkeit und Elutionsverhalten. In: Cotta H, Braun A (eds) Fibrinkleber in Orthopädie und Traumatologie. Thieme, Stuttgart, pp 18–21
31. Redl H, Schlag G, Stanke G, Hirschl A, Seelich T (1983) In vitro properties of mixtures of fibrin seal and antibiotics. Biomaterial 4: 29–32
32. Riekel B (1993) Qualitäts- und Sicherheitsanforderungen an Fibrinkleber. Symposium Fibrinklebung in der Augenheilkunde, Heidelberg, October 1993
33. Schlag G, Redl H, Turnher M, Dinges HP (1986) The importance of fibrin in wound repair. In: Schlag G, Redl H (eds) Fibrin sealant in operative medicine, vol 2. Springer, Berlin Heidelberg New York, pp 3–12
34. Shepherd JR (1989) Induced astigmatism in small incision cataract surgery. J Cataract Refract Surg 15: 85–88
35. Singer JA (1991) Frown incision for minimizing induced astigmatism after small incision cataract surgery with rigid optic intraocular lens implantation. J Cataract Refract Surg 17: 677–688

36. Steinkogler FG (1986) Fibrin tissue adhesive for the repair of lacerated canaliculi lacrimales. In: Schlag G, Redl H (eds) Fibrin sealant in operative medicine, vol 2. Springer, Berlin Heidelberg New York, pp 92–94
37. Watts MT, Collin R (1992) The use of fibrin glue in mucous membrane grafting of the fornix. Ophthalmic Surg 23: 689–690

III. ENT

Rhinologic Applications of Fibrin Glue

H. Stammberger, J. A. Jebeles, and W. Luxenberger

Abstract

Endoscopic repair of cerebrospinal fluid (CSF) leaks and meningoencephaloceles of the anterior skull base as well as optic nerve decompression have been made possible by technological and surgical technique advances. Fibrin glue, with its ability to provide tissue seals, hemostasis, and tissue support, plays an important role in these new endoscopic procedures. An endoscopic endonasal approach combined with intrathecal injection of fluorescein was used in 70 patients with a CSF fistula and/or a meningoencephalocele of the anterior skull base. Autogenous tissue grafts with fibrin glue to provide support and to create a watertight seal were used to close the dural tear and bridge any bony defects. This technique resulted in a successful repair in all patients. The endoscopic approach is also used to perform optic nerve decompression. Fibrin glue is applied to protect against development of a CSF fistula after opening the nerve sheath. Also discussed are our techniques or orbital decompression, nasal septal perforation (NSP) repair, and repair of medial blowout fractures. During our 20 years of experience with the use of fibrin glue, we have seen no evidence of disease transmission and feel it is a safe and effective product for tissue sealing and tissue coaptation.

Introduction

Fibrin glue (Tissucol, Immuno, Vienna) is a substance with many important applications in rhinologic procedures; it consists of a concentrated fibrinogen solution which is activated by the addition of thrombin and calcium chloride. The interaction of these components mimics the final steps of the coagulation cascade [1, 5]. The two components are combined during application and subsequently the fibrin glue consolidates and adheres to the surfaces to which it is applied. Fibrin glue assists in hemostasis, tissue sealing, and tissue or suture support [1, 3, 4]. Various concentrations of thrombin can be applied to alter the rate of clotting. This forms a rapidly sealing and a slower sealing variety, each with its specific role in various surgical procedures. Concentrations of thrombin at 4 NIH-U/ml create the slow clotting variety which allows time for subsequent manipulation of graft materials into the proper prior sealing. With the use of a thrombin concentration of 500 NIH-U/ml, a mixture is formed which will clot almost instantaneously upon application [5].

A variety of delivery techniques exist for the application of fibrin glue, each adapted for specific application requirements. The Duploject delivery system allows rapid and easy application, either as a stream through a catheter or as a spray. Delivery through the Duploject double syringe applicator provides thorough mixing of the components, easy single-handed application, and application in thin layers. In situations requiring coverage of large surface areas, the Duploject system may be attached to a spray head [5]. The use of the Duploject application system avoids the problems of using the sequential application which requires mixing and handling.

In otorhinolaryngology as well as in other medical fields, fibrin glue has widespread and important applications [2, 3, 6]. In this paper we limit our discussion to the uses of fibrin glue in the following rhinologic procedures: repair of CSF leaks of the anterior skull base, reduction of meningoencephaloceles, endoscopic optic nerve decompression, orbital decompression, NSP repair, and the repair of medial blowout fractures.

Methods

Repair of Cerebrospinal Fluid Leaks and/or Meningoencephalocele Reduction

Advances in endoscopic rhinologic instruments and surgical techniques have made it possible for us to repair CSF leaks and reduce meningoencephaloceles with repair of the bony defect in the anterior skull base through an endoscopic endonasal approach (Figs. 1, 2). The operative procedure begins with the injection of fluorescein dye intrathecally to assist us in localizing the area of the CSF leak [7]. Using the technique of Messerklinger and Stammberger, the anterior skull base is exposed and, if necessary, a blue light is used to identify the leakage site or the meningoencephalocele [9] (Fig. 3). The mucosa surrounding the bony defect is denuded with a curet to facilitate the attachment of the patch with the use of fibrin glue. Materials most frequently used for the repair are lyophilized dura, fascia lata, ear cartilage with perichondrium, or harvested mucosa with or without bone from the middle or inferior turbinates. At this point, the surgeon has two options: an underlay or an overlay technique (Fig. 4). The underlay technique is preferable; however, it is not always technically possible to perform, especially in the vicinity of the internal carotid artery and optic nerve. Successful results may also be achieved with the overlay technique. In the underlay technique, the dura is elevated from the margins of the defect. The slow-acting variety of fibrin glue is placed onto the patch material, which is introduced through the defect and allowed to be trapped between the dura and bony skull base. The graft is now supported by both the bony margin as well as the fibrin glue, which is critical in producing a watertight seal. This initial layer of patch material may be reinforced by a second or even a third layer of material, again secured in place by fibrin glue. In situations such as these, where tedious manipulations of graft materials are required with the nar-

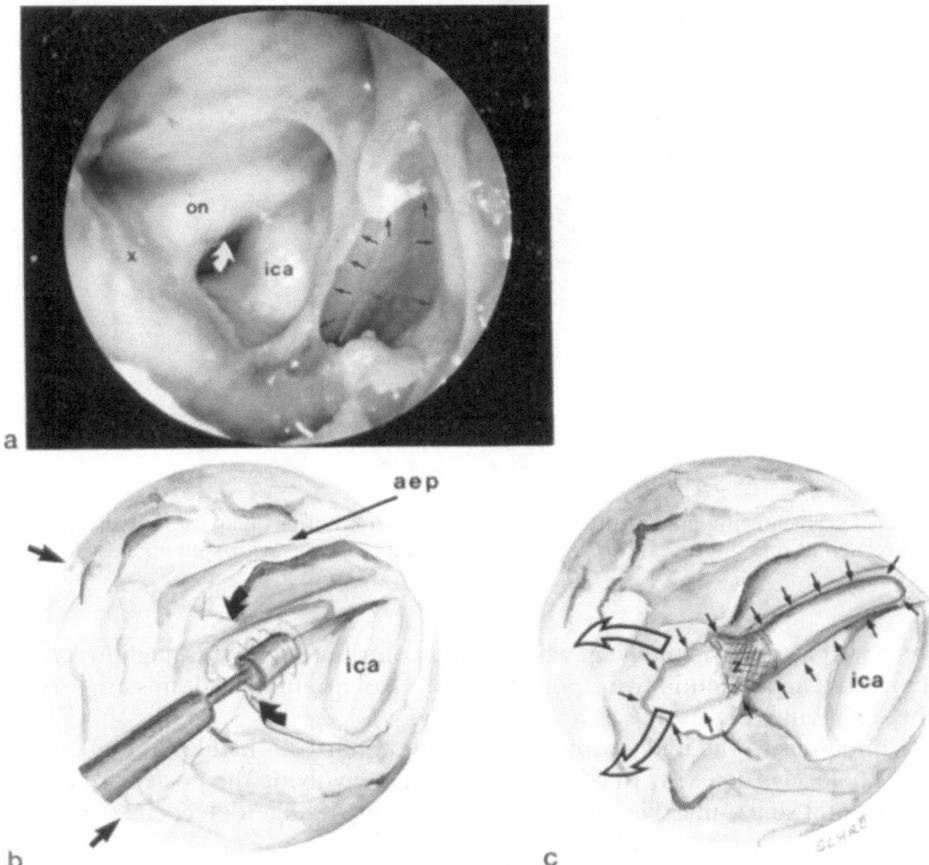

Fig. 1.a Endoscopic view of optic nerve *(on)* and internal carotid artery *(ica)* exposed in a posterior ethmoid air cell on the right side. The *white arrow* indicates pneumatization into anterior clinoid process. *x,* tuberculum opticum. *Small arrows* indicate opening into sphenoid sinus. **b** Drilling away bone of optic nerve canal from optic tubercle towards the prechiasm area. *aep,* arteria ethmoidalis posterior. *Small arrows* indicate exposed periorbita (lamina papyracea removed), *large arrows* area of optic tubercle. **c** A 180° medial decompression of the optic nerve has been accomplished *(small arrows).* Z, anulus of Zinn. *Large arrows* indicate periorbita exposed

row confines of the paranasal sinus system, the slow-acting variety of fibrin glue is indispensable. In the overlay technique, the patch material is positioned directly over the defect so that it completely bridges the area to be covered. The patch is covered with slow-acting fibrin glue before being placed in position and is held secure for 1 min, allowing the fibrin glue to clot and seal the defect. Once secured, fibrin glue is again used to reinforce the patch support. Once, the grafting is completed, the cavity is packed with Oxycel (oxidized cellulose) to further support the graft material. The packing is removed on day 7 after the operation and the nasal cavities are inspected. In the postoperative period, patients are kept in bed for 5–7 days and instructed to avoid blowing their

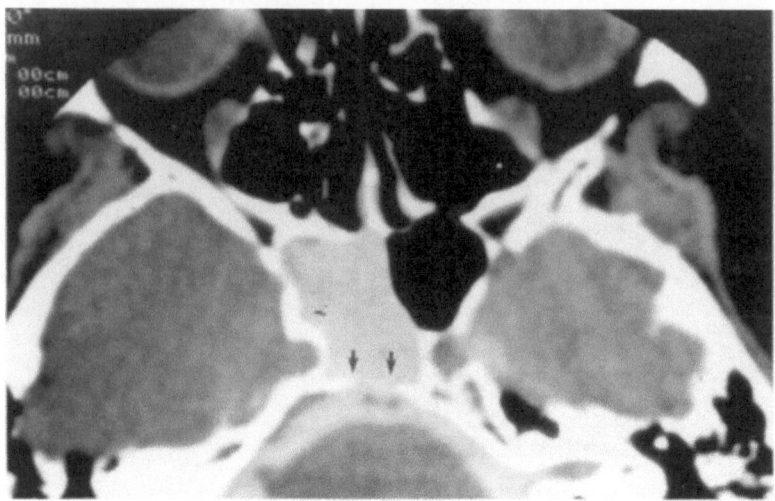

Fig. 2. CT scan showing opacification of the right sphenoid sinus in a patient with a history of recurrent meningitis. *Arrows* indicate bony defect in posterior sphenoidal wall

nose as well as other maneuvers which could contribute to increasing intracranial pressure and potentially dislodge the graft. No intralumbar drains are used in these patients (Fig. 5, 6).

Limitations to the endoscopic approach to repair CSF fistulas and meningoencephaloceles do exist. In cases with fractures involving the posterior table of the frontal sinus, massively comminuted fractures, huge defects associated

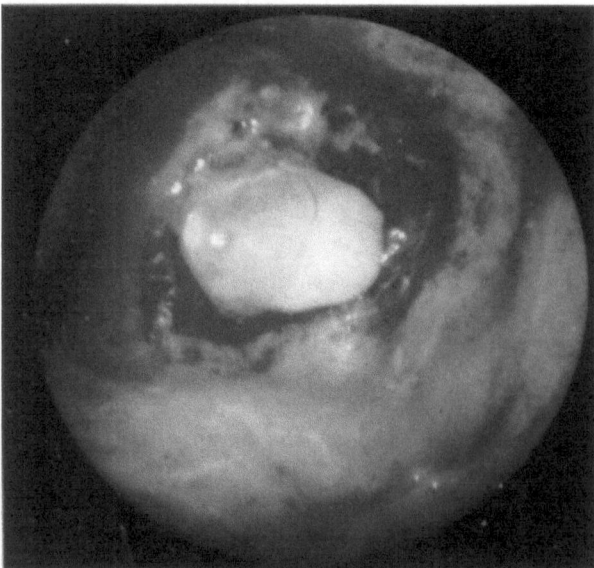

Fig. 3. Endoscopic view of the sphenoid sinus after intrathecal injection of sodium fluorescein showing a meningoencephalocele herniating into the sinus

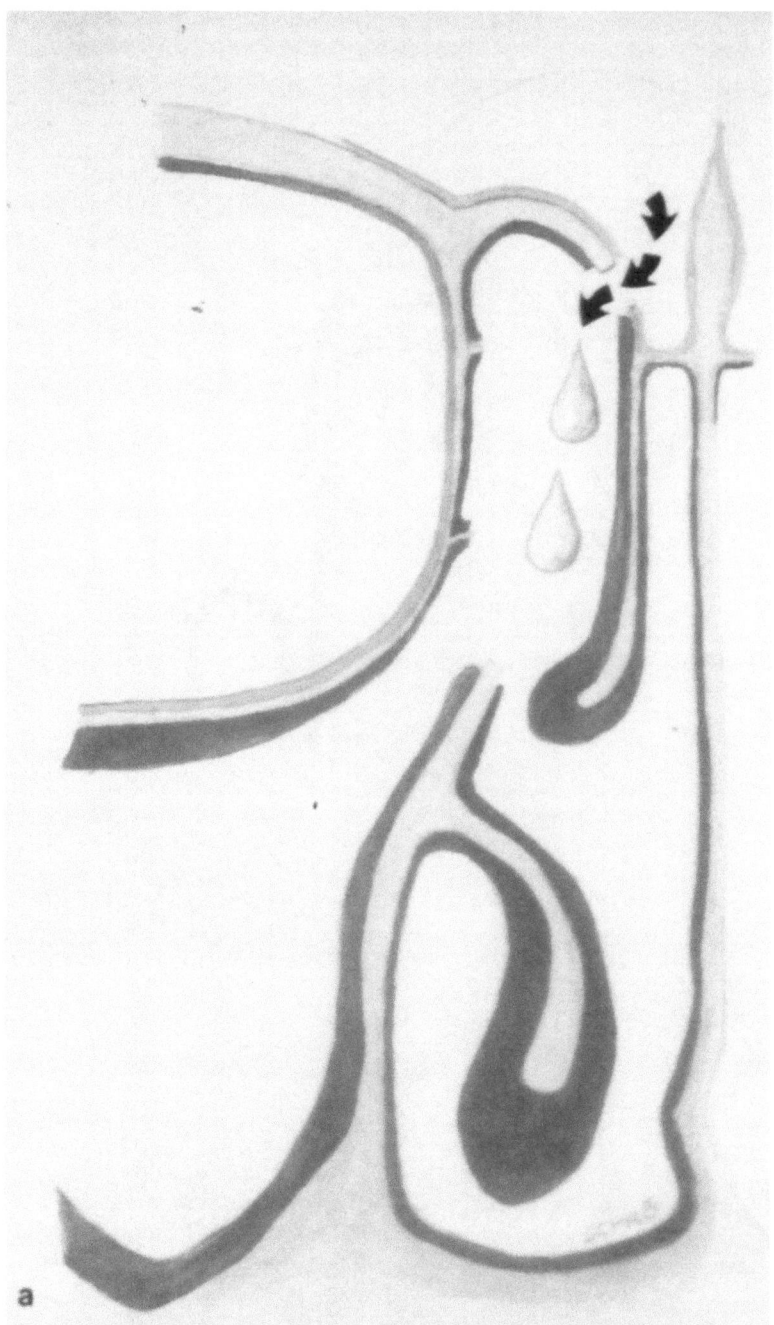

Fig. 4a. Site of cerebrospinal fluid (CSF) fistula in the anterior skull base (to be continued on page 141)

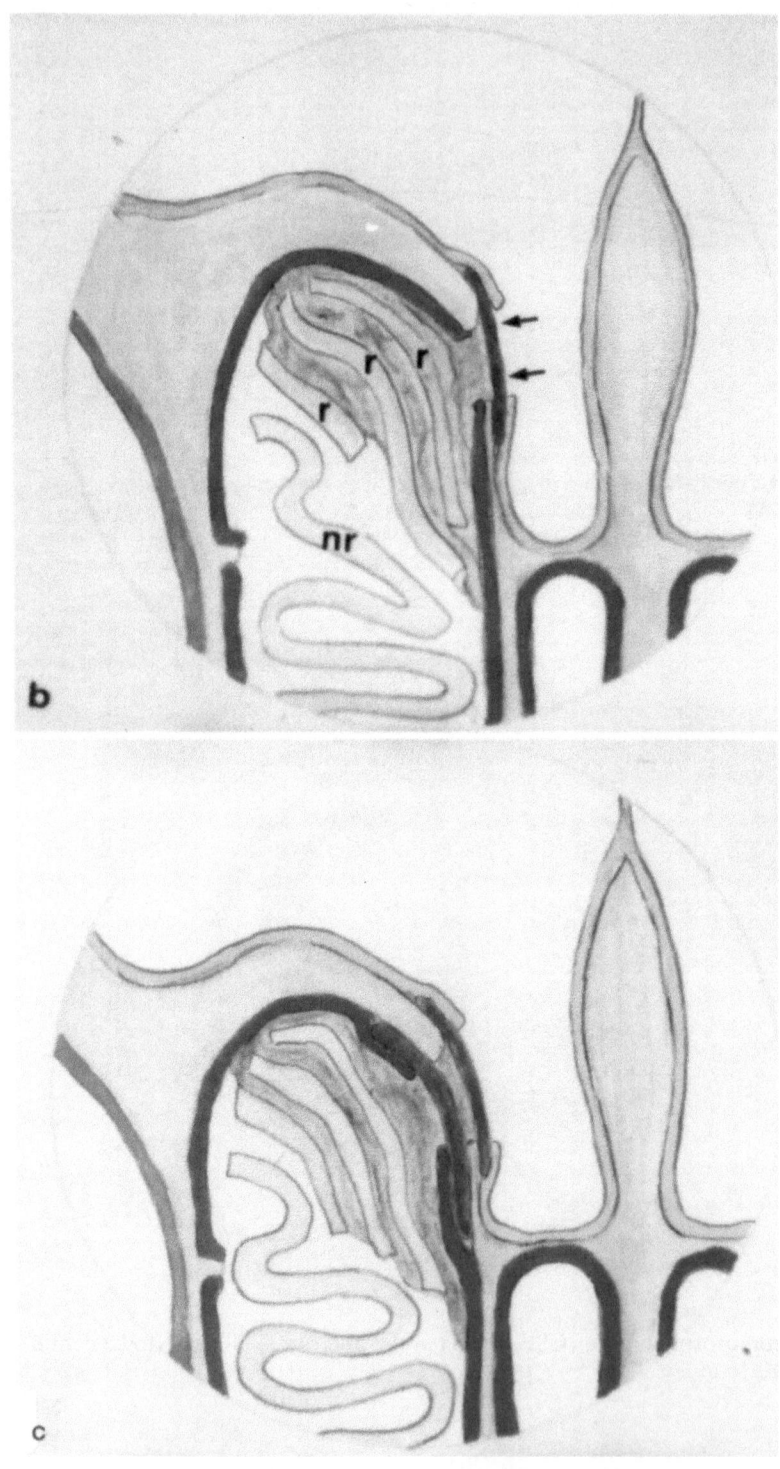

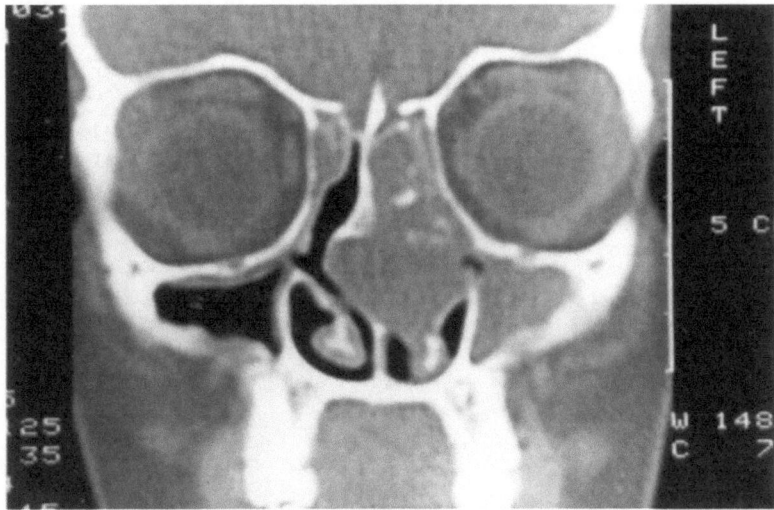

Fig. 5. Coronal CT scan of a patient after closed head trauma with herniating intracranial contents into the left nasal and paranasal sinus cavities

with large meningoencephaloceles and fractures crossing the midline, a non-endoscopic approach is used (Fig. 7, 8).

Using the above-described technique in 70 selected patients treated for repair of CSF leaks and/or reduction of meningoencephaloceles, a very high success rate has been achieved. Only six patients so far required revision surgery for failure of the initial procedure. It is of interest that all of the failures were in the early years of our experience with this technique and could have been attributed to our inexperience at that time.

Optic Nerve Decompression

In contrast to more traditional techniques of optic nerve decompression such as craniotomy or transfacial approach, the endoscopic approach to optic nerve decompression is associated with significantly less morbidity and a better cosmetic result [8]. We have performed an endoscopic endonasal optic nerve decompression on ten patients in our clinic and use fibrin glue as a routine part of this procedure. The surgical procedure includes a complete endoscopic sphenoethmoidectomy to expose the bony covering of the optic nerve from the orbital apex to the region of the optic chiasm. The bone covering the optic nerve is removed by a combination of drilling with a specially modified drill for endonasal usage and subsequent elevation of the thinned bone. The optic

---

◀ **Fig. 4b.** Fistula repair using the underlay technique. *r*, Resorbable packing; *nr*, nonresorbable packing; *blue area*, fibrin glue; *arrows*, lyophilized dura. **c** Fistula repaired using a combination of the underlay and overlay technique. *blue area*, fibrin glue

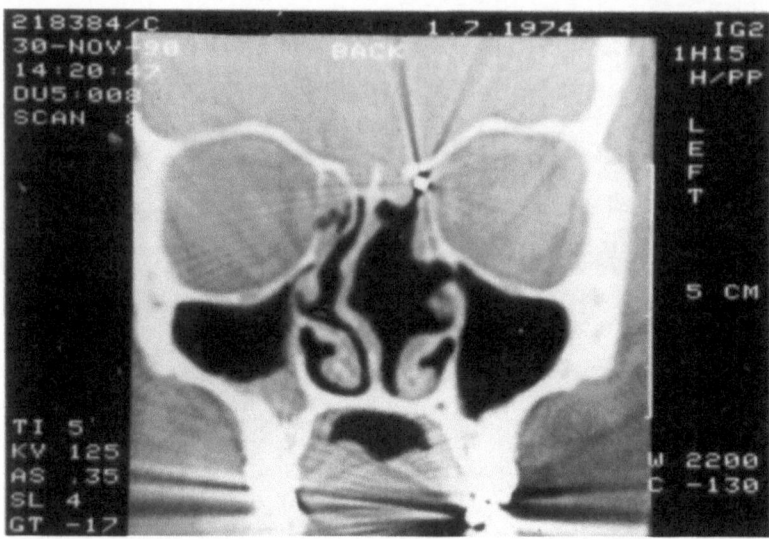

Fig. 6. Coronal CT scan of the same patient as in Fig. 5 after repair of a traumatic cerebrospinal fluid fistula and meningoencephalocele using lyophilized dura and fibrin glue

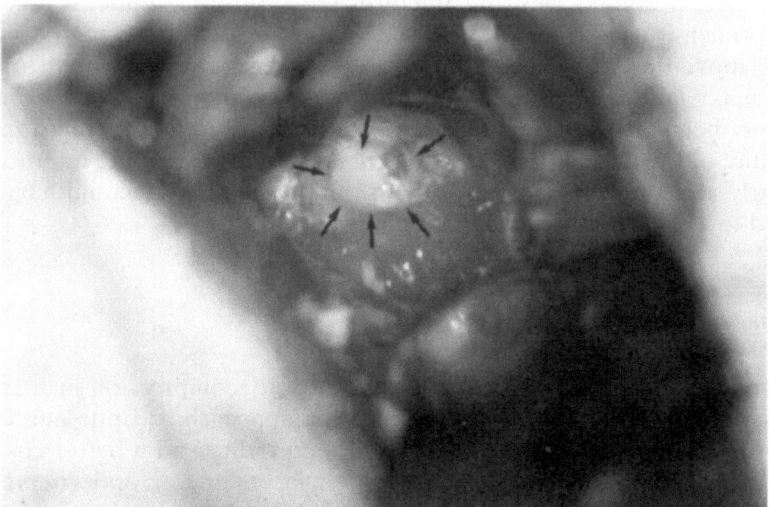

Fig. 7. External approach utilized in a patient after closed head trauma which resulted in a massively comminuted fracture of the posterior table of the frontal sinus, cerebrospinal fluid (CSF) fistula, and meningoencephalocele. Close-up view through operating microscope showing the injured area. Preoperatively, the patient had an intrathecal injection of sodium fluorescein, which is seen as the yellow color through the meninges *(arrows)*

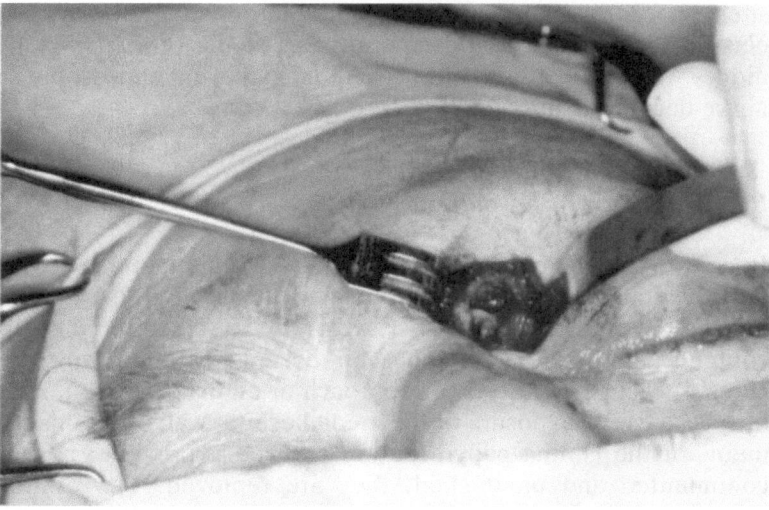

Fig. 8. Situation after repair with lyophilized dura and fibrin glue

nerve is exposed and in selected cases for further facilitation of the decompression the optic sheath is incised with a sickle knife. Care is taken to incise only the outer of the two layers of the optic sheath so as to avoid the potential CSF leak which may occur as a result of inadvertently entering the second layer; however, due to the intimate relationship of these two layers, one can never be sure that the inner layer has not been accidently violated. To avoid the potential CSF leak in this area, we routinely place fibrin glue over the incision

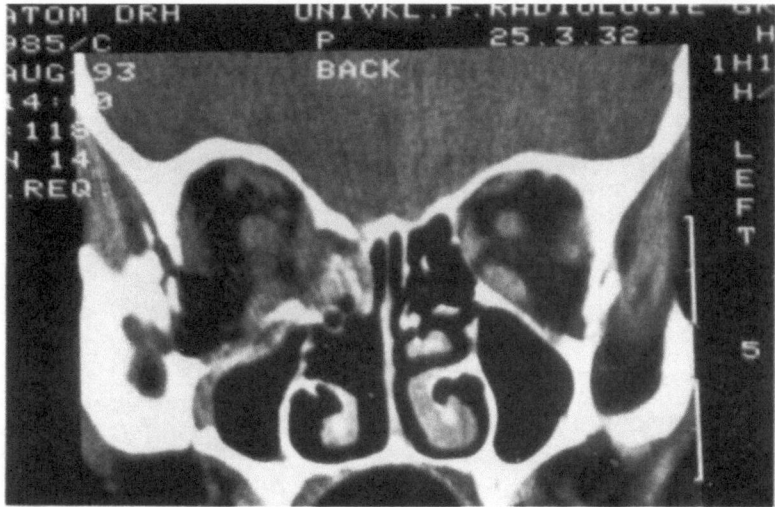

Fig. 9. Coronal CT scan of the paranasal sinuses showing a right-sided medial blowout fracture with herniation of the orbital contents

sites. The fibrin glue seals the potential dural violation, yet provides adequate elasticity for satisfactory decompression of the optic nerve. Using this technique, we have encountered no CSF leaks during endoscopic endonasal optic nerve decompression.

Repair of Medial Blowout Fracture

In cases of medial blowout fractures in which the lamina papyracea is virtually destroyed and the periorbita is violated, resulting in herniation of the orbital fat into the ethmoid sinus cavity, we prefer to reposition the herniating orbital contents and secure them in their original location with lyophilized dura (Fig. 9). Using an endoscopic approach or an external ethmoidectomy incision in special cases, exposure of the medial orbital wall is obtained. The bony fragments of the lamina papyracea are reduced if possible; however, if severely comminuted and unattached, they are removed. The orbital contents are reduced into the orbital cavity and a sheet of lyophilized dura is fashioned in the size and shape of the preexisting medial orbital wall. The lyophilized dura is placed in the position of the medial orbital wall and is secured with fibrin glue, resulting in a reduction of the displaced orbital contents and separation of the orbital and nasal cavities (Fig. 10).

We feel this technique offers several advantages over leaving the herniated contents in the sinus cavity. By reducing the contents and sealing them in place with a tissue sealant, we avoid the possibility of injury to these contents by another surgeon attempting sinus surgery in the future. This separation also protects the orbit from the contaminated sinonasal cavities, thus decreasing the potential risks of infection spreading from the sinonasal cavities into the orbit.

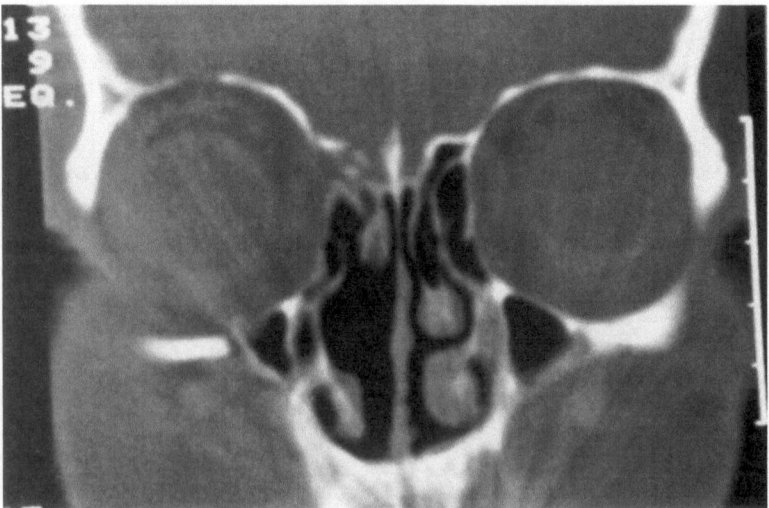

Fig. 10. Postoperative CT scan of the same patient as in Fig. 9 after repositioning of the orbital contents and reconstruction of the orbital wall with lyophilized dura and fibrin glue

Orbital Decompression

A wide range of indications for orbital decompression exists, including, but not limited to, Graves' orbitopathy, malignant exophthalmos (endocrine orbitopathy), and retrobulbar hematoma causing an increased intraocular pressure. We perform orbital decompressions by the endoscopic endonasal approach. After an ethmoidectomy is performed, the lamina papyracea is exposed. The lamina papyracea as well as portions of the orbital floor, which is the roof of the maxillary sinus, are removed to facilitate decompression. A sickle knife is used at this time to incise the exposed periorbita sinus cavities. Fibrin glue is now placed over the herniated orbital contents to form a seal and prevent the potential spread of infection from the contaminated sinonasal cavities into the orbit.

Nasal Septal Perforation Repair

Fibrin glue may play an important role in the repair of some NSP. When elevating mucoperichondrial and mucoperiosteal flaps for the repair of a large NSP, it is often difficult to maintain the proper position of the septal flaps with sutures due to the inaccessibility of the posterior aspect of the nasal cavity to conventional suturing techniques without using an open approach to the nasal cavity. Fibrin glue is extremely valuable in these situations to maintain the new position of these flaps and to provide support during the healing process. In cases of NSP repair which require a graft, whether fascia lata, turbinate mucosa, or other material, we routinely use fibrin glue to assist in holding the graft in the proper position during the postoperative healing process.

Discussion

Widespread uses for fibrin glue exist in the field of otorhinolaryngology, head and neck surgery, and other medical fields. With its ability to seal leaks and support tissues, fibrin glue is becoming more important in rhinologic procedures. In surgery where fixation of tissue flaps or grafts in areas with difficult access may be required, the use of fibrin glue is indispensable. Tissucol also plays an important role in sealing various surgical surfaces and assists in creating a watertight seal in endoscopic endonasal repair of CSF fistulas of the anterior skull base. In addition to traditional uses for fibrin glue, new applications are continually arising as advances in the field of rhinology are made.

Concern has been raised in the past regarding the transmission of viruses through the use of fibrin glue. In an attempt to eliminate the risk of viral transmission, the production process of Tissucol now includes steps to detect viral disease and an additional step of heat inactivation to destroy any viruses which were not detected in the screening process [7]. The final product is again screened prior to release [7]. Various studies have evaluated the potential risk of transmitting hepatitis B, hepatitis non-A/non-B, or the human immunodeficiency virus through the use of fibrin glue. These studies failed to show the transmission of any of these viruses by the use of fibrin glue [3, 6]. Our experience with the use of fibrin glue for over 10 years in hundreds of patients has failed to reveal the transmission of either the hepatitis virus or the human immunodeficiency virus.

The availability of both the slow- and fast-clotting varieties of Tissucol is important for the otorhinolaryngologist. Situations exist, especially in endoscopic procedures performed on the anterior skull base, where the use of the slow-clotting variety of Tissucol is required to allow ample time for manipulation of the graft materials into the proper position. In other circumstances in which rapid adhesion and support are needed and the operative conditions allow rapid coaptation of the graft materials, the rapid-acting variety can be beneficial. We feel that it is important that both varieties continue to be commercially available.

Conclusion

Technological and surgical advances have made it possible to address pathological processes of the anterior skull base by an endoscopic endonasal approach. Traditionally, these pathologic processes were approached through a craniotomy with its associated increased morbidity. In addition to anterior skull base surgery, many other rhinologic procedures benefit from the availability of fibrin glue. Fibrin glue is critical in creating watertight seals and successfully holds grafted materials in place. Long-term experience with the use of Tissucol has failed to show evidence of disease transmission. Our experience has shown Tissucol to be a safe and effective product for the sealing of tissues as well as providing a means for tissue coaptation.

References

1. Brennan M (1991) Fibrin glue. Blood Rev 5(4): 240–244
2. Cavallaro G et al. (1989) Usefulness of 2-component human fibrin glue in stabilizing vascular sutures at risk in hemodialysis. Minerva Chir. 44(21): 2241–2244
3. Draf W (1980) Experiences with fibrinogen glue in ENT surgery. Laryngol Rhinol Otol 59: 99–107
4. Eder G (1986) Preliminary results of a randomized controlled study on the risk of hepatitis transmission of a two-component fibrin sealant (Tissucol/Tisseel). In: Schlag G, Redl H (eds) Fibrin sealant in operative medicine, vol. I. Springer, Berlin Heidelberg New York, pp 51–59
5. Redl H, Schlag G (1986) Fibrin sealant and its modes of application. In: Schlag G, Redl H (eds) Fibrin sealant in operative medicine, vol. I. Springer, Berlin Heidelberg New York, pp 51–59
6. Rousou J et al. (1989) Randomized clinical trial of fibrin sealant in patients undergoing resternotomy or reoperation after cardiac operations. A multicenter study. J Thorac Cardiovasc Surg 92(2): 194–203
7. Schlag G, Turnher M, Redl H, Dinges HP (1986) The importance of fibrin in wound repair. In: Schlag G, Redl H (eds) Fibrin sealant in operative medicine. vol. I. Springer, Berlin Heidelberg New York
8. Sofferman R (1991) Transnasal approach to optic nerve decompression. Op Tech Otolaryngol Head Neck Surg 2(3): 150–156
9. Stammberger H (1991) Functional endoscopic sinus surgery. Decker. Philadelphia. pp 436–441

Spray Application of Fibrin Glue in Microsurgical Ethmoidectomy – Technique and Short-Term Results

B. BERTRAND, P. ELOY, J. JAMART, A. DOYEN, and P. ROMBAUX

Abstract

The aim of this work is to demonstrate the interest, efficiency, and safety of fibrin glue sealing immediately after ethmoidectomy. One hundred and one patients who underwent ethmoidectomy under endoscopic or microscopic control in combination with other surgical procedures when necessary (middle meatotomy, nasal septoplasty) were divided into two groups: in group 1 ($n = 80$) fibrin glue was sprayed locally by a spray catheter under 3 Pa pressure; in group 2 ($n = 91$), conventional gauze packing was used. Postoperative safety was estimated by recording the occurrence of nose bleeding according to a four-point scale. In group 1, the mean score for nose bleeding was 0.49, versus 0.63 in group 2 (not significant); in grouping absent and slight nose bleedings together and moderate and severe nose bleedings together, group 1 was significantly better than group 2 ($p = 0.007$). Postoperative patient comfort was also recorded on a four-point scale. The mean score for postoperative patient discomfort was 0.41 in group 1 and 0.77 in group 2 ($p = 0.014$). In grouping the two lowest levels of discomfort together and the two highest levels together, group 1 was again better than group 2 ($p = 0.004$).

Introduction

Hemostasis and postoperative fixation in nasal and sinus surgery are commonly performed by conventional gauze packing. Nasal packing is a very safe way to insure immediate postoperative safety for patients, but its disadvantages are well known: discomfort for several days and nights due to breathing through mouth, nasal smear retention, and in some rare cases local bacterial superinfections despite prophylactic antibiotic therapy. Furthermore, some patients are worried about nasal packing removal. Fibrin glue has been in use for many years in various fields of surgery [1] and especially in ENT surgery [2–4]. Fibrin tissue adhesive has also been successfully used to prevent or repair cerebrospinal fluid leakage in transsphenoidal microscopic surgery [5] and in endoscopic sinus surgery [6]. It has been described as an alternative to tamponage in maxillary sinus surgery [7, 8]. Techniques of vapor heating the blood products [9–13] give a very high security level against viral transmission. Up to now no viral transmission after fibrin glue application (Tissucol, Immuno, Vienna) has been reported.

The aim of this work is to demonstrate the interest, efficacy, and safety of fibrin glue sprayed in the postoperative cavities of microsurgical ethmoidectomies performed under microscopic or endoscopic control, as an alternative way for postoperative hemostasis and contention, compared to conventional nasal gauze packing.

Material and Methods

One hundred and seventy-six successive patients suffering from inflammatory chronic ethmoidal sinusitis and from nasal polyposis underwent ethmoid microscopic surgery associated with other procedures, mainly septoplasties and middle meatotomies. All the procedures were performed under general anesthesia with controlled hypotension.

Five patients (2.8%) presented with major bleedings at the end of the surgical procedure. In these five cases, sealing was impossible because of glue washout by the blood flow. These five patients were excluded from the study.

The 171 remaining patients were divided into two groups: 80 patients in the first group received fibrin glue spray and 91 patients in the second group were submitted to gauze packing. Seventy patients with full septoplasty were submitted to nasal packing for reasons of postoperative architectural stability and so were included in the second group. Two patients who had undergone very limited septoplasty were included in the first group. The other patients were randomized following a 3:1 ratio in order to obtain two numerically equal groups. Septoplasty is not involved in the surgical field of this work and does not introduce biases into the result analysis. In group 2, nasal packing was removed at day 4 after surgery.

Figure 1 shows the age and sex breakdown of patients, which is not different from other studies on chronic ethmoidal sinusitis. At the end of the operation, in group 2 sealing was carried out using a Duploject syringe and a spray catheter (Immuno, Vienna). The spray pressure was 3 Pa, sufficient to clear the surgical area of blood traces and low enough to avoid air insufflation into the blood vessels or into the anterior cerebral fossa and the orbita in case of unrecognized break of the ethmoidal roof or of the internal orbital wall. Each side needed 1 ml fibrin glue. Surgical areas were glue coated as thinly as possible.

The efficacy and safety of both groups were evaluated for the first 8 days according to a four-step scale. Postoperative nasal bleeding was classified as 0 (absent), 1 (slight), 2 (moderate), or 3 (severe). Steps for patient postoperative comfort estimation were: 0 (good or excellent), 1 (fairly good), 2 (quite bad), and 3 (bad or very bad).

The difficulty of surgery and its importance were evaluated according to the following parameters: age, perioperative bleeding, middle turbinate removal, nasal polyposis stage, surface of wounded mucosa, and combined nasal septoplasty.

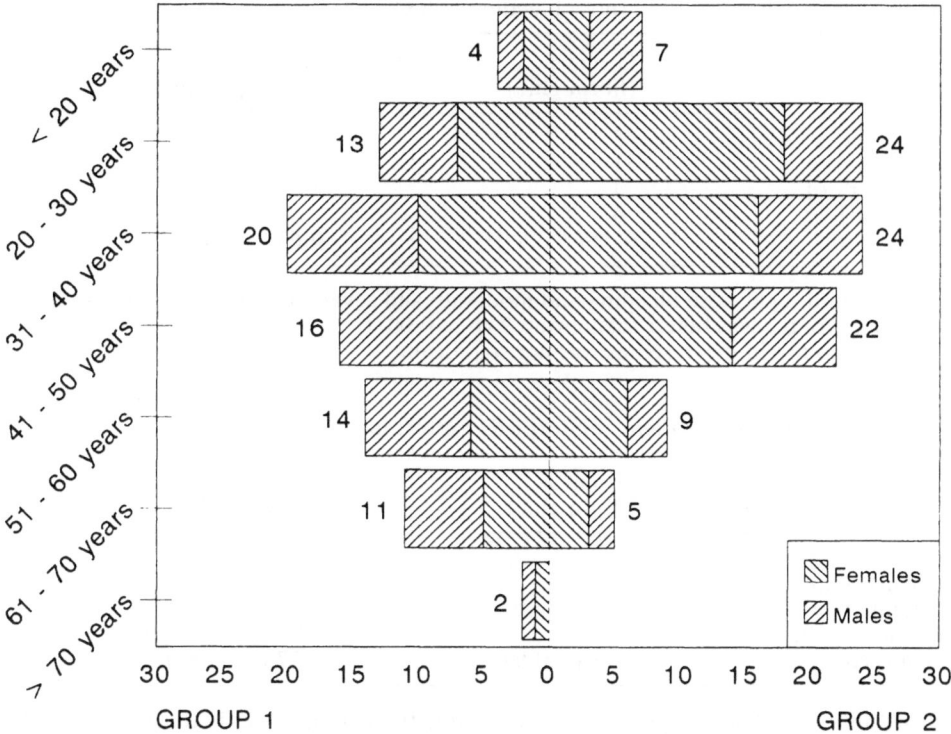

Fig. 1. Age breakdown of male and female population for each group

Scores were compared by the Wilcoxon signed rank test, qualitative variables were compared by chi squared test, and correlation between quantitative variables was made by the Spearman rank correlation test. All statistical tests were two tailed.

Results

No air insufflation in blood vessels or in the anterior cranial fossa and orbita occurred during the sealing process. Thus the sealing procedure can be considered as safe in this series. However, in our opinion this spray technique must be avoided when bone breaking of the ethmoidal roof or of the orbital wall is suspected during surgery.

No correlation was found between parameters of surgical difficulty and safety scores, with a Spearman coefficient lower than 0.116 for all the parameters including combined septoplasty.

No correlation was found for analyzing patient comfort scores and surgical parameters, the Spearman coefficient being lower than 0.062 for all the measured parameters. Chi-squared tests showed no significant difference between the two groups for surgical parameters. Groups 1 and 2 can thus be regarded as

Table 1. Postoperative safety (nose bleeding index)

Nose bleeding	Group 1 (fibrin glue)	Group 2 (gauze packing)
0 (Absent)	45	56
1 (Slight)	31	18
2 (Moderate)	4	12
3 (Severe)	0	5
Mean score[a]	0.49 ($\pm$ 0.59)	0.63 ($\pm$ 0.91)

If absent and slight nose bleeding and moderate and severe nose bleeding are grouped together, group 1 was better than group 2 ($p = 0.007$).
[a] The difference in mean scores was not significant.

Table 2. Postoperative patient comfort (discomfort index)

Patient comfort	Group 1 (fibrin glue)	Group 2 (gauze packing)
0 (Very good/good)	54	45
1 (Fairly good)	21	26
2 (Quite bad)	3	16
3 (Bad/very bad)	2	4
Mean score*	0.41 ($\pm$ 0.69)	0.77 ($+/-0.89$)

Grouping classes 0 and 1 and classes 2 and 3 together, group 1 was better than group 2 ($p = 0.004$).
* $p = 0.014$.

homogenous for statistical analysis. Results for safety are displayed in Table 1 and those for patient comfort in Table 2. In terms of safety, the difference between the two means scores in groups 1 and 2 was not significant, but when grouping together absent and slight bleeding on the one hand and moderate and severe nose bleeding on the other, the fibrin glue group was significantly better than group 2 ($p = 0.007$).

Regarding patient comfort, the fibrin glue group was significantly better than group 2 ($p = 0.014$). When analyzing classes 0 and 1 together, and classes 2 and 3 together, group 1 was better than group 2 ($p = 0.004$).

Conclusion

The following conclusions may be drawn:

1. Fibrin glue sealing in ethmoid microsurgery is at least as safe as conventional nasal gauze packing, despite the fact that nasal packing was removed at day 4 after surgery.
2. Patient comfort is significantly improved when fibrin glue is used, allowing patients to breathe normally through the nose 1 hour after surgery.

3. The sealing technique has proved to be safe in this series, but further safety rules should be followed: a pressure of 3 Pa should not be exceeded when spraying the glue and spraying should be avoided in cases of bone puncture in the ethmoidal roof or in the orbital bone area.
4. Five patients (2.8%) were not sealed because of severe bleedings during surgery.

References

1. Waclawiczek HW, Meiser G (1990) La colle de fibrine en chirurgie. Lyon Chir 86/5: 412–419
2. Lyons MB, Lyons GD, Webster D, Whecler V (1989) Adhesives in larynx repair. Laryngoscope 99: 377–381
3. Pech A, Cannoni M, Zanaret M, Thomassin SM (1988) Tissucol dans les septo-rhinoplasties. Ann Oto-Laryngol (Paris) 105: 629–634
4. Siedentop KH, Harris DM, Sanchez B (1985) Autologous fibrin tissue adhesive. Laryngoscope 95: 1074–1076
5. Van Velthoven V, Clarici G, Auer LM (1991) Fibrin tissue adhesive sealant for the prevention of CSF leakage following transsphenoidal surgery. Acta Neurochir 103/1–2: 26–29
6. Stankeiwicz JA (1991) Cerebrospinal fluid fistula and endoscopic sinus surgery. Laryngoscope 101/3: 250–256
7. Giesen K, Merten HA (1989) Application of fibrin adhesive systems in the maxillary sinus as an alternative to tamponage. Dtsch Zahnarztl 44/2: 113–115
8. Merten HA, Giesen K (1989) Use of fibrin adhesive in maxillary sinus surgery. Dtsch Z Mund Kiefer Gesicht Chir 13/3: 230–233
9. Mannucci P, Schimpf K, Abe T, Aledort L, Anderle K, Brettler D, Hilgartner M, Kernoff P, Kunschak M, McMillan C, Preston F, Rivard G, The International Investigator Group (1992) Low risk of viral infection after administration of vapor-heated factor VIII concentrate. Transfusion 32: 134–138
10. Preiss D, Eberspächer B, Abdullah D, Rosner I (1991) Safety of vapor heated prothrombin complex concentrate (PCC) Prothromplex S-TIM4. Thromb Res 63: 651–659
11. Rousou J, Levitsky S, Gonzalez-Lavin L, Cosgrove D, Weldon C, Hess P, Joyce L, Bergsland J, Gazzaniga A (1989) Randomized clinical trial of fibrin sealant in patients undergoing resternotomy or reoperation after cardiac operations. J Thorac Cardiovasc Surg 97: 194–203
12. Schimpf K (1988) Substitutiontherapie Hämophiler mit virusinaktivierten Gerinnungsfaktorenkonzentraten. In: Landbeck G, Marx R (eds) 18. Hämophilie-Symposion, Hamburg 1987. Springer, Berlin Heidelberg New York, pp 221–224
13. Turecek PL, Schwarz HP, Barett N, Polsler G, Dorner F, Eibl J, Feiba VH (1993) Immuno: Partitionning and inactivation of HIV-1. Poster presented at the international symposium on inhibitors to coagulation factors, Chapel Hill, North Carolina, USA, 3–5 November 1993

Use of Fibrin Glue in Craniofacial and Skull Base Trauma

F. X. BRUNNER and U. SCHWAB

Abstract

Traffic accidents frequently cause trauma to the midface and frontal skull base. In many cases, there are posttraumatic functional deficits, deformities, and stressful psychosocial problems accompanying facial distortions. The availability of microsurgical reconstruction techniques using tissue adhesive, preserved dura, resorbable materials, and thin rigid titanium plates for osteosynthesis place more demands on the quality of surgery in maxillofacial and skull base trauma. By means of miniplate and microplate osteosynthesis, secure stabilization of the midface can be achieved following even extensive fractures of the midface or the floor of the anterior cranial fossa. This procedure is considered a satisfactory operative treatment in terms of cosmetic and functional results. As a rule, sealing of the frontal skull base should be performed before repairing the fractures of the midface. The postoperative results depend on the extent of the primary bone or soft tissue lesions. To achieve satisfactory results in operative treatment, a team approach is necessary.

Introduction

Fifty percent of all visceral cranium fractures are associated with skull base fractures. The defects of the skull base require a tight and safe dural closure to prevent secondary meningitis. Regarding the fractures of the visceral cranium, all functional and aesthetic aspects have to be considered right away, starting with primary treatment.

Indications for Surgery and Technique

Extensive crush fractures of the midfacial and frontal skull normally require interdisciplinary cooperation between the departments of ENT, oral surgery, and neurosurgery. Isolated and central depressed fractures of the foreheadnose pillar and the anterior wall of the frontal sinus are usually taken care of by rhinosurgeons themselves [3–6].

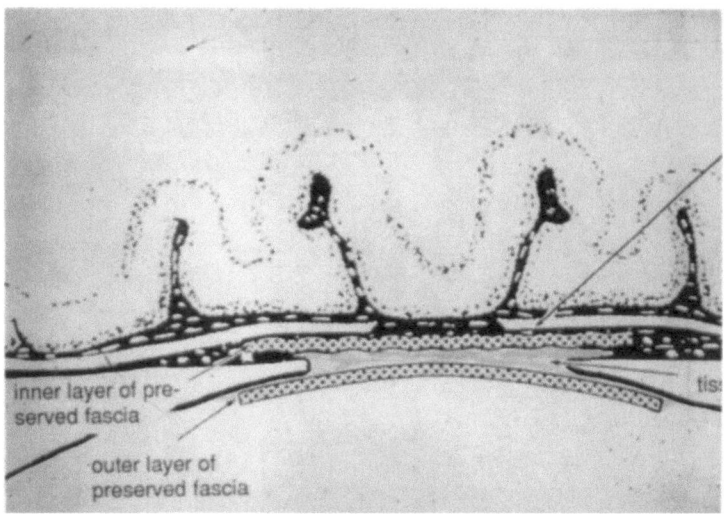

Fig. 1. Rhinosurgical technique for closure of localized dural tears of the posterior wall of the frontal sinus and the roof of the ethmoid cells

The coronal incision is the most favored surgical approach to the anterior skull base. This approach has the advantage of an exact subperiostal survey of all upper and lower midfacial fractures without having to remove any bone fragments or adding more cuts within the facial region.

In the case of soft tissue injuries within the forehead, glabella, or supraorbital rims, an approach via a Killian incision or bilateral Killian incisions may be easier to carry out and if followed by careful wound dressing is no disadvantage, especially in order to gain full access to the areas of the posterior ethmoid and sphenoid sinus.

Among the 58 patients suffering from an anterior skull base fracture who were treated in the Würzburg ENT clinic between 1986 and 1988, the most common defect was located in the area of the ethmoid roof and on the junction between the posterior wall of the frontal sinus and the ethmoid roof. A total of 31 cases showed defects in the form of bony gaps only, and 27 had a bony defect of more than 0.5 cm^2 in size. The size of the defect of the skull base, described by the radiologist using a coronal CT, was compared to the lesion found intraoperatively. A dura lesion existed in 92.4% of the cases in which the CT had already shown a gap of more than 2–4 mm and in all of the cases with a gap of more than 4 mm.

Rhinosurgical Closure of Dural Lesions

The surgical way of treating dural lesions is from the inside out. The first step consists of closing the defect within the anterior skull base. Doing this the rhinosurgical way, fascia lata, fascia of the m. temporalis, or preserved dura is

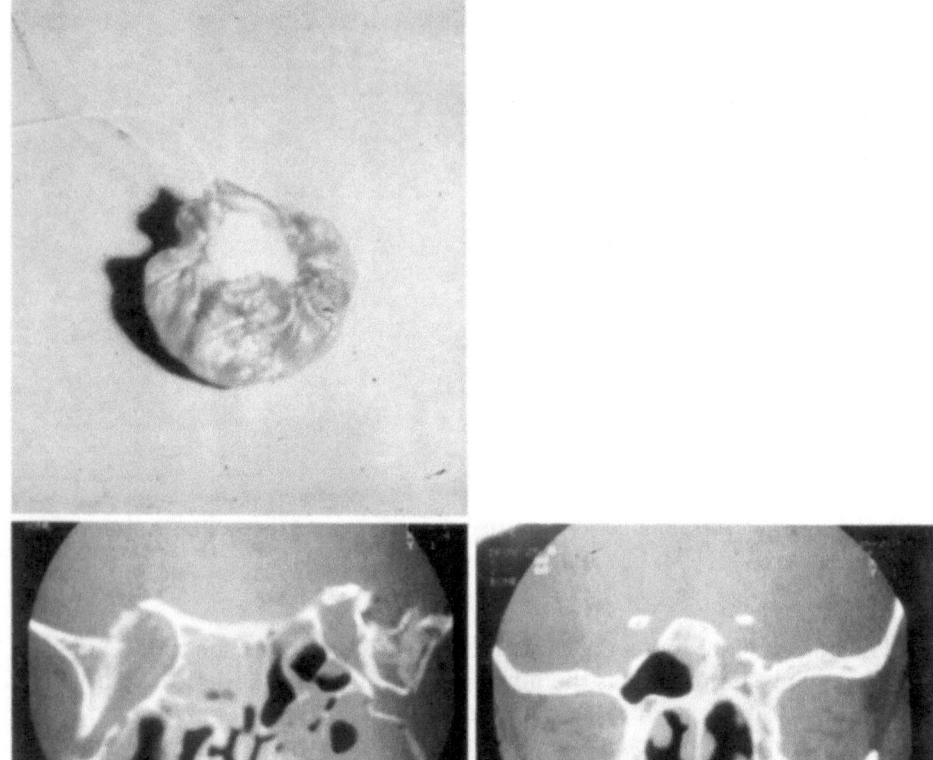

Fig. 2a–c. Rhinosurgical technique for closure of dural lesions in the area of the sphenoid sinus (according to Kley). **a** Tobacco pouch. **b** CT scan of a clinical case preoperatively. **c** CT scan of same case 9 months postoperatively

used to cover the defect or, even more efficient, a double layer of two fascia transplants is used and attached with fibrin glue (Fig. 1). The tight sealing of cerebrospinal fluid leaks within the area of the roof or posterior wall of the sphenoid sinus often causes a major problem. Kley [6] suggested a sealing technique using a "tobacco pouch" consisting of fascia lata filled with gelatine sponges. It can also be recommended that the tobacco pouch packing be covered with fibrin glue and stuck in place (Fig. 2). Provided that the leakage within the roof or posterior wall of the sphenoid sinus can be totally surveyed under the microscope, a cover of fascia lata coated with fibrin glue will do. Extensive fractures and depressions within the area of the os frontale are often associated with vast crush fractures of the posterior wall of the frontal sinus. In these cases, dural lesions and subdural hematomas are common, thus making a primary or secondary interdisciplinary treatment involving neurosurgeons necessary.

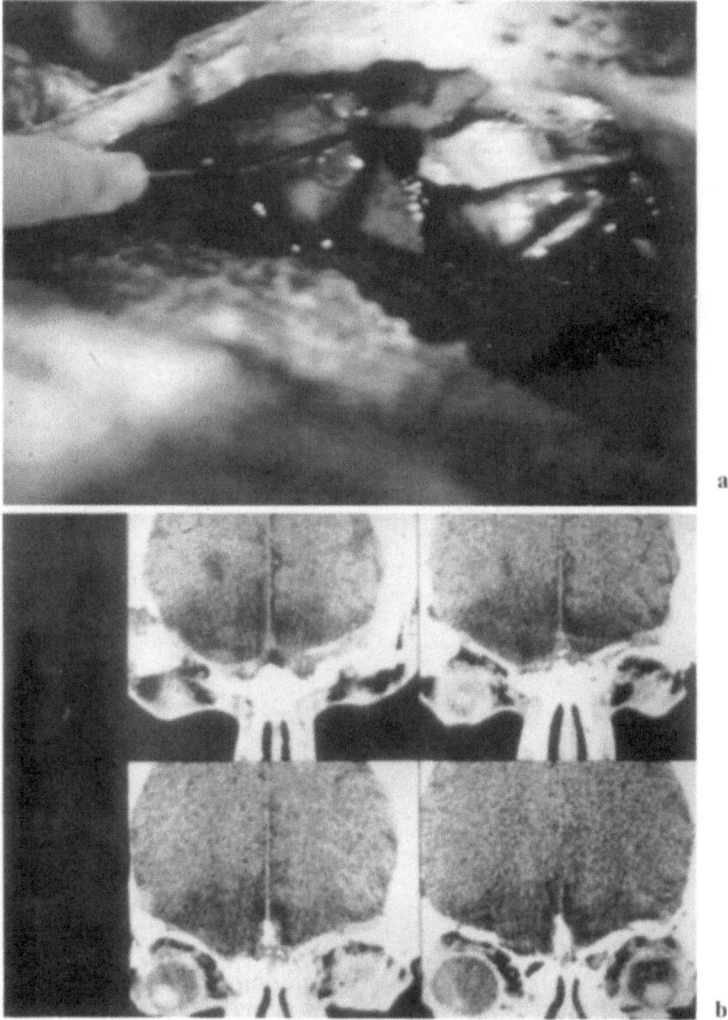

Fig. 3. a Reconstruction of the floor of the anterior skull base after complete cranialization of the frontal sinus; application of bone chips, bone meal, and fibrin glue. **b** CT scan
6 months postoperatively showing complete bony restoration

The surgical approach chosen in these cases is via a frontal or frontotempo-
ral bone lid performing a craniotomy. There is also the possibility of an intradural or an extradural approach. In cases of an excessively large crush defect of
the posterior wall of the frontal sinus, reconstruction is no longer possible and
a "cranialization" of the frontal sinus is therefore necessary. Tears of the dura
are fixed using sutures or fibrin glue. Bone edges on the transition of the former frontal sinus towards the tabula interna of the os frontale have to be
smoothed down in order to avoid overhangings and to give the brain and the
dura the chance to use up the entire newly gained space. The mucosa of the

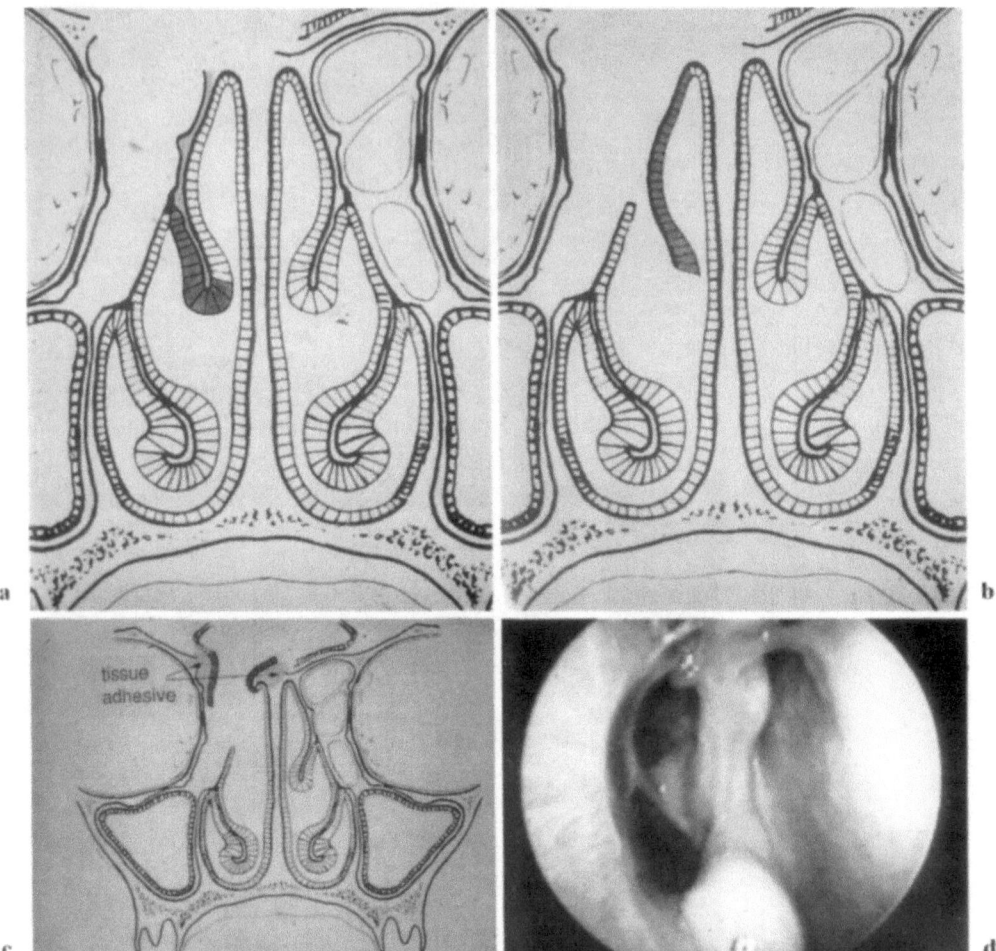

Fig. 4a–d. Rotating flap using the anterior parts of the middle nasal turbinate for creation of a wide and epithelialized new frontonasal canal. **a–c** The bony lamina *(yellow)* has to be removed; flap *(green)* and free, transplanted mucosa *(red)* of the lateral turbinate parts are attached with tissue adhesive. **d** The endoscopic control 6 weeks postoperatively shows wide openings to the frontal sinus and the ethmoid cavity

frontal sinus must be entirely removed. For sealing towards the nose and the ethmoid roof a pediculated flap consisting of periost and muscle–periost, fibrin glue, bone meal, and bone chips of the former frontal sinus with all mucosa removed are used.

In the last 5 years this technique, combining rhino- and neurosurgical treatment, has been used very successfully in the head clinic in Würzburg (Fig. 3).

Drainage of the Frontal Sinus and Ethmoid Cell System

In most of the cases of midfacial and anterior skull base fractures, the frontal sinus and ethmoid cell system remain pneumatised. In order to avoid mucoceles later on and therefore inflammation as well, a broad, fully epithelialized access to the frontal sinus, the ethmoid cells, and the nose has to be created.

For a crush fracture of the upper bony septum, associated with corresponding lesions of the mucosa, the construction of a median drainage according to Mayer is suggested. In cases of no major fractures in the upper parts of the septum, this method should not be applied, in order not to cause more instability in the area of the forehead–nose pillar, which is to be reconstructed. Since there is already a bony crush within the area of the nose and glabella, any further bony instabilization should be avoided. In such cases, the present author found a modification of the Uffenorde flap [2, 8], already altered by Berendes and Minnigerode [1, 7] to be most convenient. A rotating flap is created, using the mucosa of the anterior parts of the middle concha, and tipped sideways and up, epithelializing the access to the frontal sinus and ethmoid cells, before carrying out the osteosynthesis of the forehead–nose pillar (Fig. 4).

If there are thick external bone walls narrowing the drainage canals of the frontal sinuses, bone must be reduced in the area of the nasofrontal junction. Nevertheless, it is important to avoid extensive thinning in order to still be able to obtain a stable bony consolidation.

Fibrin glue is used for the attachment of the mucosa–periost flap of the frontal parts of the middle turbinate.

Conclusion

The use of a microscope for surgery, the availability of high-resolution techniques in radiology, modern methods of osteosynthesis, and fibrin glue have considerably improved the precision of many rhinosurgical operations. In the area of the skull base, the fibrin glue makes a reliable fixation of free and pediculated transplants of fascia and muscle–periost flaps possible. This provides a tight sealing of the dura in traumatology as well as in tumor surgery. In special cases bone meal, fibrin glue, and free bone transplants are used in the bony reconstruction of the skull base and parts of the cup. Long-term drainage and ventilation of the frontal sinus after loss of the natural efferent duct often poses a problem, and post-traumatic scarred and bony obliterations in particular predispose for inflammatory complications.

Epithialization of newly obtained efferent ducts of the frontal sinuses, using mucosa flaps from surrounding areas, and their reliable attachment with fibrin glue have proved to be very efficient.

References

1. Berendes J (1956) Doppelter autoplastischer Verschluß größerer Duradefekte in Nähe der Mittellinie bei Liquorrhoea nasalis. HNO 6: 220
2. Boenninghaus HG (1967) Rhinologische Eingriffe bei der Versorgung frontobasaler Frakturen. Z Laryngol Rhinol 46: 110
3. Brunner FX, Kleine BI (1987) Frakturen des zentralen Mittelgesichts und der Rhinobasis – operative Versorgung – postoperative Nachsorge – Komplikationsmöglichkeiten. HNO 35: 106
4. Brunner FX, Kley W, Plinkert P (1988) Anatomical studies and a correlative management of facial skeleton and skull base injuries with bone plate fixation. Arch Otolaryngol 113: 61
5. Brunner FX (1989) Trauma des zentralen und lateralen Mittelgesichts und der Rhinobasis. Med Welt 30: 133
6. Kley W (1968) Die Unfallchirurgie der Schädelbasis und der pneumatischen Räume. Arch HNO Heilkd 191: 1
7. Minnegerode B (1967) Zur Technik der extraduralen rhinochirurgischen Deckung von Liquorfisteln nach frontobasalen Schädelverletzungen. Monatsschr Ohrenheilkd 101: 441
8. Uffenorde W (1952) Anzeige und Ausführung der Eingriffe an Ohr, Nase, Hals. Thieme, Stuttgart

Use of Fibrin Glue in Rhinoplasty

F. DISANT, A. MORGON, and J. LEBLOND

Abstract

The term "reshaping rhinoplasty" is a good designation for the new techniques of rhinoplasty using cartilage grafts and fibrin glue.

The open technique allows a complete reshaping of the cartilage structures, but it needs extensive dissection of the skin cover. We use fibrin glue to obtain good repositioning of the skin. Fibrin glue provides more effective support of the mobile part of the nose than an external system. It makes it possible to obtain a good fixation of the skin in its new position in cases in which the dorsum has to be lifted after an extensive reduction of the vault.

Introduction

The concept of reshaping rhinoplasty has replaced those of reduction rhinoplasty and augmentation rhinoplasty. The aim is to obtain at the end a natural nose shape with the aesthetic subunits such as the dorsum, the tip, and the infratip lobule clearly recognizable.

Regardless of whether we use a dissimulated approach or an open approach, the main challenge is to obtain a good fixation of the skin to the remodelled cartilagenous structure. Skin trophicity is an important factor, especially its thickness and elasticity. The precise adaptation of the skin to the new cartilagenous shape is important, too. The absence of any cavity with blood or fluid between skin and cartilage cannot be obtained with a suction system such as, for instance, the one used in ear reconstruction with a rib cartilage graft.

The classical external holding systems of the dorsum skin are not effective for the tip. Indeed, the difference in rigidity between the skin and the cartilage of the tip is much less than between the thin skin of the dorsum and the hard osseous layer. For the dorsum, any external pressure system is effective. If it can be used, the technique of atraumatic rhinoplasty with minimal dissection of the skin is the best method. The conditions are totally different when an open approach is chosen with a whole dissection of the lobule skin.

We describe four situations in which fibrin glue can be used:

1. Remodeling graft in a minimal rhinoplasty
2. Filling graft for correction of saddle noses
3. Reshaping rhinoplasty of the tip with an open approach
4. Rhinolifting without skin reduction

Remodeling Graft of the Dorsum

The remodeling graft of the dorsum is used in minimal rhinoplasty to give the dorsum a natural form after suppressing the hump and making the "in fractures" (i.e., fractures of the bony vault from the exterior of the nose to the interior) improves the natural rectangular aspect of the dorsum. The best material to use is alar cartilage, obtained after the reduction of lateral crus by a transcartilaginous incision.

The fat is taken from the cartilages, which are then glued together; the graft is pressed and mixed with fibrin glue to obtain a soft slice thicker than a fascia temporalis layer and resistant to stretching. This material is placed under the skin from the radix to the supratip area. The skin is fixed to the graft with glue and the result can be evaluated immediately. If the graft seems too thin, we can get a multilayered graft using septal cartilage. This type of graft is soft and can be modeled through the skin if its shape is not satisfactory. This type of graft is very effective to mask the small irregularity of the long vault after the reduction of the hump.

Filling Graft with Binding Material

A filling graft with binding material composed of cartilage and fibrin glue is used for moderate saddle noses, for which a bony graft is not necessary. All the chips of septal cartilage are mixed together with fibrin glue and pressed so that they are homogeneous and soft.

Modeling of this binding material is easy. The shape can be adapted to the deformation. The graft is positioned under view control and then remodeled, if necessary, through the skin for a few minutes, until the best possible shape is obtained. Fibrin glue fixes the graft to the skin and the remaining structures, so the result can be seen immediately. An overcorrection is recommended, because this type of binding material will partially resorb during the first postoperative months.

The coarseness of grain of the graft surface must be adapted to the trophicity of the skin in order to avoid cartilage chips protruding under the skin in the months following the operation. We have been using this technique for 4 years now and it has proved satisfactory.

Reshaping Rhinoplasty by Open Approach

The reshaping of the tip with cartilagenous graft fixed on the tip or under the tip does not improve the shape of the nose if the grafts become immerged in an enlarged area of scar tissue. The consequence is a structureless tip of the nose. Among the factors leading to the subcutaneous scar tissue, postoperative bleeding is certainly the worst, especially after the fat has been taken from the cartilages.

In such situations, the use of fibrin glue is certainly a step forward in terms of technique. A better shape can be expected, because several important factors contributing to success have been improved:

- Hemostasis
- Skin–cartilage linkage
- Fixation of the graft
- Immediate analysis of the shape

Rhinolifting Without Skin Reduction

Rhinolifting requires good sliding of the dorsum skin upward. The external binding techniques are effective in elevating the tip, but they are not sufficient for sliding the skin with a shortening of the nose, even if the bony and cartilagenous structures have been reduced correctly. Fibrin glue enables us to fix the lifted skin in its new position, and the tip is thus stretched up and the labial angle of the nose increases. The angle and the shortening of the nose can be evaluated immediately. This technique is sometimes too effective and with elderly patients, there is a risk of creating unaesthetic wrinkles near the radix or shortening the nose too much.

Conclusion

Whatever type rhinoplasty is used – normal rhinoplasty, reshaping rhinoplasty, or open approach – the use of fibrin glue improves the fixation of the skin to the new cartilagenous structure, reduces the risk of an interstice and thus the risk of hematoma, ensures a better tip shape, and allows to quickly see whether the new design of the nose is correct. The application of this biomaterial gave new impetus to our practice of rhinoplasty.

Suggested Reading

1. Vincentiis M, Ruoppolo G, Gallo A (1986) The use of fibrin sealant in ear, nose and throat surgery. In: Schlag G, Redl H (eds) Fibrin sealant in operative medicine, vol 1. Springer, Berlin Heidelberg New York, pp 86–90
2. Pech A, Cannoni M et al. (1988) Le Tissucol dans les septorhinoplasties. Ann ORL (Paris) 105 (8): 629–634
3. Wullstein SR (1979) Die Septumplastik bzw. submuköse Septumresektion ohne postoperative Nasentamponade. HNO 27: 322–324

Use of Fibrin Glue in Intracranial Procedures Following Acoustic Neuroma Surgery: Application in Facial Nerve Reconstruction and Prevention of Cerebrospinal Fluid Rhinorrhea

J. KANZAKI, R. SHIOBARA, and T. O-UCHI

Abstract

Favorable results were obtained by using fibrin glue in the reconstruction of the facial nerve sacrificed during acoustic neuroma surgery. Good results were also obtained in intracranial anastomosis by transposing the superficial petrosal nerve (SPN) and partly splitting it to lengthen it, so that the nerve could be repaired by end-to-end anastomosis rather than grafting. The use of fibrin glue also enabled a reduction in the number of stitches necessary in hypoglossal-facial nerve anastomosis to two thirds the usual number.

Among the methods of obliteration of the surgical defect after tumor removal in AN surgery, the incidence of CSF leak was lowest, i.e., less than one third that with previous methods using only muscle, when both abdominal fat and pedicled temporalis muscle were used in combination with fibrin glue and lumbar drainage was carried out at the same time.

Introduction

The present report discusses the application of fibrin glue (Tisseel; Immuno, Vienna) in the reconstruction of the facial nerve sacrificed during acoustic neuroma (AN) surgery and in the prevention of postoperative cerebrospinal fluid (CSF) rhinorrhea.

Materials and Methods

Intracranial Facial Nerve Anastomosis

At the present time, we at Keio University School of Medicine are using the extended middle cranial fossa (EMCF) approach for AN surgery [6]. Regardless of the approach chosen, however, it is often difficult in AN surgery to reconstruct the sacrificed facial nerve by intracranial suturing, including grafting. While there are some reports in the literature on the direct anastomosis of the facial nerve [3, 5], other surgeons have been using a modified version [2] of Dott's [1] intracranial–extratemporal anastomosis technique because of its technical simplicity.

In recent years, consequent to the wide propagation of its use and based on advances in basic [9, 10] and clinical [4, 11] research, fibrin glue has come to be applied in nerve repair. Fisch, for example, has reported on his sutureless technique, which involves the use of fibrin glue with collagen splints [4]. We, too, have been using fibrin glue in nerve repair. In these cases, we have mostly combined a rerouting technique with transposition of the superficial petrosal nerve (SPN) in order to repair the nerve by end-to-end anastomosis whenever possible and avoid grafting [8]. Our results are presented below.

Prevention of Cerebrospinal Fluid Rhinorrhea

In EMCF approach type III, in which hearing preservation is attempted, it is necessary only to obliterate the internal auditory canal. In EMCF approach types I and II, however, in which hearing preservation is not carried out, there is also the need to obliterate the defect resulting from labyrinthectomy. We carried out various methods of obliteration in 274 cases of AN surgery. The results are compared in Table 1.

Techniques

Facial Nerve Anastomosis

In 53 cases the facial nerve was severely damaged or sacrificed during surgery and intracranial facial nerve anastomosis was carried out in 15 cases either by direct end-to-end anastomosis or using rerouting (Table 2). In the rerouting technique, the SPN and the facial nerve (from its labyrinthine portion to its horizontal portion) were decompressed, and the facial nerve was translocated from the facial canal.

Among the 14 cases of AN in which intracranial facial nerve anastomosis was carried out, the facial nerve was repaired by suturing in eight cases and with fibrin glue in six cases. Repair was carried out by suturing in the one

Table 1. Incidence of cerebrospinal fluid (CSF) leakage in different methods of obliteration

Group	Total (*n*)	Incidence of CSF leak	
		(*n*)	(%)
FM + PTM + Biobond	134	21	15.7
FM + PTM + FG	93	15	16.1
FM + PTM + FG + LD	11	2	18.2
Abdominal fat + PTM + FD + LD	24	1	4.2
Others	12	1	8.3
Total	274	40	14.6

FM, free muscle; PTM, pedicled temporalis muscle; FG, fibrin glue; LD, lumbar drainage.

Table 2. Facial nerve reconstruction

	Intracranial	Intratemporal
A. End-to-End		
a Direct	5	0
b_0 Rerouting	7	0
b_1 Rerouting +	1	0
Transposition (GPN) +		
Splitting		
b_2 Rerouting +	1	1
Transposition (GPN)		
B. Graft		
GPN	1	
GAN	0	1
Total	15	2

GPN, greater petrosal nerve; GAN, greater auricular nerve. a, b_0, b_1 and b_2 see Fig. 1

case of meningioma and with fibrin glue in the two cases of intratemporal lesions (one case of petrous cholesteatoma and one case of facial neuroma). In the latter case, the greater auricular nerve was grafted and attached with fibrin glue. In three of the six cases in which fibrin glue was used, the SPN was transposed and anastomosed to the distal end of the facial nerve (Fig. 1).

Hypoglossal–facial nerve anastomosis was carried out in 36 cases. In 19 of these cases, reinforcement with fibrin glue made it possible to carry out anastomosis with two less than normal.

Obliteration

Pedicled temporal muscle was used to obliterate the surgical defect in all our cases. Biobond was used as adhesive in 134 cases, while fibrin glue was used in 128 cases. To obliterate the middle ear cavity after removal of the incus, pieces of free temporal muscle were placed in the defect and stabilized with fibrin glue in some cases, while pieces of abdominal fat were used in place of the free muscle tissue and stabilized with fibrin glue in the more recent cases. In our most recent cases, we filled the defect with abdominal fat, covered the surface of the middle cranial fossa with pedicled temporal muscle, and simultaneously carried out lumbar drainage. The patients were classified into five groups according to the obliteration method, and the incidences of CSF leak were examined.

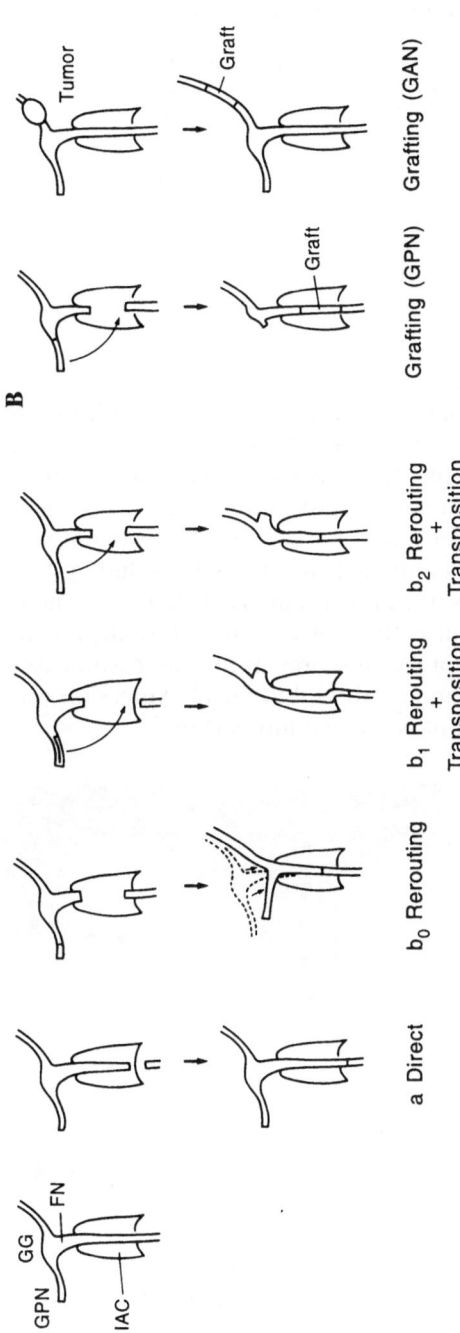

Fig. 1A, B. Various techniques used in intracranial and intratemporal facial nerve anastomosis. **A** End-to-end anastomosis. **B** Graft. *GPN*, greater petrosal nerve; *GG*, geniculate ganglion; *IAC*, internal auditory canal; *FN*, facial nerve

Table 3. Results of facial nerve anastomosis using two different techniques

Technique	Success	Failure	No evaluation	Total
Suture	6	3	0	9
Fibrin glue	5	1	2	8
Total	11	4	2	17

Results

Facial Nerve Anastomosis

The results of facial nerve anastomosis either by suturing combined with fibrin or by a sutureless technique in 15 cases of intracranial anastomosis and two cases of intratemporal anastomosis are shown in Table 3. The two unsuccessful cases with the suture technique were one case of facial nerve anastomosis on the brain stem side and another involving a badly damaged facial nerve. Facial movement was judged to have improved in all cases of repair with fibrin glue, excluding two cases in which postoperative follow-up was too short for analysis. One case, however, was classified as unsuccessful because there was only a low degree of improvement. The postoperative facial expression scores in the successful cases were grades III–IV by the House-Brackmann method, but facial expression was more natural than with hypoglossal–facial nerve anastomosis (Fig. 2).

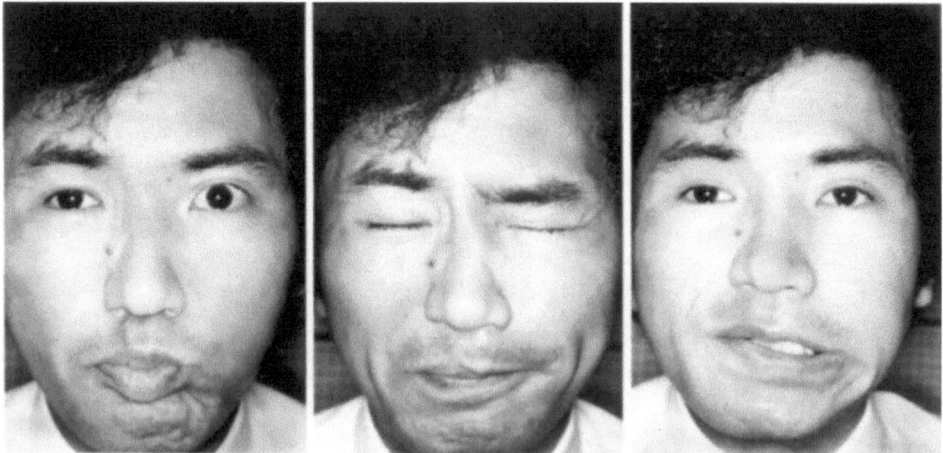

Fig. 2. Facial movement 6 years after right intracranial facial nerve anastomosis. Rerouting and transposition of split greater petrosal nerve GPN as in Fig. 1b₁

Cerebrospinal Leakage

The incidence of CSF leakage was lowest in the group in which abdominal fat and pedicled temporal muscle was used in combination to obliterate the defect, fibrin glue was used for stabilization, and lumbar drainage was carried out at the same time (Table 1).

Discussion

The direct suturing of the intracranial facial nerve is often technically difficult and time-consuming. In contrast, anastomosis using fibrin glue is simple and quick. We have been able to achieve favorable results by using fibrin glue on the ends of the resected nerve and stabilizing with the dura of the internal auditory canal (IAC) or fascia or free muscle tissue.

For the prevention of CSF leakage in AN surgery, we have found that the method we have recently been using, involving the use of abdominal fat, is most effective. With this method, the incidence of CSF leakage, which had been approximately 15 % by previous methods of obliteration [7], decreased to 4.2 %. When CSF leakage did occur, the leak was managed with only conservative treatment in two thirds of the cases; less than 5 % of the total number of cases required surgical treatment for CSF leakage. In three of five cases of slight CSF leakage, the leak was able to be stopped by the transtympanic injection of fibrin glue. Therefore, we feel it may be worthwhile to attempt this technique before carrying out surgical treatment in cases of slight CSF leakage.

References

1. Dott NM (1958) Facial paralysis – restitution by extra-petrous nerve graft. Proc R Soc Med 51: 900–902
2. Draf W, Samii M (1982) Intracranial-intratemporal anastomosis of the facial nerve after cerebellopontine angle tumor surgery. In: Graham MD, House WF (eds) Disorders of the facial nerve. Raven, New York, pp 441–449
3. Drake CG (1963) Intracranial facial nerve reconstruction. Arch Otolaryngol 78: 456–460
4. Fisch U, Dobie RA, Gmur A et al. (1987) Intracranial facial nerve anastomosis. Am J Otol 8: 23–29
5. Jaaskelainen J, Dykko I, Blomstedt G et al. (1990) Functional results of facial nerve suture after removal of acoustic neuroma: analysis of 25 cases. Neurosurgery 27: 408–411
6. Kanzaki J, Shiobara R, Toya S (1991a) Classification of the extended middle cranial fossa approach. Acta Otolaryngol (Stockh) [Suppl] 467: 6–16
7. Kanzaki J, Ogawa K, Tsuchihashi N et al. (1991b) Postoperative complications in acoustic neuroma surgery by the extended middle cranial fossa approach. Acta Otolaryngol (Stockh) [Suppl] 467: 75–79
8. Kanzaki J, Kunihiro T, O-Uchi T et al. (1991c) Intracranial reconstruction of the facial nerve. Acta Otolaryngol (Stockh) [Suppl] 467: 85–90
9. Medders G, Mattox DE, Lyles A (1989) Effects of fibrin glue on rat facial nerve generation. Otolaryngology Head Neck Surg 100: 106–109

10. Nishihara S, McCaffrey TV (1989) Repair of motor nerve defects: comparison of suture and fibrin adhesive techniques. Otolaryngol Head Neck Surg 100: 17–21
11. Wigand ME, Thumfart W (1982) Fibrin seal for supralabyrinthine facial nerve repair. In: Graham MD, House WF (eds) Disorders of the facial nerve. Raven, New York, pp 477–483

Partial and Total Reconstruction of the Auricle

H. WEERDA and R. SIEGERT

Abstract

In the last 15 years we have operated on 500 patients with auricular defects or malformations. We report about reconstruction of small defects after trauma or tumor excision of the helix, antihelix, lobule, and concha in a one-stage procedure as well as the procedures for reconstruction of partial defects and the total loss of the auricle. Our special techniques involving replantation of freshly avulsed parts of the auricle are demonstrated using fibrin glue for the reconstruction. Different methods of construction are demonstrated for first-, second-, and third-degree microtia. The risk of losing free grafts has declined considerably since fibrin glue came into use. Some examples show the outcome several months after completion of surgery.

Material and Methods

Cancer of the external ear accounts for 10% of all malignant skin tumors. There is no difference in the reconstruction of defects after tumor surgery or after trauma. Small tumor defects of the rim can be closed by our modification of the Gersuny technique by a single operation. This procedure combines a reductive technique with a sliding helix and a crescent excision; the closure produces minimal auricular deformity (Fig. 1). Small parts of the helical border are reconstructed by local flaps from the pre- and retroauricular region. A defect in the antihelical region is covered with a retroauricular flap and the helix has to be transposed for a short time. The flaps are sutured and additionally glued into position. In surgery involving reconstruction of parts of the concha, we like to use a full-thickness skin graft, taken from one of the auriculocephalic sulci, which is glued to the rough surface. Alternatively, a pedicled flap or a retroauricular myocutaneous island flap may be used. For the reconstruction of large subtotal defects we use large, bilobed rotation–transposition flaps. To prevent shrinkage, a defect-filling support of rib cartilage has to be inserted.

Reconstruction of parts of an auricle or a whole auricle necessitates reconstruction with rib cartilage and skin from the surrounding area. The upper part of the auricle is reconstructed with rib cartilage and skin of the surrounding area in two or three stages (Fig. 2A, B). A pattern of the patient's healthy ear

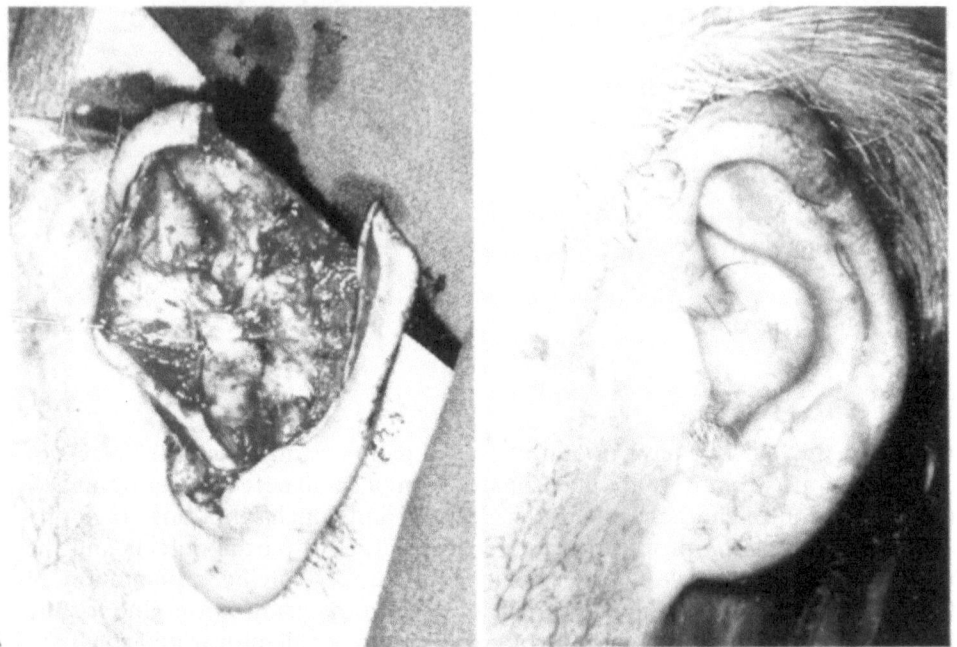

A   B

Fig. 1. A Resection of a tumor of the auricular rim. **B** Reconstruction with a sliding helix (Gersuny technique)

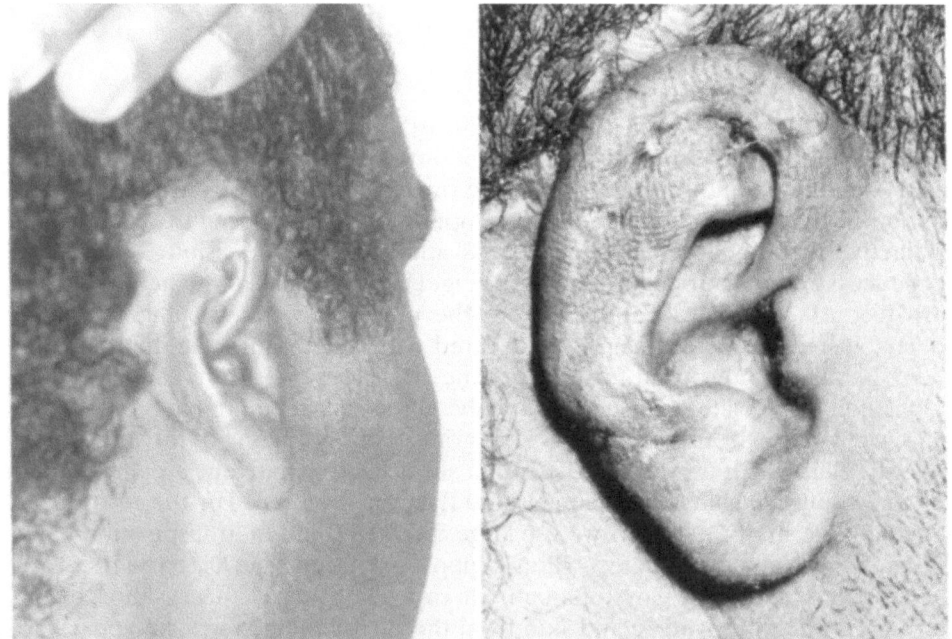

A   B

Fig. 2. A Avulsion of the middle and upper part of the pinna. **B** Reconstruction with an autogenous rib cartilage support and skin from the surrounding area

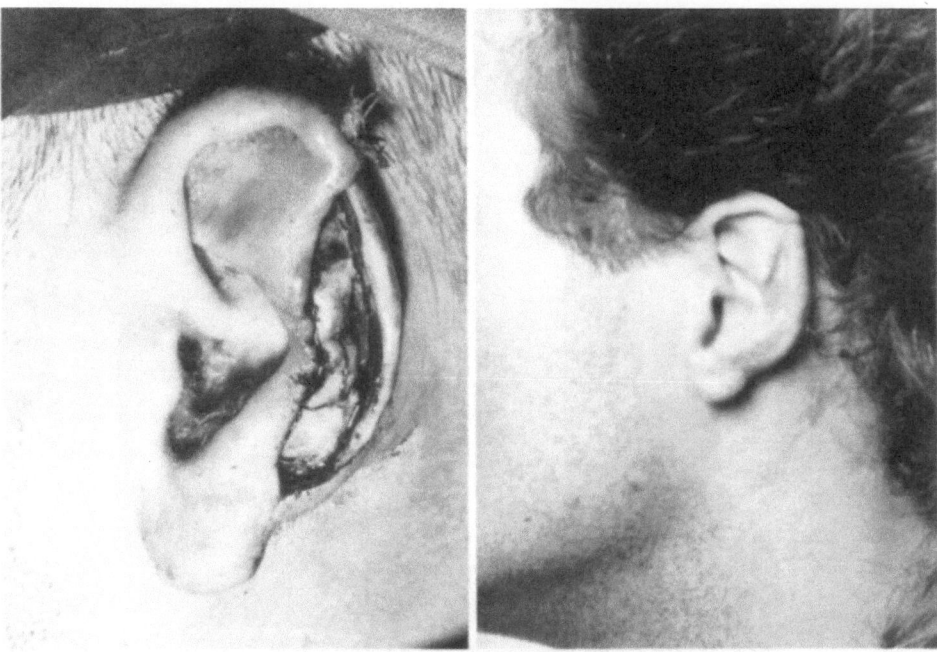

A   B

Fig. 3. A The rib cartilage support is sutured to the auricular stump after loss of the middle part of the auricle. **B** Result some weeks after reconstruction of the auricle

is used in excising a supporting structure of rib cartilage [1]. One of the patients we treated had been bitten by a dog, and necrosis of the median part of the auricle occurred after reimplantation. In the first stage of surgery, the necrosis was removed and a support of rib cartilage was stitched to the auricular cartilage with resorbable sutures (Fig. 3A). A retroauricular flap was mobilized. Next, the flap was sutured to the auricle stump with fine sutures, and the helix was shaped with mattress sutures. Four weeks later the support, together with its envelope of connective tissue, was separated from the mastoid. A previously obtained full-thickness skin graft was attached behind the auricle with fibrin glue and was then sutured at once to the anterior skin of the auricle. Figure 3B shows the result after three reconstructive procedures.

The lower half of an ear can be reconstructed by the Gavello flap technique. The reconstructive procedure and flap formation is mapped out in advance on photographs. Cutting along the hairline, we mobilize the flap from the back of the neck, and with the flap we sheathe the rib cartilage support [2]. With this method we repair the lobule, too.

A female patient had lost all of one auricle in a serious car accident. The skin in the ear region was coarse, barely mobile, and permeated with scars and the auditory canal was closed. This case illustrates our procedure for reconstructing an auricle under fairly adverse conditions (Fig. 4A). An autogenous rib cartilage was excised with the help of a pattern and the auricle support was carved (Fig. 4B). A large skin pocket had to be formed and the cartilage sup-

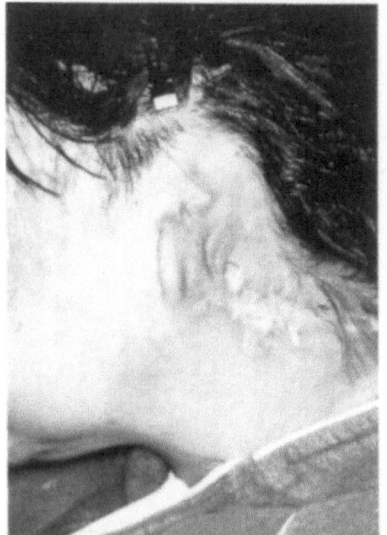

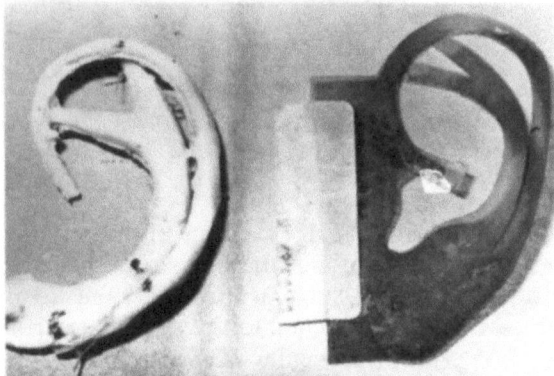

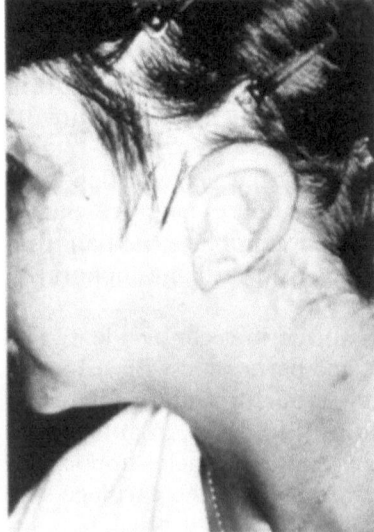

Fig. 4. A Situation after loss of the
entire auricle in a car accident. **B** The
pattern from film of the healthy ear
serves as a model for the autogenous rib
cartilage support. **C** Result some months
after reconstruction

port was worked into place. The helix was attached with glue and shaped with mattress sutures. Fibrin glue stanched bleeding quickly and insured a close fit of skin to cartilage support. In a second stage, the auricle was elevated and a fullthickness skin graft from the buttocks was inserted and glued and sutured to the postauricular surface. We obtained a good result with the third stage of surgery (Fig. 4 C).

Conclusion

In conclusion we have found fibrin sealing to be a valuable aid in plastic reconstructive surgery. Since we started using fibrin glue, we have fixed about 300 free grafts and all were successful.

References

1. Converse JM (ed) (1977) Reconstructive Plastic Surgery, 2nd ed.: vol. 3. Saunders, Philadelphia
2. Weerda H (1989) Reconstructive surgery of the auricle. Facial Plast Surg 5: 399–410

Mastoid Cavity Filling for Bone Reconstruction with a Mixture of Fibrin Glue and Ceramic Granules

M. Bagot d'Arc, P. Corlieu, and G. Daculsi

Abstract

After initial experimental studies in canine mastoid cavities with regard to the use of macroporous biphasic calcium phosphate (MBCP) ceramics, we used MBCP granules in combination with Tissucol (Immuno, Vienna) fibrin adhesive in humans to obliterate radical mastoidectomy cavities immediately after open procedures or in reoperations to fill older cavities. MBCP granules (60 % hydroxyapatite, 40 % tricalciumphosphate, Triosite, Zimmer) are bioactive and osteogenic. Fibrin glue (Tissucol) is used to fix the granules during the packing process to prevent formation of dead spaces between the granules and to promote cell growth and osteointegration. Since 1982, 42 cases have been treated in this manner. The operative technique as well as the anatomical and functional results after a medium-term follow-up period are described. Postoperatively, the middle ear has remained dry in all patients, and no recurrent cholesteatoma has been observed. When, after several months, stapes reconstruction was performed in ten patients, biopsies of the granules were obtained for histological and ultrastructural examination and microanalysis. MBCP granules are well tolerated and remain stable. Histological results demonstrate the bioactivity and osteoconduction of this material along with partial transformation of MBCP granules into lamellar bone after several months.

Introduction

Thanks to their chemical composition and crystalline structure, calcium phosphate (CaP) ceramics are quite similar to bone [1, 2]. They are bioactive and induce ionic exchanges with surrounding tissues capable of accelerating osteogenesis [3–5]. However, bony colonization is strongly related to the nature of proteins in contact with ceramic particles.

Polymerized fibrin and fibronectin, which are contained in fibrin sealant, are well known for their osteogenic properties [6]. They can play an important role in synergy with bioactive ceramics [7].

In 1988, in collaboration with Gersdorff, we published the first results obtained with a mixture of CaP and fibrin glue [8]. The mastoid cavity of dogs was filled, one side with CaP alone and the other side with CaP mixed with fibrin glue. Tolerance was excellent on both sides, bus healing was different. With CaP alone, we only observed the formation of osteoid tissue, whereas with fibrin sealant and CaP there was perfect osteointegration with a true haversian bony colonization.

In radical mastoidectomy cavities, we are faced in clinical practice with the problem of monitoring and of recurrent infections; after obtaining this first experimental result, we first applied the technique of mastoid cavity filling in humans in 1987.

Materials and Methods

Between 1987 and 1992, 42 patients were selected in a prospective open clinical trial. A total of 23 men and 19 women between the ages of 16 and 56 years (average age, 31 years) were enrolled.

Eighteen patients underwent a radical mastoidectomy with immediate reconstruction after exeresis of a cholesteatoma and 24 were reoperated, having experienced complications of radical mastoidectomy several years before.

Operative Technique

First, we gently lifted the skin of the posterior wall of the mastoid cavity; then, after exeresis of cholesteatoma, if present, we carefully drilled until reaching healthy bone capable of stimulating osteogenesis.

To fill the cavity, we used Triosite (Xomed, USA), a macro- and microporous biphasic CaP composed of two parts of tricalciumphosphate (TCP) to three parts hydroxylapatite (HA). Both are bioactive ceramics: TCP is highly resorbable and rapidly promotes osteogenesis, and hydroxylapatite is fairly nonresorbable and ensures mechanical stability [9].

We used 1 g triosite in 1-mm granules mixed with 1 ml fibrin sealant (Tissucol; Immuno, Austria). Tissucol was prepared with low-concentrated thrombin (4 IU/ml) allowing slow setting. Both products are fully mixed in a receptacle and form a kind of plastic bone cement [10]. This mixture was placed in the cavity in small quantities using a spatula and carefully compacted to avoid the formation of dead spaces.

Since the mixture retains its plasticity whatever the form, it was easy to fill the mastoid cavity until the posterior wall of the external auditory meatus had been reshaped (Fig. 1).

A large piece of autologous temporal fascia was then applied over the entire area. Finally, a tympanoplasty was performed with a second fascia by an underlay technique and the cutaneous meatal flap was replaced over the fascia (Fig. 2).

At the end of the procedure, an expandable packing was placed in the external auditory meatus for 1 week.

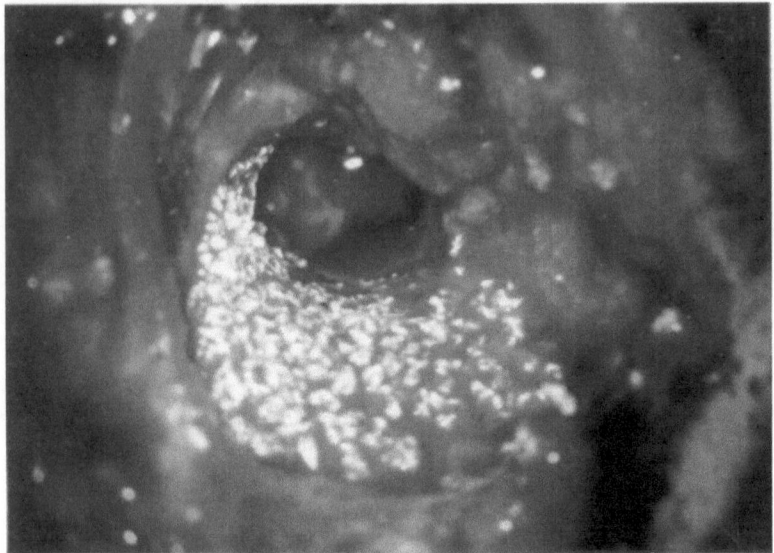

Fig. 1. Mastoid cavity filling with ceramic granules mixed with fibrin glue. Immediate aspect

Results

A total of 42 patients were operated on with this technique, but only 35 of them had a sufficiently long period of follow-up (>6 months) to allow us to present the results. The average follow-up was 32 months (range, 6–65 months).

During the first few postoperative months, the patients were observed weekly. In 23 out of 35 patients, we observed a serous otorrhea during the first 20 days with migration of some granules. This could have been due to the release of excess thrombin and needed regular microsuction. This migration led to a partial resorption of ¼ of the original volume and did not modify the clinical results.

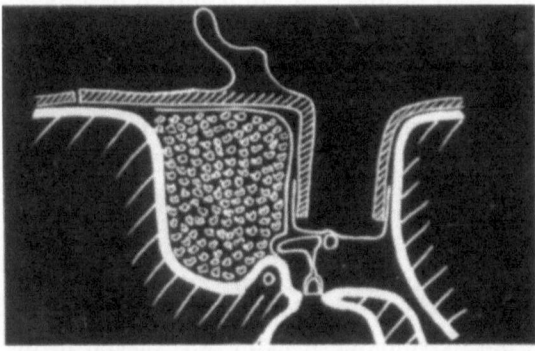

Fig. 2. Total mastoid cavity filling covered by a fascia

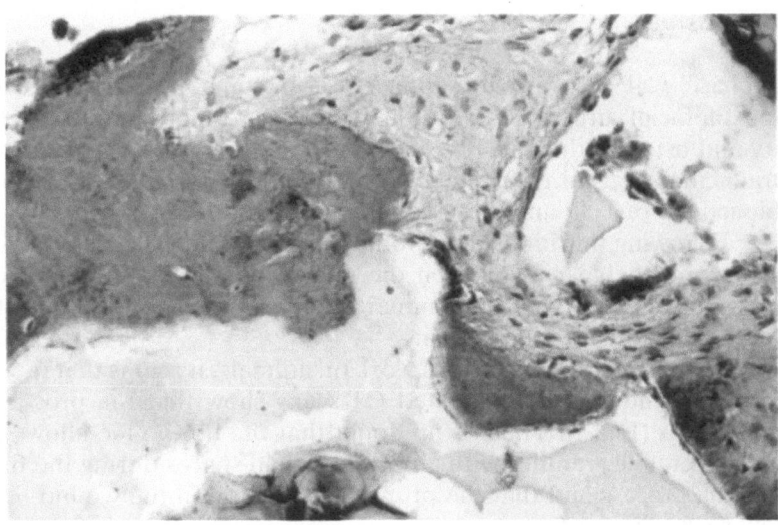

Fig. 3. One year after implantation: mineralization occurs around the granules and inside the macropores

The skin of the posterior wall directly in contact with the mixture was easily observed under the microscope. In 54 % of cases its appearance was normal after 2 weeks and in 96 % after 1 month, showing good tolerance of this material by the skin. After 3 months the posterior wall skin looked normal in color and thickness and did not subsequently change.

All the ears operated on in which regular episodes of otorrhea had occurred before surgery remained dry afterwards. This was a great change for these patients, who previously had to have several aural infections a year.

Eight months to 1 year later, a biopsy of the filling material was performed during a second surgical stage for ossiculoplasty in 11 cases. In the filled area the ceramic granules were found to be embedded in a dense, smooth and milky-white bony substance, resistant to pressure [11]. Hammer and chisel were necessary to extract the block specimens. The ostogenesis was more intense on the periphery than in the center. Analysis in polymerized lumen revealed lamellar bony structures in strong contact with the ceramic granules. This mineralization occurred around the granules and inside the macropores. Haversian lamellar bone appeared inside the spaces between the granules (Fig. 3).

Transmission electronic microscopy showed the coalescence of the bone – mineralized matrix with the ceramic crystals. No trace of fibrin sealant was seen at this stage.

Discussion

Biphasic CaP ceramics are clinically used for bone repair in orthopedic and maxillofacial surgery [12, 13]. The histologic results demonstrate their bioactivity and osteoconduction. We have observed that the granules decrease in size, traducing a partial resorption during the first 2 months in relation to the high bioactivity of TCP and the greater stability of HA [14].

Following this biodegradation process, osteoblastic cells invade the macropores and the spaces between the granules. True bone, characterized by the presence of osteocytes and a mineralized matrix, then appears with a remodeling similar to haversian systems.

According to our previous work on animals, it seems that the bone appears after 2–3 months, but repeated CT scans show that the process slows down afterwards (Fig. 4). There is no doubt that the fibrin glue allows good fixation of the ceramic granules with absence of dead spaces during the first step of the healing process and that the properties of fibrin in the wound-healing process favor osteointegration.

Conclusion

The mixture of biphasic ceramic granules and fibrin glue is easy to use for filling the mastoid cavity, providing good anatomical results. It provides a partial osteogenesis, which guarantees the stability of the assembly, as proved by the long-term histologic results.

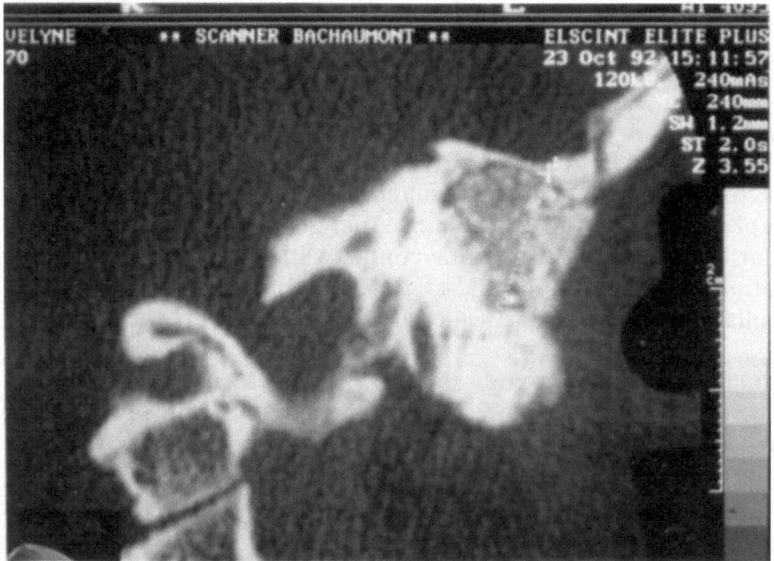

Fig. 4. CT scan control 1 year after implantation: the implant is easy to identify with a thin osteolysis at the interface with the living bone

In our hands, this material constitutes a significant step forward in middle ear surgery, in comparison with the classical techniques used to reconstruct the ear after a radical mastoidectomy [15–19].

References

1. Jarcho M (1981) Calcium phosphate ceramics as hard tissue prosthetics. Clin Orthop 157: 259–263
2. Osborn JF (1980) The materials science of calcium phosphate ceramic. J Bioeng 1: 108–111
3. Metseger DS, Driskell TD, Paulstrud JR (1982) Tricalcium phosphate ceramic. A resorbable bone implant: review and current status. J Am Dent 105: 1035–1038
4. Daculsi, Legeros RZ (1988) In vivo transformation of biphasic calcium phosphate ultrastructural and physical characterization. J Biomed Mat Res 47: 253–257
5. Jarcho M, Kay JF, Drodeckj HP (1976) Tissue, cellular and subcellular events at bone ceramic hydroxylapatite interface. J Bioeng 1: 79–83
6. Schlag G, Redl H, Turnher M, Dinges HP (1986) The importance of fibrin in wound repair. In Schlag G, Redl H (eds) ED. Fibrin sealant in operative medicine, vol 1. Springer, Pub, Berlin Heidelberg New York, pp 3–12
7. Blayney AW, Erre JP, Dhem A, Cazals Y (1987) Experimental mastoid cavity obliteration with hydroxyapatite tricalcium phosphate (Zimmer/Xomed) and fibrin glue (Tissucol/Immuno). Interfaces Med Mech 13: 34–39
8. Gersdorff M, Franceschi D, Bagot d'Arc M, Dhem A, Daculsi G (1988) Revalidation of radical mastoidectomy cavities. Reconstruction with bone dust and biomaterials. Clinical and experimental study. In: Babighian G, Feldmann H (eds) Transplants and implants in otology. Kugler, Amsterdam, pp 69–72
9. Nery EB, Legeros RZ, Lynch KL, Kalbleisch J (1988) Tissue response to biphasic ceramic with different ratios of hydroxyapatite and b-tricalcium phosphate. J Dent Res 67: 178–183
10. Bagot d'Arc M, Corlieu P, Daculsi G (1992) Revalidation of radical mastoidectomy cavities with macroporous biphasic calcium phosphate granules. Clinical study. In: Yanagihara N, Suzuki J (eds) Transplants and implants in otology. Kugler, Amsterdam, pp 145–146
11. Daculsi G, Bagot d'Arc M, Corlieu P, Gersdorff M (1992) Macroporous biphasic calcium phosphates. Efficiency in mastoid cavity obliteration. Experimental and clinical findings. Ann Otol Rhinol Laryngol 101(8): 669–674
12. Passuti N, Daculsi G, Rogez JM, Martin S, Bainvel JV (1990) Macroporous calcium phosphate ceramics performances in human spine arthrodesis. Clin Orthop Relat Res 67: 234–239
13. Legeros RZ (1988) Calcium phosphate material in restorative dentistry: a review. Adv Dent Res 2: 164–167
14. Klein CP, Driessen AA, De Groot K, Van der Hoof A (1983) Biodegradation behavior of various calcium phosphate materials in bone tissue. J Biomed Mater 17: 769–784
15. Palva T (1963) Surgery of chronic ear without cavity. Arch Otolaryngol Head Neck Surg 77: 570–580
16. Portmann M (1986) Traité de technique chirurgicale ORL et cervico-faciale. Masson, Paris, pp 223–230
17. Tos M (1978) Reconstruction of old radical cavities. Clin Otolaryngol 3: 255–261
18. Perkins R (1976) Tympanomastoid reconstruction: an operative procedure for anatomical and functional restoration of the radicalized ear. Laryngoscope 86: 416–430
19. Reck R (1985) Rekonstruction der hinteren Gehörgangswand mit Ceravitalprothesen. HNO 33: 162–165

Fibrin Sealing in Tympanoplasty

R. Frank and G. Stange

Abstract

In microsurgery of the ear, fibrin sealing is used in many indications; these include stapedioplasty, tympanoplasty, reconstruction of the ossicular chain, plastic surgery of the external auditory meatus, and fluctuant hearing loss [2, 4, 7, 11].

Introduction

The operative possibilities in microsurgery of the ear increased with the introduction and use of fibrin sealing. Supplementary microsurgical techniques such as fixation of the shea-Teflon-thorp and the vein on the oval window membrane [3, 6, 10] became possible by using fibrin glue. Fibrin sealing (Tissucol Duo S, human fibrinogen, human thrombin, steam-treated) is now used in many indications, including the following [2]:

1. Stapedioplasty
   a) Vein fascia transplantation of the oval window membrane
   b) Fixation of the stapes substitute
   c) Sealing of the transmeatal incision
2. Tympanoplasty
   a) Subtotal defects of the tympanic membrane
   b) Reconstruction of the lateral attic wall
   c) Reconstruction of the posterior external auditory meatus
3. Reconstruction of the ossicular chain
   a) Anvil interposition
   b) Stapes elevation
   c) Columellization
4. Plastic surgery of the external auditory meatus
   a) Skin transplantation
5. Fluctuant hearing loss
   a) Vein fascia transplantation of the round window membrane
   b) Vein fascia transplantation of the oval window membrane
   c) Fistula syndromes

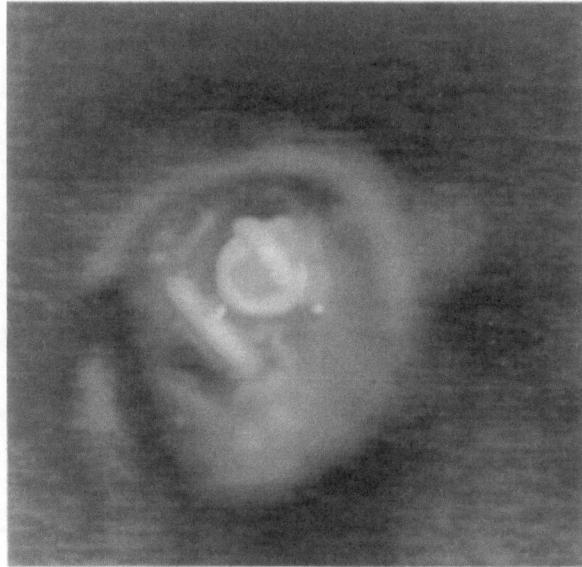

Fig. 1. Fixation of a shea-Teflon-thorp after stapedectomy with fibrin seal

The use of fibrin seal makes operation techniques easier and shortens the operation duration, permitting immediate graft stabilization in the right position.

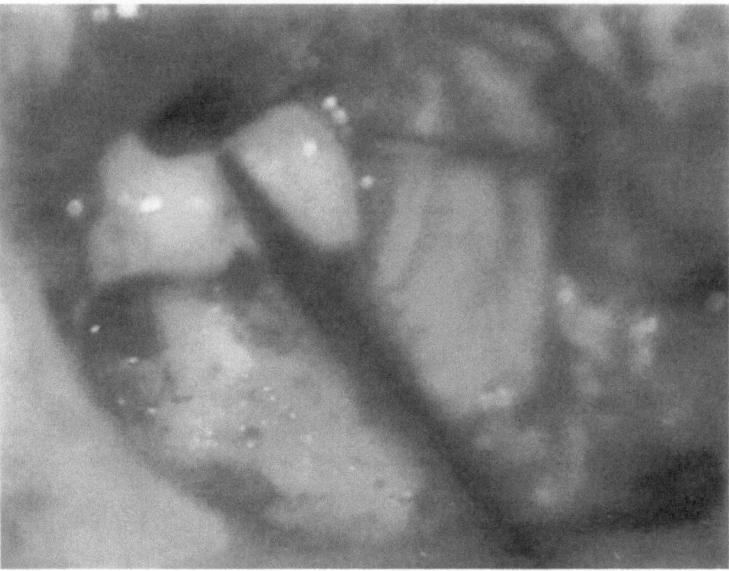

Fig. 2. Reconstruction of the lateral attic wall with cartilage and the fixation with fibrin seal shows optimal stabilization

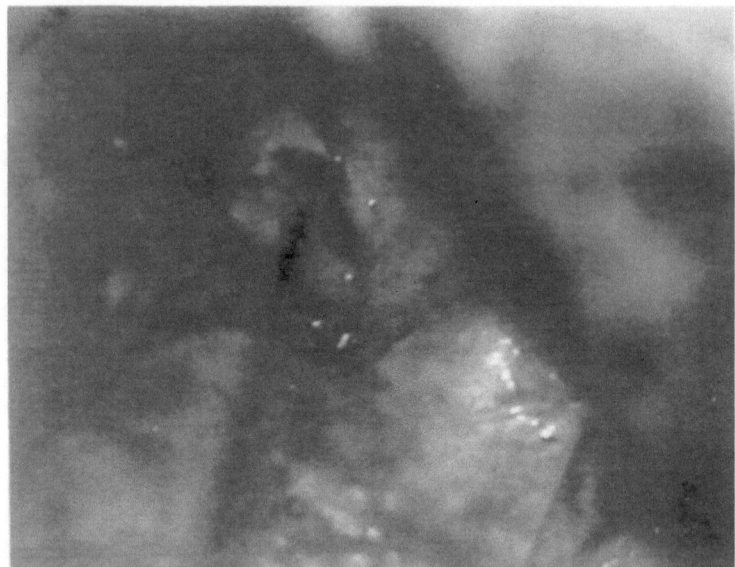

Fig. 3. Columealization with malleus in reconstruction of the ossicular chain and fixation with fibrin glue

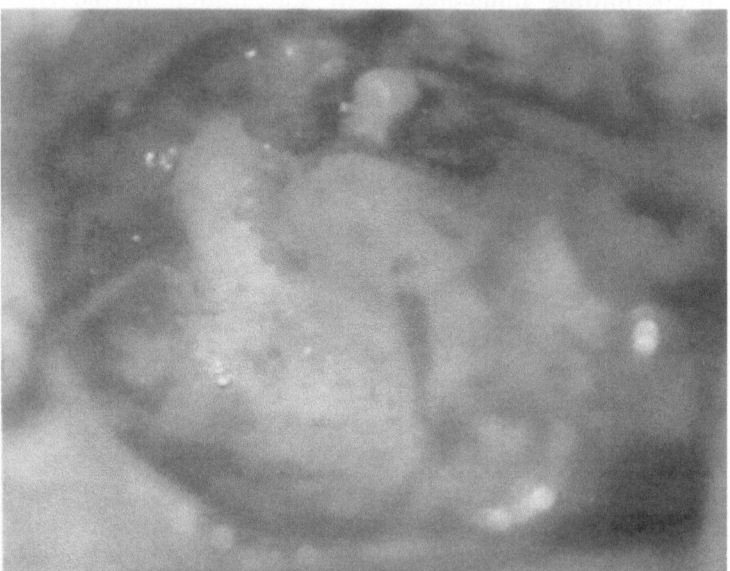

Fig. 4. Secure fixation of a malleus head in stapes elevation with fibrin sealant

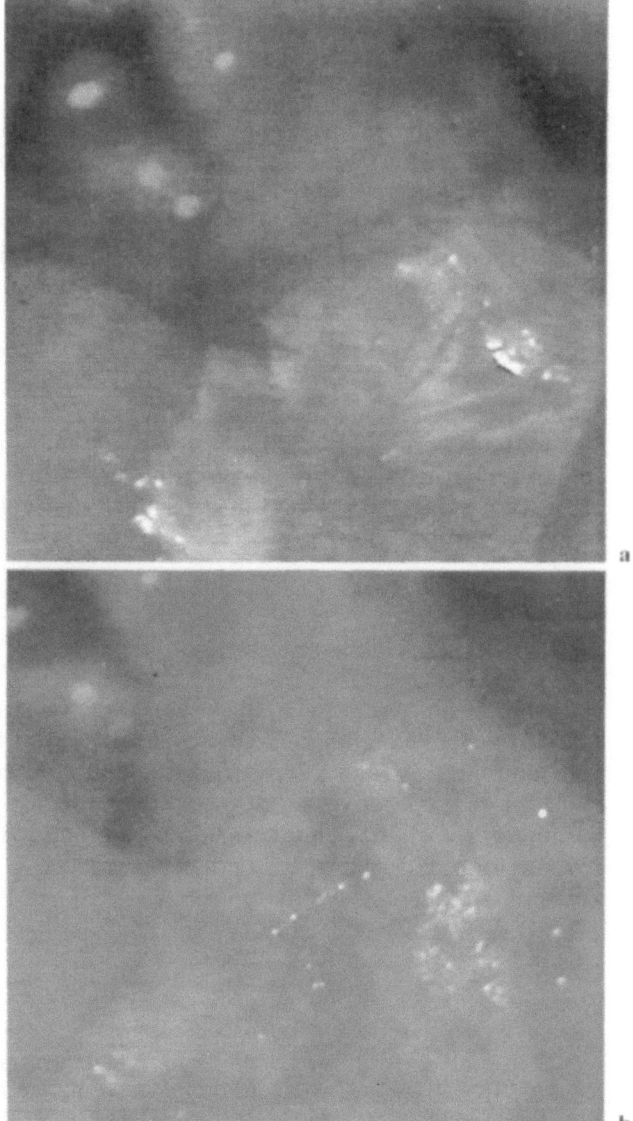

Fig. 5a, b. Covering a fistula of labyrinth with a piece of vein **(a)** and fixing it with fibrin glue **(b)**

Material and Methods

In stapedectomies, use of fibrin glue in the fixation of a vein or fascia transplant after opening the oval window membrane and the fixation of a shea-Teflon-thorp (Fig. 1) shows advantages and results in a better postoperative hearing gain, as it does in the fixation of the transmeatal incision [9, 10].

In tympanoplasties with subtotal defects, we use fibrin seal for fixing the temporal fascia or sometimes heterografts; it allows immediate graft stabilization. In cholesteatoma surgery and in the reconstruction of the pneumatic system by rebuilding the mastoid cavity, the posterior wall, and the lateral attic wall (Fig. 2), fibrin sealant in combination with cartilage makes adaption and stabilization unproblematic [8].

In ossicular chain reconstruction, anvil interposition, columellization (Fig. 3), and stapes elevation (Fig. 4) show no problems if fibrin seal is used. A secure interposition and fixation in the correct position with one drop of fibrin sealant is guaranteed [5, 6, 9].

Healing without complications in plasties of the external auditory meatus has become possible with the use of fibrin sealant. The risk of postoperative stenosis is no longer present. Skin transplants were fixed with fibrin sealant and tamponated to prevent shifting; after 1 week no stenosis, granulation formation, or secondary healing was found. This kind of operation can now be done on an outpatient basis thanks to fibrin glue.

Patients with fluctuant hearing loss and leaks in the oval or round window membrane or fistulas of the labyrinth (Fig. 5a, b) no longer have relapses. The fixing of a vein or transplant at the site of the leak is now done without problems using fibrin glue.

Results and Discussion

By using fibrin seal in microsurgery of the ear, considerable progress has been made; operative techniques already in use could be performed more successfully and new efficient microsurgical techniques were made possible.

Our postoperative results following the use of fibrin sealant in microsurgery of the ear are characterized by a functional improvement in hearing, a low rate of reperforations and adhesive processes, and better wound healing in cases of complicated tympanoplasties.

References

1. Bebear JP, Bagot d'Arc M, Portmann M (1986) Remarks on the daily use of Tissucol (Tisseel) during 5 years in otology and otoneurosurgery. In: Schlag G, Redl H (eds) Otorhinolaryngology in fibrin sealant in operative medicine, vol 1. Springer, Berlin Heidelberg New York, pp 63–67
2. Elies W (1994) Perilympathischer Druckverlust – Hauptursache des M. Ménière und anderer cochleo-vestibulärer Störungen? 11th Cochlea-symposium Halle, 21–24 Apr 1991, Wernigerode (in press)
3. Frank R, Stange G (1992) Results of different stapedectomies of the last 15 years; abstract of the Politzer Society international conference: otology in the 90's: trends and perspectives, 15–21 March 1992, Cortina d'Ampezzo, Italy, abstract, p 65
4. Stange G (1975) Bindegewebe-Siliconfolien-Plastiken bei Adhäsivprozessen des Mittelohres. Arch Otorhinolaryngol 211: 163–171
5. Stange G (1980) Mikrochirurgische Ohroperationen als Vorbereitung zur hörprothetischen Versorgung. Audiol. Akust 19: 62–82
6. Stange G (1982) Veränderungen des Tinnitus in der postoperativen Phase bei Otosklerose und feuchtem Tubenmittelohrkatarrh. Laryngol Rhinol Otol 61: 128–131

7. Stange G (1983) Das akut und das chronisch erkrankte Ohr. Therapiewoche 33: 259–276
8. Stange G, Esser G, Schuhnicht R, Adam D, Löw J, Krieger M, Woischwill J, Berghorn K (1981) Kindliche Ohrerkrankungen. Therapiewoche 31: 7169–7191
9. Stange G (1919) Die Chirurgie der Mittelohrerkrankungen beim Erwachsenen. TW Kopf Hals 1: 48–53
10. Stange G, Frank R (1990) Résultats des diverses stapédoplasties. Communication LXXXVIIe Congres Français d'Oto-Rhino-Laryngologie et de Pathologie Cervico-Faciale, 8–11 Oct 1990, Paris
11. Zöllner F (1966) Behandlung der chronischen Mittelohrentzündung und ihre Folgen. In: Berendes J, Link R, Zöllner F (eds) Hals-Nasen-Ohrenheilkunde, vol III/2, Thieme, Stuttgart, pp 1226–1336

Compound Prosthesis and Cartilage Layer: Two New Applications of Fibrin Sealing in Reconstructive Middle Ear Surgery

H. Schobel

Abstract

The purpose of this short chapter is to demonstrate two of the more important concepts resulting from more than 40 years of experience in reconstructive middle ear surgery, i.e., the compound prosthesis and the cartilage bed method.

Introduction

In reconstructive middle ear surgery, ENT surgeons all over the world are faced with the following problems:

1. Healing a chronic inflammation process which encompasses all the structures and spaces of the middle ear and the adjacent organs
2. The permanent reconstruction of hearing
3. Avoiding the well-known postoperative and late problems and complications such as secretory mastoid cavities, retraction pockets, and the occurrence of cholesteatoma recurrence.

Whereas specialists all over the world are united in far-reaching agreement concerning the first issue mentioned above, which refers to the healing of the complex chronic inflammation process, they differ considerably with regard to the methods employed in order to ensure an optimum reconstruction of hearing, to avoid late complications, and, last but not least, to obtain results that are both stable and permanent. Consequently, the numerous procedures suggested form a very varied spectrum. This multitude of methods is indicative of the fact that surgeons are still searching for a superior approach.

Forty years of international experience in reconstructive middle ear surgery have led to the use of a variety of surgical techniques with regards to access to the middle ear, either endaurally or postauricularly. The radical nature of the procedures performed also differs widely. Materials and techniques used for reconstruction of the ossicular chain and tympanic membrane are many, and good, permanent surgical results often depend on the pathological conditions encountered in the middle ear and mastoid. The experience of the ear surgeon and the choice of his technique play an important role in the outcome of many procedures.

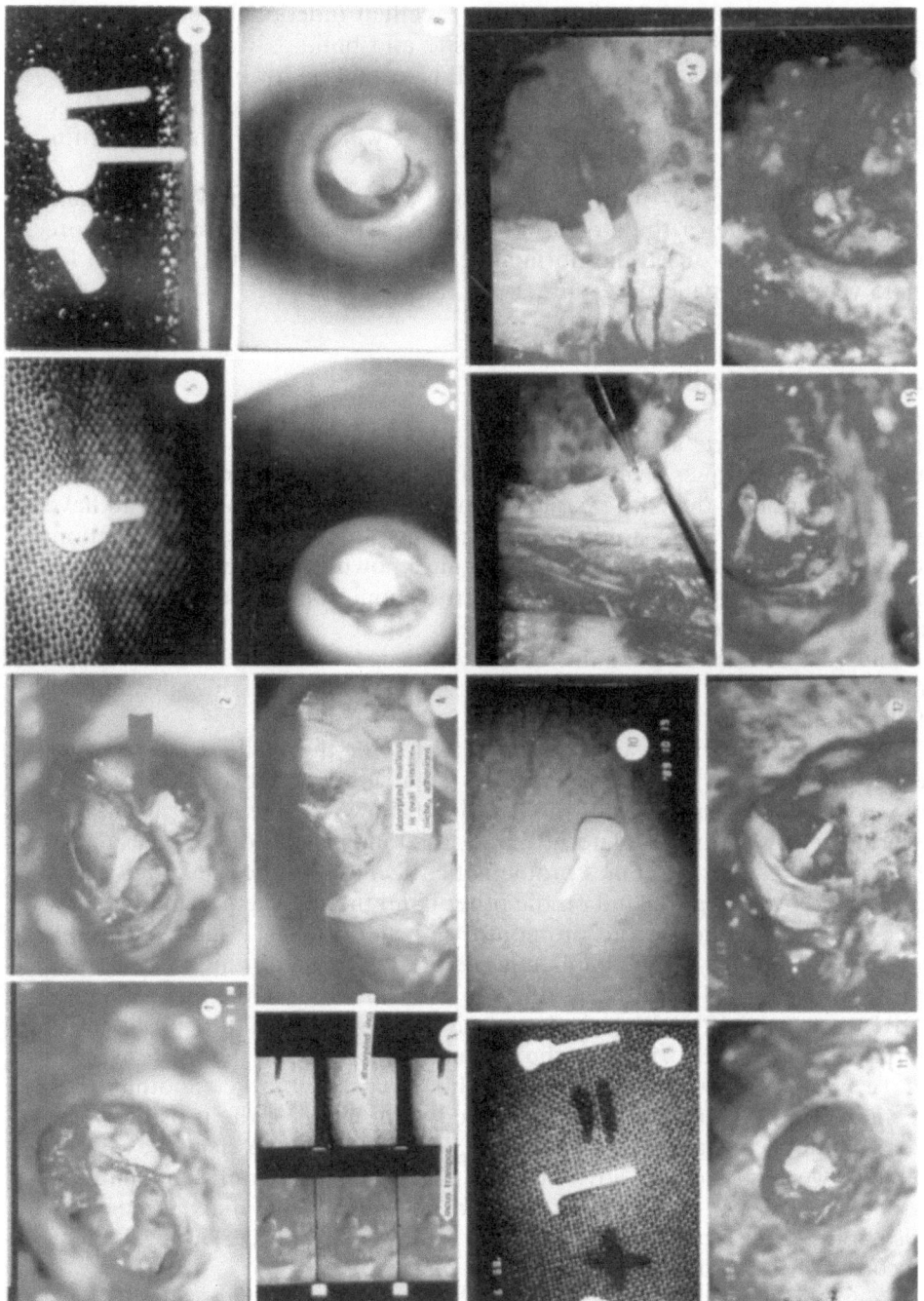

Fig. 1. (1–16) See text for details

It has been observed that immediate, excellent functional results may disappear due to reactions of connective tissue and bone as well as shifting of transplants or implants due to scarring, callus formation, or bone absorption.

Naturally, the results of all middle ear procedures depend to a very large extent on the function of the eustachian tube, which often cannot be influenced.

The present author, initially stimulated by the work of Wullstein and Zöllner, has led one of the largest otologic departments in Austria for more than 30 years and has used the fibrin adhesive Tissucol (Immuno, Vienna) for over 15 years in tympanoplasty surgery.

Material and Methods

The following report, supported by two figures, shows two of the present author's own techniques. Here, very good permanent results can be obtained on reconstruction of the entire ossicular chain, especially in patients who have previously had radical mastoid surgery and have limited eustachian function. The figures point out the problem of certain known procedures and the way they have been solved. They also show an example of the functional results which can be achieved.

Thus, I would first like to describe my concept of a compound prosthesis, which is used in cases in which the total ossicular chain is missing; in addition, I shall present the cartilage bed method.

Autologous materials such as the incus rest or the malleus have proved without doubt to be the best suited for the reconstruction of the ossicular chain, if the stapes is preserved (Fig. 1a, b). If, however, the stapes is missing, the insertion of autologous materials, e.g., the long process of the incus or the handle of the malleus, becomes problematic, because on the one hand it may be deformed by resorption and on the other hand there is the possibility of callus development either at the promontory or at the facial canal. Adhesions hindering the mobility of the implanted material in the oval window constitute a third obstacle (Fig. 1c, d). By using alloplastic materials in the form of a total (TORP) or partial (PORP) ossicular replacement prosthesis, the problems of resorption or fixation due to the formation of callus may be avoided (Fig. 1e, f). In using alloplastic materials, however, we observed another problem, namely extrusion, which also occurred if the head of the prosthesis was covered with a cartilage disc (Fig. 1g, h). To solve these ossicular extrusion problems, we combined the advantages of bioactive glass ceramic and autologous bone grafts. We used healthy remnants of autologous malleus heads or incus bodies, occasionally conserved bone, and bone cubes cut out of the mastoid cortex of the same patient.

Figure 1i shows a malleus and a TORP. We used the head of the malleus and the shaft of the TORP and joined these parts to form the so-called compound prosthesis, which can also be seen in Fig. 1j.

Figure 1k shows a compound prosthesis consisting of a mastoid cortex cube in a right middle ear with the external canal wall up. Figure 1l shows a compound prosthesis consisting of the malleus head and a Macor strut, anchored between the footplate and the tympanic membrane graft in a left middle ear. To prevent the prosthesis from falling down, the system of the tent pole is used, as is shown in Fig. 1l. The creation of a sufficiently deep tympanic cavity is very helpful here. Figure 1m, n shows the preparation of the compact cube from the mastoid cortex.

Compound prostheses, which have been used by us in more than 400 tympanoplasties since 1987, may be implanted in either "canal wall up" or "canal wall down" procedures. In Fig. 1o, a remnant of the ossicular chain, the malleus handle, is still present, and in Fig. 1p, the compound prosthesis is being installed in a middle ear, following a radical mastoidectomy procedure. It is important to create a sufficiently deep tympanic cavity so that adhesions cannot develop between the new eardrum and the promontory and facial canal. Moreover, it is essential that the prosthesis is erected at a 90° angle to the footplate and that normal footplate mobility is not impaired. Tympanic membrane perforations, bony adhesions with the facial canal, and the absorption of the bony part of the prostheses have not been observed over a 5-year period.

Regarding the functional results in cases with good tubal function, good mucous lining, and the compound prosthesis remaining erect at a 90° angle to the mobile footplate, we have succeeded in obtaining excellent results, comparable to the best results ever achieved in otosclerotic surgery, as can be shown by comparing the audiograms of a 70-year-old man on the left and on the right. The latter was taken almost 4 years later (Fig. 2a, b). In some cases with initial good functional results and later deterioration of hearing, however, we found that the prosthesis was inclined either to the facial canal or to the promontory. For this reason we modified the eardrum transplant. For the substitution of the eardrum, not fascia but a perichondrium flap from the tragus with a cartilage circle or ring is used. In the centre of this circle (ring), the head of the compound prosthesis has to be anchored by means of Tissucol. In this way the postoperative inclination of the compound prosthesis can successfully be prevented (Fig. 2c, d). One of the main causes of failures of tympanoplasties is the impaired function of the eustachian tube (Fig. 2e). Air absorption in the middle ear takes place via the mucosa. If the mucosa surface is enlarged and the tubal function is impaired, it is obvious that the air should be absorbed more rapidly and negative pressure in the middle ear should increase much faster. Thus, the first consequence of the impaired function of the eustachian tube is a retraction pocket, and the next a new cholesteatoma. Therefore, it becomes uncertain whether it really makes sense to create an air-filled antrum, lined with mucosa, by reconstructing the bony canal wall. These previous experiences and observations form the basis for our concept of a partial obliteration of the mastoid, namely the creation of a cartilage bed in the attic and the use of the compound prosthesis. Figure 2f illustrates this concept. A longitudinal section through the external canal is shown. Because of the removal of cholesteatoma, the ossicular chain and the entire posterior canal wall are missing. On the left, the eustachian tube orifice is indicated. On the footplate, covered with a piece of fascia, is the compound prosthesis, and in the attic to the far right, dorsal to the horizontal canal, a layer of cartilage chips, colored yellow, can be

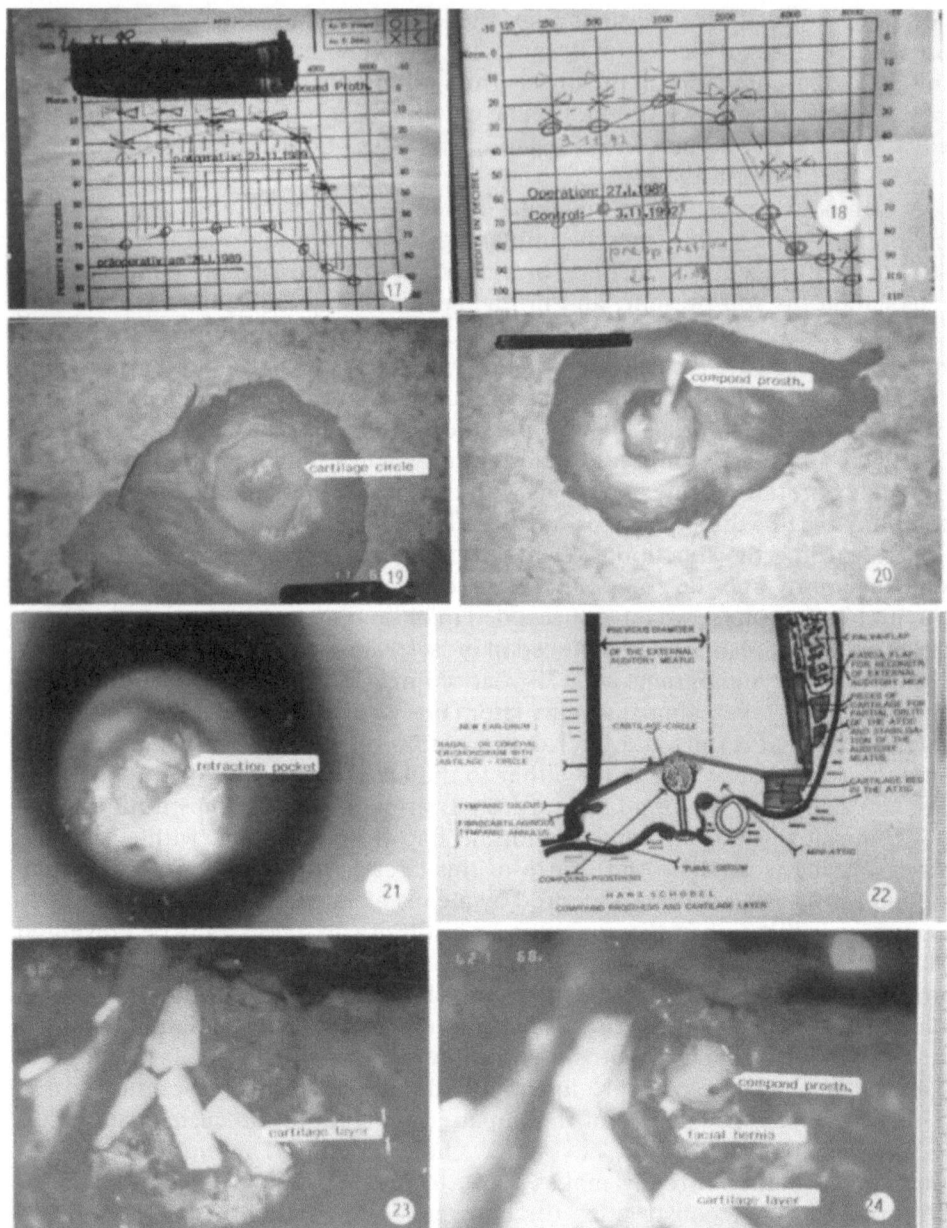

Fig. 2. (17–24) See text for details

seen. The red tympanic membrane graft has been tucked into the deepened sulcus tympanicus anteriorly, thus obtaining not only an acute anterior tympano-meatal angle, but also good healing of the anterior border of the tympanic membrane graft. It rests both upon the head of the compound prosthesis, where it is stabilized by the surrounding cartilage circle, and upon the cartilage bed in the attic.

Hence the air-filled middle ear has become separated from the non-aerated mastoid, and the tympanic membrane graft can vibrate on both sides of the prosthesis. The air-filled space, bordered by the head of the prosthesis, the facial nerve canal, the horizontal semicircular canal, the cartilage bed, and the tympanic membrane graft, is, from a functional point of view, of decisive importance. We have named this space the mini attic. Dorsally, the external canal is reconstructed with fascia and cartilage, and the mastoid cavity is partially obliterated with cartilage only or with cartilage and Palva flap.

This system offers the following advantages: the bradytrophic cartilage hardly changes its form, and therefore the lateralization of the tympanic membrane graft does not occur. All complications that may originate from the classical mastoid cavity, namely an inflammation with desquamation, granulations, retraction pocket, and cholesteatoma, are avoided as far as possible. Because of the separation and the obliteration of the antrum, the middle ear contains much less air-absorbing mucosa, which is important in cases with reduced tubal function. Figure 1 g, h shows examples of cartilage beds and a compound prosthesis in a right ear. These pieces of cartilage, taken either from the tragus or from the concha auris, are stabilized and fixed by means of Tissucol. The permanent functional result of this operation is shown in Fig 2 a, b.

In conclusion the most important goals in the use of the compound prosthesis and the cartilage layer are as follows:

– To reconstruct the middle ear according to its normal anatomy as far as possible
– To avoid any known problems of the open mastoid cavity
– To prevent retraction pockets as well as recurrent cholesteatomas
– To prevent subsequent lack of hearing by changes in the position and the direction of the prosthesis

References

1. Schobel H (1965 a) Probleme der Wiederherstellungschirurgie nach Otitis media. Monatsschr Ohrenheilkd 99: 503
2. Schobel H (1965 b) Vorschläge zu drei aktuellen Problemen der rekonstruktiven Mittelohrchirurgie. Arch Ohren Nasen Kehlkopf Heilkd 185: 510
3. Schobel H (1966) Ricostruzione dell'orecchio dopo otite media, interventi radicali e timpanoplastiche. Giornale dell'Accademia di Medicina di Torino, anno CXXIX, fasc 1–12
4. Schobel H (1968 a) Erfahrungen bei tympanoplastischen Nachoperationen. Monatsschr Ohrenheilkd 102: 699
5. Schobel H (1968 b) La recconstruccion del oido en la otitis media y colesteatoma. Rev Otolaringolog VIII: 320–330
6. Schobel H (1968 c) Die Rekonstruktion des Ohres nach früherer Radikaloperation oder Tympanoplastik. Arch Ohren Nasen Kehlkopf Heilkd 191: 788
7. Schobel H (1969) Die Rekonstruktion der Schalleitung. Monatsschr Ohrenheilkd 103: 319–320

8. Schobel H (1974) Bewährte und neue Rekonstruktionsmöglichkeiten des Schalleitungsapparates. Monatsschr Ohrenheilkd 108: 84
9. Schobel H (1979) Einige Ursachen des Mißerfolges bei der Tympanoplastik. Laryngol Rhinol Otol 58: 583
10. Schobel H (1984) Tympanoplastik 1983. In: Majer E, Zrunek M (eds) Aktuelles in der Otorhinolaryngologie 1983. Thieme, Stuttgart, p 21
11. Schobel H (1985a) Tympanoplastik bei und nach Komplikationen. In: Majer EH, Zrunek M (eds) Aktuelles in der Otorhinolaryngologie 1984. Thieme, Stuttgart, p 247
12. Schobel H (1985b) Erfahrungen bei tympanoplastischen Nachoperationen. In: Majer EH, Zrunek M (eds) Aktuelles in der Otorhinolaryngologie 1984. Thieme, Stuttgart, p 245
13. Wullstein H (1960a) Principles of tympanoplasty. Arch Otolaryngol 71: 329
14. Wullstein H (1960b) Indication for tympanoplasty. Arch Otolaryngol 71: 380
15. Wullstein H (1960c) Results of tympanoplasty. Arch Otolaryngol 71: 478
16. Zöllner F (1957) Hörverbessernde Operationen bei entzündlich bedingten Mittelohrveränderungen. Arch Ohren Nasen Kehlkopf Heilkd 171: 1
17. Zöllner F (1966) Behandlung der chronischen Mittelohrentzündung und ihrer Folgen. In: Berendes J, Link R, Zöllner F (eds) Hals-Nasen-Ohrenheilkunde, vol III/2. Thieme, Stuttgart, 1226

Use of Bovine Heterologous Cartilage and Fibrin Sealant in Middle Ear Reconstructive Surgery

F. Piragine, P. Bruschini, S. Berrettini, G. Segnini, and S. Sellari-Franceschini

Abstract

We report our experience in using cartilage heterografts and fibrin sealant in middle ear reconstructive surgery. The heterologous cartilage drawn from cattle of selected breeding was sterilized and preserved in 70 % alcoholic solution. Eighty-nine patients operated on were followed for at least 12 months. Follow-up ranged from 12 months to 3 years. Heterografts were used in 47 "canal up" techniques (12 reconstructions of defects in the posterior and superior aspects of the external ear canal and 41 columellas), 28 "canal down" techniques, and 11 anatomical and functional rehabilitations of radical cavities. Fibrin glue was used in all cases to achieve sticking of cartilage fragments.

A good anatomical result with an intact tympanic graft and no signs of inflammation and retraction were observed in 74 cases (86 %). In 12 cases a retraction of the new eardrum and a protrusion of the cartilage strut was noted. No extrusion was observed. As far as function is concerned, the mean postoperative air-bone gap was 11.1 dB and the mean hearing gain was 26.3 dB.

Heterologous cartilage could provide a good alternative to autologous and homologous cartilage grafts. Compared to homologous grafts, bovine cartilage heterografts are easily accessible and they present no viral risk. Fibrin glue improves the results because it promotes an early and correct sticking of all fragments used in middle ear reconstructive surgery.

Introduction

Since 1981 fibrin sealant has been routinely used in our department in different operations of ENT surgery [2, 8, 11]. As far as middle ear surgery is concerned, fibrin glue has proved to be very useful in myringoplasty, ossiculoplasty, tympanoplasty, stapedectomy, middle ear reconstruction in radical cavities, cochlear implants, and repair of facial paralysis (end-to-end anastomosis, repair by nerve graft). Fibrin glue is useful in sticking tympanic grafts, stabilizing the new chain (ossicles, cartilage, or biocompatible implants), reconstructing the lateral aspect of the attic, closing labyrinthine or dural fistulas, and dealing with perioperative accidents such as perilymph gusher [1, 7–12].

To date no satisfactory method has been devised to reconstruct the ossicular chain. Until 1987 we used Plastipore prostheses – total (TORP) or partial (PORP) ossicular prostheses – using a cartilage slide between the prosthesis and tympanic grafts, stuck by fibrin glue. However, long-term follow-up revealed a high incidence of extrusion in contrast to the good functional results observed in the first postoperative period [14]. Therefore, we preferred to use homologous ossicles and we experimented with stored, lyophilized allografts collected by cortical substance of long bones]3]. Unfortunately, at present the large diffusion of viral diseases has stopped our research into homografts and we are looking for different materials.

Cartilage heterografts are frequently used in facial plastic and reconstructive surgery to correct bone or cartilage defects, but they are not currently used in otologic surgery. The fate of cartilage implanted in the middle ear has been the subject of interesting studies. No evidence of foreign body or rejection phenomena has been reported, but in a few cases absorption and replacement by fibrous tissue has been observed [4–6, 13, 15]. Furthermore, experimental studies suggest that heterologous cartilage presents the same structural and immunologic characteristics as homologous cartilage [5].

In this study we report the results of using cartilage heterografts and fibrin glue in middle ear reconstructive surgery.

Material and Method

Rib and xiphoid cartilage was taken from cattle of selected breeding. After dissection of the subcutaneous tissue and perichondrium, blocks of cartilage were placed in an antibiotic solution for 3 days and then in a 70 % ethyl alcoholic solution, where they were preserved for 20 days before utilizing. The alcoholic storage causes the coarctation and the degeneration of chondrocytes, preserving the organic matrix. A microbiologic examination is performed after 2 weeks; the alcoholic solution is changed every 3 weeks. Before use, cartilage was removed from the alcoholic solution by a sterile technique and put through several washings of Ringer's lactate solution to remove residual alcohol.

One hundred and nineteen cartilage heterografts were implanted into the middle ear from 1989. We report the results of 86 selected cases which were followed for at least 12 months. Cases that failed due to relapse of pathology were excluded. Follow-up ranged from 1 to 3 years. Heterografts were utilized in 47 "canal up" techniques (12 reconstructions of defects in the posterior and superior wall of the external ear canal and 41 columellas), in 28 "canal down" techniques, and in 11 middle ear reconstructions in radical cavities. Two surgical techniques were performed in order to reconstruct radical mastoid cavities. In seven cases we reconstructed an open cavity with obliteration of the mastoid, and in four cases we reconstructed a closed cavity with an aired mastoid (Fig. 1). In all cases we used rapid glue with or without the Duploject (Immuno, Vienna). If we had to seal cartilage pieces into the mastoid cavity in order to fill it, we used the Duploject because the procedure is faster. Otherwise, if we had to stick structures close to the oval window, the fibrinogen solu-

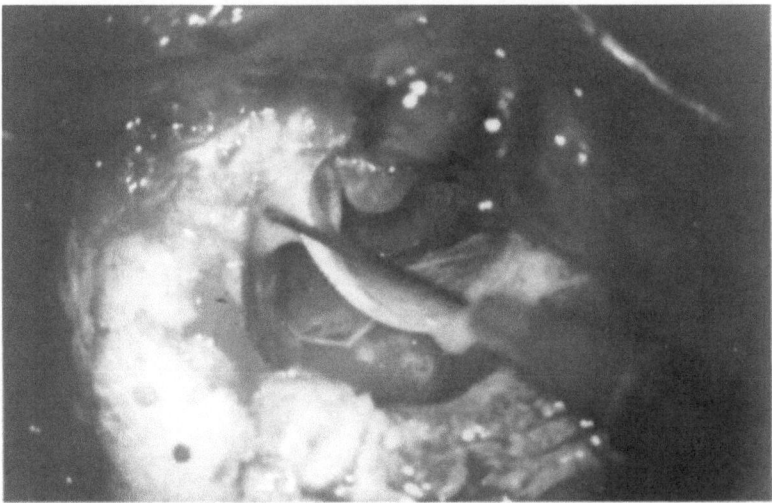

Fig. 1. Middle ear reconstruction in radical cavity to obtain a closed cavity with an aired mastoid cavity. Cartilage fragments are sealed with fibrin sealant

tion was applied first and any excess solution was removed by suction. When we were sure that just the areas to be glued were covered by fibrinogen, the thrombin solution was applied.

Results

Cartilage was used to reconstruct the epitympanic wall, tympanic frame, and epitympanic mastoid roof as well as for ossiculoplasty and partial mastoid obliteration. In all cases fibrin glue was used to stick cartilage to the cavity walls or to the tympanic graft and to keep in the correct position all the fragments used in middle ear reconstruction in radical cavities.

Some cartilaginous columellae were removed after more than 1 year. Such operations enabled us to observe the good tolerance of the graft in vivo and to carry out further histologic examinations. The heterografts appeared to be coated by a normal mucosa. The histologic findings revealed a normal and intact cartilaginous matrix, lined by fibrous tissue and mucosa with no evidence of chondrocytes (Fig. 2).

Tympanic graft intact with no signs of inflammation and/or retraction was considered a good result. We observed good anatomical results in 74 cases. In the "canal down" technique and in middle ear reconstruction in radical cavities we were satisfied when the cavity presented a normal epithelization. In 12 cases (five "canal up" techniques, five "canal down" techniques, and two middle ear reconstructions), we observed a retraction of the eardrum and a protrusion of the cartilage strut. In two "canal down" techniques we observed a total eardrum retraction. No signs of inflammation or extrusion were observed (Table 1).

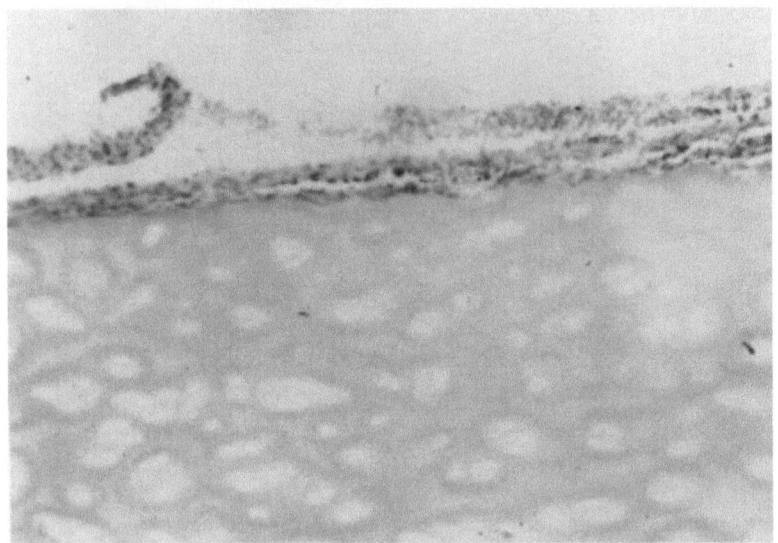

Fig. 2. Bovine cartilage removed after 1 year: normal and intact cartilaginous matrix, no evidence of chondrocytes. EE, ×250

In the 41 cases operated on using a "canal up" technique, the mean preoperative air-bone gap was 37.4 dB, the mean postoperative air-bone gap was 11.1 dB, and the mean hearing gain was 26.3 dB. In 25 cases (61%) the postoperative air-bone gap was under 10 dB, in 11 cases (27%) it was between 11 and 20 dB, and in five cases (12%) it was between 21 and 30 dB.

Table 1. Anatomical results

	Closed technique		Open technique		Reconstruction of radical cavities		Total	
	(n)	(%)	(n)	(%)	(n)	(%)	(n)	(%)
Intact new eardrum, normal epithelium	42	89	23	82	9	82	74	86
Retraction of new eardrum	5	11	5	18	2	18	12	14
Extrusion, reperforation	–	–	–	–	–	–	–	–
Total	47	100	28	100	11	100	86	100

Discussion

Cartilage grafts and fibrin glue were well tolerated in all cases. No host versus graft reaction and no inflammatory reaction or exuberant fibrosis were observed. When the heterologous cartilage was used for ossicular reconstruction, no extrusion was observed, not even in cases with a serious retraction of the eardrum. The heterografts removed were not stuck to the middle ear walls and their general appearance remained unchanged. No vascular proliferation, inflammatory reaction, or resorption was noted. In the 41 cases operated on using a "canal up" technique we obtained satisfactory results, probably because of the structural properties of cartilage: heterologous cartilage has some properties, e.g., firmness and elasticity, which we considered better than in homologous cartilage.

The availability of large pieces of cartilage allows us to perform every kind of reconstruction in middle ear surgery. Compared to biocompatible implants, heterologous cartilage presents no extrusion problems. Compared to homologous grafts, bovine cartilage heterografts are easily accessible and they present no viral risk.

Although this is a series with too short a follow-up to draw definitive conclusions, it can nevertheless be stated that bovine cartilage is well tolerated in the middle ear. Fibrin glue was very important in all cases involving sealing of cartilage fragments. We have never seen infection or immunologic reaction due to fibrin glue and thus advise the use of bovine cartilage and fibrin glue in all reconstructions of middle ear surgery.

References

1. Berrettini S, Bruschini P, Sellari-Franceschini S, Bottoni S (1985) Un caso di Geyser perilymph risolto con colla di fibrina. Riv Orl Aud Fon 5: 165–167
2. Bruschini P, Berrettini S, Sellari-Franceschini S, Segnini G, Costantino L, Piragine F (1990) Aritenoidectomia e aritenoidectomia con emicordectomia sottomucosa nel trattamento delle paralisi cordali bilaterali in adduzione. Otorinolaringologia 40:447–451
3. Bruschini P, Berrettini S, Segnini G, Sellari-Franceschini S, Bocci S, Piragine F, Gersdorff M (1991) Omotrapianti ossei liofilizzati nella chirurgia ricostruttiva dell'orecchio medio. Acta Otorhinolaryngol 11: 159–165
4. Don A, Linthicum FH (1975) The fate of cartilage grafts for ossicular reconstruction in tympanoplasty. Ann Otol Rhinol Laryngol 84: 187–191
5. Ersek R, Hart W, Greer D (1984) Processed bovine cartilage: an improved biosynthetic implant for contour defects. Ann Plast Surg 12: 397–401
6. Kerr AG, Smyth GDL (1972) Histologic study of transplanted ossicles and cartilage homografts. Otolaryngol Clin North Am 5: 183–194
7. Piragine F, Bruschini P, Sellari-Franceschini S, Berrettini S (1983) L'uso della colla di fibrina (Tissucol) nella chirurgia ricostruttiva dell'orecchio medio. Riv Orl Aud Fon 3: 143–146
8. Piragine F, Bruschini P, Sellari-Franceschini S, Berrettini S (1984) L'impiego del Tissucol in cofochirurgia: analisi degli interventi eseguiti nella Clinica ORL di Pisa. Riv Orl Aud Fon 4: 77–83
9. Piragine F, Bruschini P, Sellari-Franceschini S, Berrettini S (1985) Die Anwendung des Fibrinklebers in der Mikrochirurgie des Ohres: eine Analyse der Eingriffe in der HNO-Klinik Pisa. HNO 33: 159–161

10. Piragine F, Bruschini P, Sellari-Franceschini S, Berrettini S (1986) Reconstruction of the open mastoidectomized ear: two surgical techniques. In: Schlag G, Redl H (eds) Fibrin sealant in operative medicine, vol. 1. Otorhinolaryngology. Springer, Berlin Heidelberg, pp 140–146
11. Piragine F, Bruschini P, Berrettini S, Sellari-Franceschini S, Grossi P (1988) Utilizzazione del tissucol congelato (DUO) in alcuni interventi di partinenza otorinolaringoiatrica. Riv Orl Aud Fon 8: 37–40
12. Piragine F, Bruschini P, Berrettini S, Sellari-Franceschini S, Grossi P, Segnini G (1990) Una tecnica di ricostruzione di orecchio medio in cavità di radicale. Videotology 3: 9–16
13. Schuknecht HF, Shi SR (1985) Surgical pathology of middle ear implants. Laryngoscope 95: 249–258
14. Sellari-Franceschini S, Piragine F, Bruschini P, Berrettini S (1987) TORPS and PORPS: causes of failure. Am J Otol 8: 551–552
15. Steinbach E, Pulsakar A (1981) Long-term histological fate of cartilage in ossicular reconstruction. J Laryngol Otol 95: 1031–1039

Pharyngeal Fistulas Following Total Laryngectomy Treated with Dilatation and Fibrin Sealant

S. Sellari-Franceschini, G. F. Menconi, G. Segnini, P. Bruschini, S. Berrettini, A. Janni, C. A. Angeletti, and F. Piragine

Abstract

The formation of pharyngeal fistulas is the most frequent complication after total laryngectomy. A wide resection of the pharynx, preoperative radiotherapy, a poor nutritional status, diabetes, wound infections, postoperative bleeding, and operative mistakes are possible causes.

Sometimes a small pharyngeal fistula may persist in spite of medical and surgical treatment. This may be the consequence of a stenosis, which is often present below or at the same level as the fistula. The stenosis is maintained by the tension developed during swallowing so that the fistula becomes the preferential route of salivary flow and this delays its healing. We have devised a method of treatment of pharyngeal fistulas by means of dilatation of the hypopharynx tract combined with the use of fibrin sealant. The main stages of this method are as follows: (a) endoscopic brushing of the fistula edges and tramitis; (b) dilatation of the stenosis using a Savary bougie; (c) injection of fibrin sealant into the fistula lumen and infiltration in the submucous area. In the cases reported we obtained adequate patency of the hypopharynx and the closure of the fistula at the first treatment.

Introduction

The pharyngocutaneous fistula is the most frequent complication following total laryngectomy. Its incidence varies from 6% to 66% [9, 17]. The different rates are due to the various operative techniques and to the grading of tumors. As T3 and T4 tumors require an extended resection of the pharyngeal wall, they undoubtedly contribute to the increase in the rate of pharyngocutaneous fistulas [9, 21]. In irradiated patients, the rate varies from 5.9% to 87% [9, 12, 15, 18, 25], while in non-irradiated patients, fistulas occur in about 8% of cases [15]. If surgery is performed within 6–8 weeks after radiotherapy, the incidence of complications is lower than in cases operated on after a longer period of time [2, 15]. Moreover, after radiotherapy, a combined neck dissection may increase the incidence of fistulas [15]. A poor nutritional status, alcoholism, diabetes, a postoperative low level of hemoglobin (less than 12.5 g per 100 ml), immune deficits, preoperative tracheostomy, postoperative bleeding, and wound infections can likewise favor the development of pharyngocutaneous fistulas [1, 5, 9, 11, 16, 18]. As far as fistula dimensions are concerned, Bellinger [3], in his classification of pharyngostomas, stated that fistulas with a diameter of less than 8 mm should not be treated primarily with surgery. Moreover, some authors confine treatment to medication for fistulas with a diameter of less than 5 mm [24], while others wait for spontaneous healing in fistulas with a diameter of less than 1 cm [21]. Finally, Murakami et al. [20] suggested that even the smallest fistulas should be treated with rotation or transposition flaps.

The review of literature shows that approximately two thirds of fistulas close spontaneously in nonirradiated patients. The vitality of neck tissue is in fact more important than the dimensions of fistula [4, 26]. In somewhat less than one third of cases, spontaneous healing of the smallest fistulas usually takes 4 weeks [4], but a fistula may heal in 2–3 months [13, 18, 24] or may persist for more than 6 months [9].

As pharyngocutaneous fistulas occur most frequently 10–15 days after a laryngectomy, it is advisable to perform a contrasting X-ray study of the hypopharynx on days 7–10 postoperatively, before removing the nasogastric tube [8, 19]. If a fistula is impending or present, it may be enough to leave the nasogastric tube in place [15] or insert a salivary bypass tube [10, 19, 27] until the fistula heals spontaneously. Furthermore, an hypercaloric enteral nutrition together with an adequate pressure dressing around the neck may help the healing process [21, 22]. A low-pressure dressing may delay the attachment of the skin flap to the underlying tissues, just as too tight a dressing may cause decubitus lesions of the enteral tube on the mucosa [6, 26].

Many methods have been utilized in order to prevent infections and to favor the fistula closure: salivary drain [21], iodinated gauze [27], argentum nitricum [7, 14], Betadine solution [7, 9], neomycin [14], aureomycin [19], zinc peroxide [21], pellidol, fissan [23], curettage of the whole fistula tramitis in pharyngoscopy [18] and closure with stitches [15, 16].

Fistulas usually form from the upper edge of the pharyngeal suture and appear at the lower edge of the cutaneous flap near the tracheostomy [15]. The pharyngoesophagus junction is the most critical area for the presence of many stitches and in view of the anatomical shrinking that usually occurs in this digestive tract [21]. A functional shrinking may occur because during swallowing the contraction of the tongue muscles is in one direction and the contraction of the pharyngeal constrictor muscles is in the opposite one [14]. Moreover, spontaneous healing of fistula may cause a stenosis [20] or a diverticulum with further trouble in swallowing [14].

The aim of this paper is to describe a method utilized to close fistulas by means of dilatation of the hypopharyngoesophagus tract combined with the injection of fibrin glue into the fistula tramitis.

Materials and Patients

Three patients developed a pharyngocutaneous or esophagocutaneous fistula after surgery for larynx, hypopharynx, or upper cervical esophagus cancer. The fistulas were treated with picric acid and iodinated gauze for 4–6 weeks without any results. An endoscopic procedure was therefore used in order to obtain the closure of the cervical salivary fistulas. The main stages of this method were as follows:

1. Brushing of fistula edges and tramitis with an endoscopic brush
2. Dilatation of the stenosis utilizing a Savary bougie (5–15 mm in diameter) introduced by means of a driving probe
3. Injection of human fibrin glue (Tissucol; Immuno, Vienna) directly into the fistula lumen as well as infiltration into the submucous area around the fistula, utilizing an endoscopic needle (21 G/13 mm).

Fibrin glue with a coagulation time shorter than 10 s (obtained with 500 IU lyophilized thrombin) was injected through the skin orifice (1 cc) as well as through the mucous one (1 cc). Fibrin glue with a coagulation time of a few minutes (obtained with 4 IU lyophilized thrombin) was injected into the submucous area of the fistula (1 cc) utilizing an endoscopic needle.

The following endoscopes were utilized: a FB19H flexible fiberoptic bronchoscope and a FG29H flexible esophagoscope. The procedure was performed by means of a Wolf 5370 CCD Endocam television system. A nasogastric tube was maintained for 24 h after the procedure and corticosteroid therapy (2 mg betamethasone once a day) was established for 15 days.

Case 1

A 55-year-old man underwent total hemipharyngolaryngectomy, left lateral subtotal thyroidectomy, and neck dissection in December 1988. A few days after the operation, the patient underwent further surgery due to the detachment of the cutaneous flap as a result of bleeding. After the second operation, a pharyngostoma appeared as a result of tissue necrosis. In March 1989, a reconstruction of the pharyngeal wall was performed, with the outcome of a pharyngoesophagus stenosis and cutaneous fistula. In May 1989, an endoscopic dilatation was performed, with no results in another hospital. In accordance with our protocol, the fistula was treated with human fibrin glue and dilatations were performed with a Savary bougie (2–7 mm in diameter). A tube for enteral feeding (Flexiflo) was placed in position. At the following check, after 7 days, the fistula had closed, the tube was removed, and a new dilatation with Savary (caliber 7–9) was performed.

On the same day, the patient started eating again with a semisolid diet. The patient is now following treatment with periodical dilatations to maintain a diameter of about 12.8 mm.

Case 2

A 70-year-old woman underwent total laryngectomy, thyroidectomy, and cervical esophagectomy in July 1989 for an extrinsic carcinoma of the larynx. In August 1989, the patient showed a serious esophageal stenosis (2–3 mm in

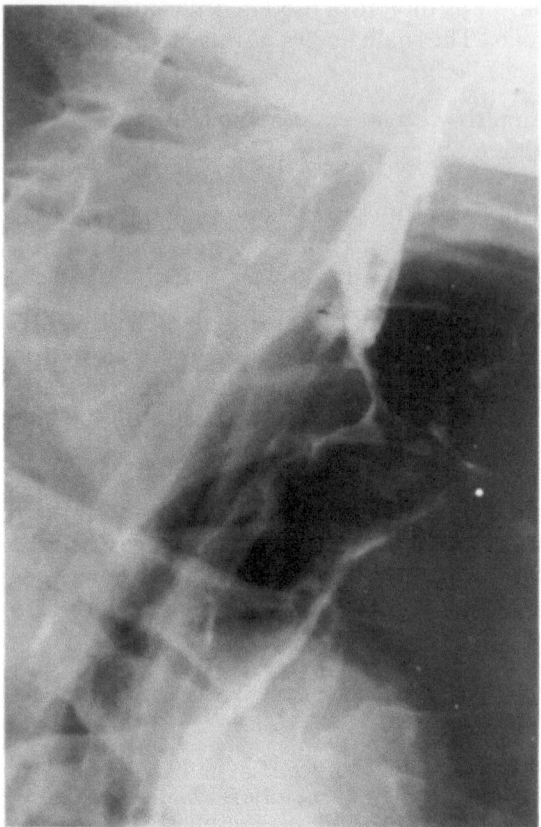

Fig. 1. A small fistula between the pharynx and the posterior aspect of the tracheostomy

diameter) combined with a cutaneous fistula. She was treated with human fibrin glue and dilatations with Savary, in accordance with our protocol. After 1 week the fistula had closed completely, the enteral tube was removed, and a new dilatation with Savary (caliber 5–9) was performed. For a period of 2 months the patient underwent periodic dilatations every 10–15 days. In November 1989, the stenotic tract reached a diameter of about 13 mm.

Case 3

A 65-year-old man, affected by a systemic vascular disease, underwent total laryngectomy and left radical neck dissection. Five days after the operation, an infiltration of saliva was found under the flap and a large fistula rapidly developed.

Fifteen days after the operation, the patient underwent further surgery in order to stitch the esophagus to the hypopharynx and to cover this area with a transposition flap. Ten days after the second operation, a small anterior fistula developed (Fig. 1). It was treated for 4 weeks with picric acid, iodinated gauze,

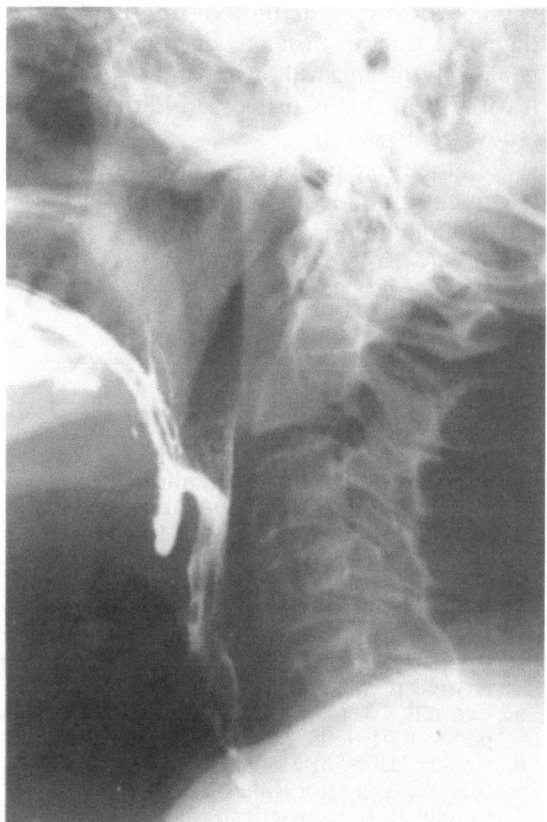

Fig. 2. An anterior neopharyngeal diverticulum remains after the closure of the pharyngotracheal fistula at the junction between the base of the tongue and the neopharynx

and compressive dressing. In accordance with our protocol, after removing the enteral tube, the patient was treated with fibrin glue and dilatations (up to 8–9 mm). The enteral tube was then placed in position again for 24 h. Since the patient ate enough, he was dismissed with corticosteroid therapy and no enteral tube the day after surgery. After two other dilatations at intervals of 7 days, the esophagus reached a diameter of 12 mm, the fistula healed, and the patient ate regularly (Fig. 2).

Discussion and Conclusion

One of the factors which causes the development of a cutaneous fistula is the tension that occurs during swallowing, because of the contraction of the tongue muscles in one direction and the contraction of the pharyngeal constrictors in the other one [25]. Stenosis of the esophagus is often present below or at the same level as the fistula, which is probably maintained by the tension developed during swallowing. The fistula becomes the preferential route of salivary flow and this delays its healing. On the basis of these considerations, we have devised a method of treating fistulas. We suggest widening the natural digestive tract in order to decrease the pressure against the pharyngoesophageal walls during swallowing and to promote the closure of the fistula by sealing it with fibrin glue. Corticosteroid therapy is also established in order to prevent a new cicatrization.

In the three patients reported, we obtained closure of the fistula at the first treatment and adequate patency of the esophagus for semisolid alimentation. Further dilatations were performed to reach regular alimentation. No more cutaneous fistulas developed.

References

1. Andre P, Pinel J, Laccourreye P (1964) Incidence des techniques de fermeture et de drainage sur les suites opératoires en chirurgie pharyngée et laryngée. (A propos de 108 interventions). Ann Otolaryngol 81: 315–326
2. Bahadur S, Kacker SK (1985) Etiology and management of pharyngeal fistulae following laryngectomy. In: Meyers E (ed) New dimensions in otorhinolaryngology-head and neck surgery, vol. 2. Elsevier Science, Amsterdam, pp 395–397
3. Bellinger CG (1971) Classification of pharyngostomas: a guideline for closure. Plast Reconstr Surg 47: 54–60
4. Briant TDR (1975) Spontaneous pharyngeal fistula and wound infection following laryngectomy. Laryngoscope 85: 829–834
5. Centrell RW (1978) Pharyngeal fistula: prevention and treatment. Laryngoscope 88: 1204–1208
6. Conley JJ (1956) Management of pharyngostoma, esophagostoma and associated fistulae. Ann Otol Rhinol Laryngol 65: 76–91
7. Connel JF Jr, Roussellot LM (1964) Povidone-iodine. Extensive surgical evaluation of a new antiseptic agent. Am J Surg 108: 849–855
8. De Jong PC, Struben WH (1970) Pharyngeal fistulae after laryngectomy. J Laryngol Otol 84: 897–904
9. Dedo DD, Alonso WA, Ogura JM (1975) Incidence, predisposing factors and outcome of pharyngocutaneous fistulas complicating head and neck cancer surgery. Ann Otol Rhinol Laryngol 84: 833–840
10. Hicks JN, Peters GE (1982) A saliva shunting technique for low anterior neck pharyngeal fistulas after laryngectomy. An emergency procedure. Laryngoscope 92: 594–595
11. Horgan EC, Dedo DD (1979) Prevention of major and minor fistulae after laryngectomy. Laryngoscope 89: 250–260
12. Joseph DL, Shumrick DA (1973) Risks of head and neck surgery in previously irradiated patients. Arch Otolaryngol 97: 381–384
13. Kent SE, Liu KC, Das Gupta AR (1985) Post-laryngectomy pharyngo-cutaneous fistulae. J Laryngol Otol 99: 1005–1008
14. Kirchner JA, Scatliff JH (1962) Disabilities resulting from healed salivary fistula. Arch Otolaryngol 75: 60–68
15. Kleinsasser O (1988) Tumors of the larynx and hypopharynx. Thieme, Stuttgart, pp 190–206
16. Lavelle RJ, Maw AR (1972) The aetiology of post-laryngectomy pharyngo-cutaneous fistulae. J Laryngol Otol 86: 85–93
17. Lundgren J, Olofsson J (1979) Pharyngocutaneous fistulae following total laryngectomy. Clin Otolaryngol 4: 13–23
18. Maw AR, Lavelle RJ (1974) An evaluation of the causes and management of pharyngocutaneous fistulae. Min Otorinolaringol 24: 75–81

19. Montgomery WW (1986) Current modifications of the salivary bypass tube and tracheal T-tube. Ann Otol Rhinol Laryngol 95: 121–125
20. Murakami Y, Ikari T, Haraguchi S, Okada K, Maruyama T, Tateno M (1988) Repair of salivary fistula after reconstruction of pharyngoesophagus. Arch Otolaryngol 114: 770–774
21. Myers EN (1972) The management of pharyngocutaneous fistula. Arch Otolaryngol 95: 10–17
22. Narne S, Ancona E, Tremolada C, Bardini R, Peracchia A (1987) Carcinoma dell'ipofaringe e dell'esofago cervicale: risultati del trattamento chirurgico. Dal 1967 al 1984. Abstract 74, Congr Naz SIO e Ch. C-F, Milano, 27–30 Maggio 1987
23. Naumann HH (1978) Kopf- und Hals-Chirurgie, vol 1: Hals. Thieme, Stuttgart, p 268
24. Raman R, Ariayanayagam C (1987) Closure of orocutaneous and pharyngocutaneous fistulas. Plast Reconstr Surg 79: 310
25. Smits RG, Krause CJ, McCabe BF (1972) Complications associated with combined therapy of oral and pharyngeal neoplasm. Ann Otol Rhinol Laryngol 81: 496–500
26. Stell PM, Cooney TC (1974) Management of fistulae of the head and neck after radical surgery. J Laryngol Otol 88: 819–834
27. Vogel DH, Strong MS (1978) Use of a T-tube in management of a pharyngeal fistula after laryngectomy. Plast Reconstr Surg 62: 573–575

Minimally Invasive Surgery with a New Distending Diverticuloscope and Use of Fibrin Sealing for Endoscopic Laser Dissection of Zenker's Diverticulum

H. Weerda and K.-H. Ahrens

Abstract

In the treatment of the pharyngeal pouch, diverticulectomy and endoscopic diverticulotomy are generally accepted forms of treatment. The latter can lead to severe bleeding and mediastinitis. Therefore, we have enlarged the preoperative diagnosis by a digital substraction angiography (DSA) of the aortic arch. Simultaneous contrast filling of the pouch enables us to find out the exact position of the blood vessels in relation to the bar. Our development of a spreadable diverticuloscope, the use of a CO_2 laser and an operation microscope guarantees best endoscopic working conditions. Postoperative sealing of the edge of the wound with fibrin glue reduces possible postoperative bleeding and mediastinitis, the risks of which we further reduced by antibiotic prophylaxis and tube feeding for 8 days. During and after the treatment of 15 patients, not a single complication has arisen.

Introduction

Zenker's diverticulum is a special type of pharyngocele. Mucous membrane from the hypopharynx folds out through a muscle gap in Killian's triangle over the lower part of the cricopharyngeal muscle.

Cinematography shows the preferred filling of the sac of the diverticulum. After relaxation of Killian's muscle, the chyme flows into the compressed esophagus, which is displaced ventrally by the diverticulum. In the case of growing processes, oral feeding can become impossible, as in one case of a giant diverticulum in a 90-year-old patient.

Nowadays, two different methods are mainly applied to treat this disease: (1) diverticulectomy with myotomy of the Killian's muscle via an external approach and (2) endoscopic diverticulotomy with splitting of the threshold between the esophagus and the sac of the diverticulum, which was developed by Mosher in 1917 [1].

The main complications of diverticulectomy via an external approach are paralysis of the recurrent laryngeal nerve, wound healing impairments, and mediastinitis.

Mediastinitis and, in rare cases, arterial bleedings from aberrant vessels have been observed in endoscopic splitting of the threshold. The fear of these

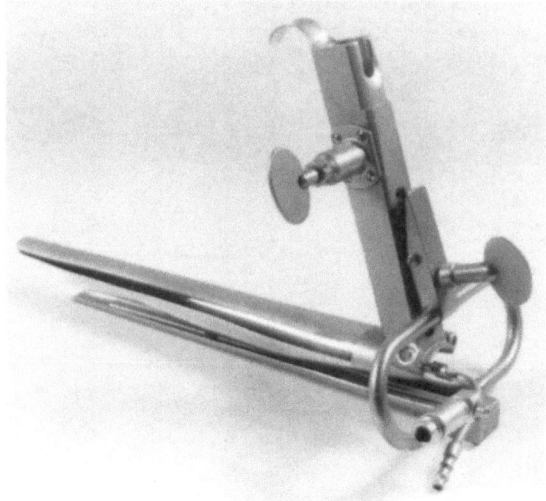

Fig. 1. New distending diverticuloscope (K. Storz, Tuttlingen, Germany)

fatal bleedings is the reason why many surgeons restrict the application to high-risk patients.

Comparing the mortality rates of both methods, external diverticulectomy presents a risk twice as high as that of endoscopic diverticulotomy. When performing endoscopic splitting of the threshold, these risks can be minimized by an enlarged preoperative diagnostic, the development of better instruments, and a sophistication of surgical techniques with a new distending diverticuloscope (Fig. 1) [2].

Methods

After diagnosis of Zenker's diverticulum, we perform a digital substraction angiography of the cervical vessels with simultaneous inspection of the diverticulum to exclude aberrant vessels in the threshold of the diverticulum. Alternatively, we use a Doppler sonographic evaluation of these vessels.

Because of the bad viewing conditions in closed pipes, we developed a special distending diverticuloscope (Fig. 1), which creates optimal viewing and working conditions, especially in the case of nontactile laser-surgical splitting of the threshold.

The two branches, one positioned above the other, are placed in the esophagus and the sac of the diverticulum. This distending diverticuloscope can be opened in its front and back part. Thus it allows an optimal adaptation to different patients and different sizes of diverticuli.

After insertion of the instrument and putting the support on a vertically adjustable table, the two branches are spread in the diverticulum and in the esophagus respectively. Then, the threshold of the diverticulum hovers and is easily surveyed between the esophagus on top and the spread sac of the diverticulum underneath (Fig. 2).

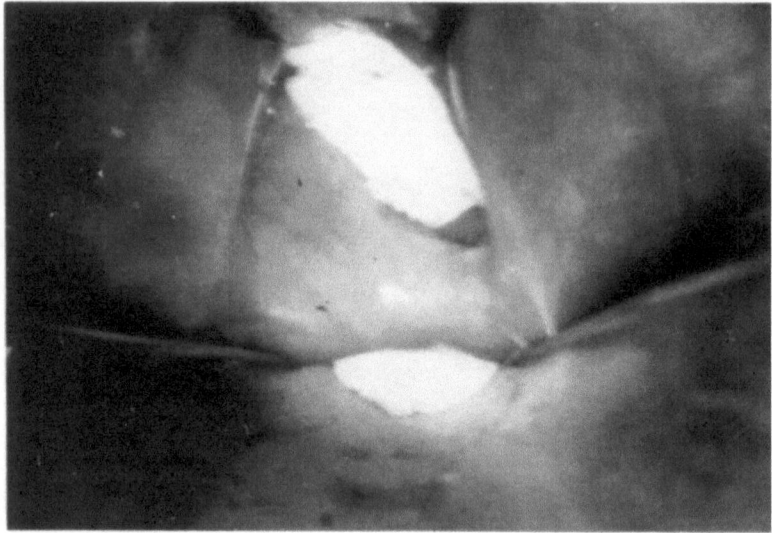

Fig. 2. Threshold of the diverticulum hovers between the spread branches of the distending diverticuloscope

Before performing laser-surgical splitting of the threshold, an efficient flue is installed at the lower leaf. After covering the face with moist cloth and inserting a moist compress into the esophagus (Fig. 2), the actual threshold splitting is not very time consuming.

Microscopically, the separation of the muscle fibers of the Killian's muscle can be clearly seen. The nontactile cutting with the CO_2 laser guarantees an optimal overview and does not cause heavy bleeding.

After threshold splitting, the entrance of the esophagus on top and the posterior wall of the diverticulum form one common compartment.

To cover the mediastinum, the surrounding mucous membrane should be glued with fibrin glue over the cut threshold of the diverticulum.

Via a flexible tube we press fibrin glue (Tissucol Duo S, human fibrinogen, human thrombin, steam-treated) directly into the wound. Then the mucous membrane of the diverticulum and the esophagus are adapted directly above the wound. Thus the initially gaping wound is reduced to a minimal lesion of the mucous membrane, which helps to prevent mediastinitis.

The postoperative follow-up kinematography, which we perform approximately 1 month after the intervention, shows a free flow of contrast medium in comparison to the preoperative finding with a distinct retention of chyme. The small rest depot drains without problems through the open sphincter of the esophagus. It causes no functional complaints.

Conclusion

The endoscopic splitting of the threshold, as described, presents a good alternative to external diverticulectomy. A great advantage of this minimally invasive and therefore tissue-preserving intervention is the minimal strain to the usually elderly patient, as well as short hospitalization time and lower complication rates.

References

1. Mosher HP (1917) Webs and pouches of the esophagus. Surg Gynecol Obstet 25: 175–197
2. Weerda H, Schlenter W, Ahrens K-H, Bach-Quang M (1988) A new distending diverticuloscope for endoscopic treatment of Zenkers diverticulum with CO_2-laser. Arch Otorhinolaryngol 245: 384

Fibrin Sealing in Endolaryngeal Surgery

H. E. ECKEL

Abstract

The application of fibrin sealant in endolaryngeal surgery may have various objectives. The main goal in patients with bleeding disorders is to compensate for impaired primary hemostasis.

A second objective is the fixation of mucosal flaps, thus obviating the need for endolaryngeal sutures.

A further application concerns the laser resection of larynx carcinoma. This recent surgical approach often requires the removal of important parts of the endolaryngeal structures and exposure of the thyroid lamina to ensure complete resection of the tumor. The formation of granulation tissue and webs in the area of the anterior commissure is a frequent complication of such operations and even intensive postoperative treatment can not effectively reduce this troublesome disruption of wound healing in the larynx. The effect of fibrin sealing of endolaryngeal wounds was studied in 59 patients following laser resection of larynx carcinoma and 32 patients following resection of granulation tissue and webs in the anterior commissure. Sealing of endolaryngeal wounds and especially of exposed cartilage was found to improve regular epitheliziation and to reduce the formation of webs. These results confirm experimental findings showing that the wound healing process can be accelerated if the wound is covered by a fibrin clot. Local infections or adverse reactions were not observed. Fibrin sealant has good adhesive properties and the sealed wounds have shown an optimal healing tendency. Primary wound healing was found to be both superior to and more rapid than the healing of endolaryngeal wounds managed without fibrin sealant.

Introduction

The application of fibrin sealant in endolaryngeal surgery may have various objectives. The main goal in patients with bleeding disorders is to compensate for impaired primary hemostasis. As suturing and electrocoagulation are both traumatic to the vocal cords and not reliable, wound sealing is the best method for the prevention of postoperative bleeding in patients with impaired hemostasis who undergo endolaryngeal surgery [8, 18, 24].

A second objective is the fixation of mucosal flaps, thus obviating the need for endolaryngeal sutures. This technique is frequently applied in endoscopic lateral cordopexy, submucous cordectomy, or arytenoidectomy for the treatment of bilateral abductor paralysis of the vocal cords [3, 21–22]. These endoscopic procedures have proved to be more effective and less traumatic than extralaryngeal surgery. The muscosal flaps are best secured in the desired position by the use of fibrin glue.

A further application concerns the laser or EHT resection of larynx carcinoma [4, 6]. This recent surgical approach often requires the removal of important parts of the endolaryngeal structures and exposure of the thyroid lamina to ensure complete resection of the tumor. The formation of granulation tissue and webs in the area of the anterior commissure is a frequent complication of such operations. Even intensive postoperative treatment cannot effectively reduce this troublesome disruption of wound healing in the larynx.

Surgical Concept

Since the first applications of the carbon dioxide laser for the treatment of carcinoma of the larnyx by Strong and Jako [27], the use of the laser has found wider acceptance in treating this condition, as pointed out by Steiner [24–26], Rudert [22], and others [10, 17]. Our present indications for laser surgery of larynx carcinoma are glottic, supraglottic, and subglottic carcinomas up to stage T2. In our view, indications for palliative laser surgery are rare, since a total laryngectomy, usually in combination with a neck dissection and a postoperative radiotherapy, allows a curative approach even to very extended cancers of the larynx.

Endolaryngeal laser surgery is not a solitary management for the treatment of larynx carcinomas. Additional therapy includes neck dissections in patients with metastatic lymphadenopathy and postoperative radiotherapy in individual cases. Up to now there have been some reports on endolaryngeal laser surgery for T1 and a few on T2 cancers of the larynx, but only limited information is so far available on the results of laser surgery for T2 tumors of the glottis and for supraglottic tumors [17, 24–26].

Since 1986 we have developed four different categories of laser partial larynx resections according to the differing locations and sizes of glottic tumors [6, 28]. These types of resection are also used for glottic tumors showing subglottic extension.

For carcinoma in situ, a type I excision is performed to resect the vocal cord mucosa, leaving the vocal muscle intact (Fig. 1a). The excision thus corresponds to conventional microlaryngoscopic decortication of the vocal cords. It starts at the arytenoid regions and proceeds to the anterior commissure. The lesion is thus completely removed for histological study. The outcome is a scar formation that replaces the vocal cord mucosa, leaving an anatomically and functionally close to normal larynx.

A T1a tumor requires a type II resection (Fig. 1b): one vocal cord is resected completely, leaving the anterior third of the other vocal cord and the

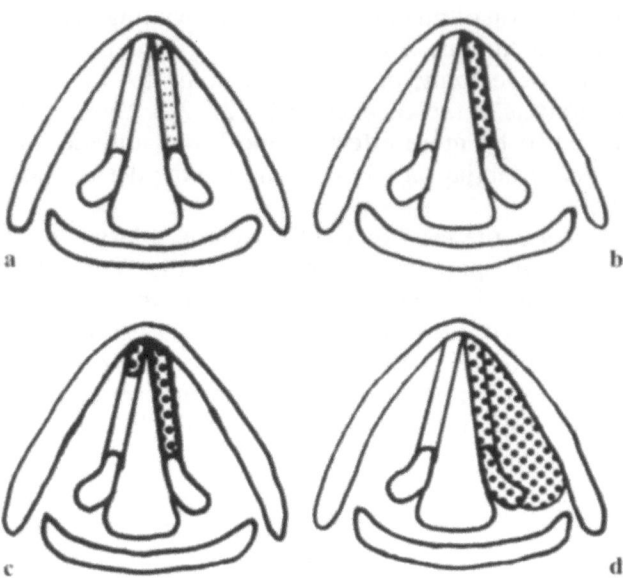

Fig. 1a–d. Endolaryngeal resections. **a** Type I (decortication of the vocal cord). **b** Type II (simple cordectomy). **c** Type III (extended cordectomy). **d** Type IV (resection of vocal and false cord)

arytenoid intact. The resection equals a conventional cordectomy in extent of the excision. T1b tumors are managed by a type III resection including the anterior commissure and Broyle's ligament down to the thyroid cartilage, to the subglottic region including the cricothyroid membrane, and the upper margin of the cricoid cartilage as a borderline (Fig. 1 c). The extension of the en bloc excision reaches up to the arytenoid cartilage or can even include it, with preservation of the posterior mucosa. A T2 tumor requires a type IV resection ("laryngeal exenteration") including all the endolaryngeal structures down to the thyroid and cricoid cartilage and to the cricothyroid membrane as well as to the arytenoid cartilage, which can be included on one side (Fig. 1 d). The excision can be more extended in the craniocaudal extent than conventional frontolateral partial laryngectomies, while the cartilaginous framework is left intact.

Type III and IV resections may include an arytenoidectomy of one side if the extension of the tumor requires it, and may be performed uni- or bilaterally. The resected specimen is mounted to a cork plate and anatomically marked according to the excision area for pathological and histological investigations. Troublesome granulation tissue formation can be markedly diminished by using fibrin glue to seal the exposed cartilage. This also contributes to minimizing postoperative bleeding [14].

A supraglottic cancer can be treated by endolaryngeal laser surgery as well, but up to now there have been an insufficient number of cases to establish resection types comparable to the glottic cancer laser resections. There is only minor postoperative discomfort and swallowing problems, and a tracheotomy is usually not required.

As any partial larynx resection for carcinoma has a certain risk of recurrence, regular and intensive follow-up investigations are absolutely necessary. Therefore, microlaryngoscopic examinations under general anesthesia with multiple biopsies are performed 6 and 12 weeks after resection. Laryngoscopy with a 90° zoom endoscope and cytological smear as well as voice and speech investigations are carried out. Optional examinations include sonography of the throat and neck biopsies under local anesthesia, flexible endoscopy, and an endoscopic methylene blue deglutition analysis.

Patients and Methods

The effect of fibrin sealing of the endolaryngeal wounds was studied in 59 patients following laser resection of larynx carcinoma. In a second trial, 32 patients had granulations and webs removed during control microlaryngoscopy. The resulting wounds were coated with fibrin glue (Tissucol Duo S, human fibrinogen, human thrombin, steam-treated) in all these patients and the effect on wound healing was judged 6 weeks later at a second microlaryngoscopic evaluation.

The two components were usually applied separately (fibrinogen first, followed by a layer of thrombin), but can be used simultaneously by means of the Duplocath application catheter device with separated injection canals. This device has been custom designed for the use in minimally invasive surgery and has proven to be a simple and reliable tool for the application of fibrin glue in endolaryngeal surgery. Excess fibrin glue is suctioned at the end of the sealing process, and a 5-min period should be allowed between the end of the sealing procedure and extubation at the end of the surgical intervention. Otherwise, the fibrin net may be disrupted by the ventilation tube as it slides back out of the trachea, resulting in an insufficient sealing result. The amount of fibrin glue needed to cover the endolaryngeal wounds ranges from 0.5 to 1 ml.

Results

The amount of granulation tissue and the formation of webs in the anterior commissure was judged during routine control microlaryngoscopy 6 weeks after transoral laser resection of glottic carcinoma. A total of 32 patients had their endolaryngeal wounds covered with fibrin glue at the end of the surgical procedure and 28 were left without wound sealing. In the first group, the amount of granulation tissue and the incidence of webs was clearly lower than in the control group (Fig. 2). Of the 32 patients who had their wounds covered with fibrin sealant following the resection of granulation tissue and webs, 14 showed a clear improvement of the healing process on reassessment, 18 were found unchanged, and none had deteriorated (Fig. 3). Local infections or adverse reactions were not observed, although fibrin glue is an ideal culture medium for bacteria.

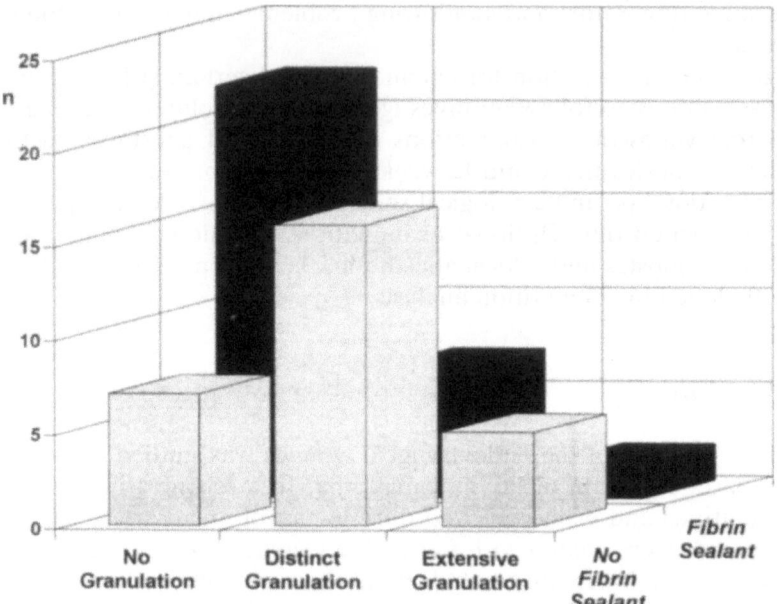

Fig. 2. Endolaryngeal granulation tissue 6 weeks after transoral resection of larynx carcinoma ($n = 59$)

Discussion

From 1972 onwards, there has been a number of reports on the use of endolaryngeal laser surgery for the treatment of larynx carcinomas. While most of them dealt with the treatment of small cancers of the vocal cords [2, 7, 9, 13, 14, 16, 29], some suggested that more extended cancers of the larynx

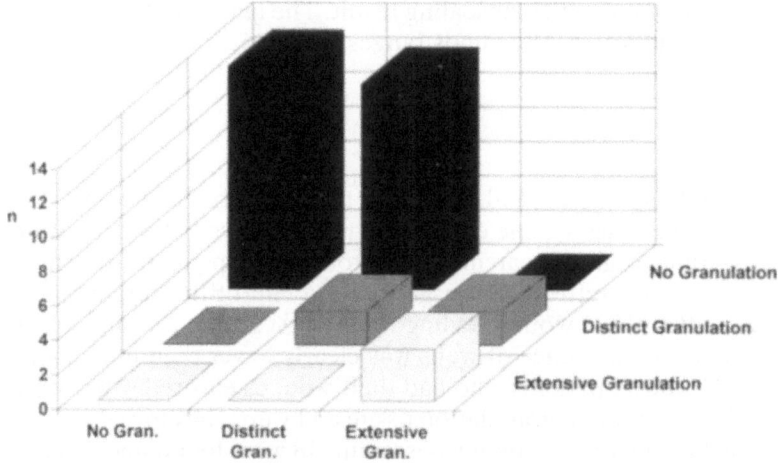

Fig. 3. Wound healing following resection of granulations and wound sealing ($n = 32$) (x-axis = preoperative findings)

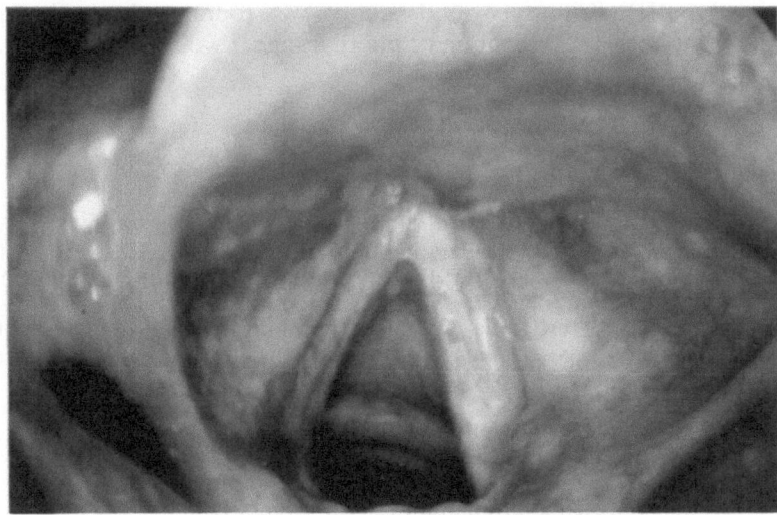

Fig. 4. Endolaryngeal aspect following endolaryngeal resection type II

could also be accessible to laser surgery [6, 17, 25]. Ahead of all other investigators, Steiner [24–26] stated that transoral laser removal even of extensive neoplasms is not only an oncologically safe procedure, but can lead to excellent results, as healthy mucosa from the margins of the wound migrates over the defect and finally covers it. One of the problems of this surgical approach is that open wounds that are left to secondary healing have a tendency to grow granulation tissue, which delays and complicates regular epithelization. Sealing of the endolaryngeal wounds and especially of the exposed cartilages was found to improve this epitheliziation process and to reduce the formation of webs [5]. These results confirm experimental findings showing that the wound healing process can be accelerated if the wound is covered by a fibrin clot [1, 12, 20, 23]. These experimental findings suggest that the fibrin net in a wound appears to act as a scaffold for migrating fibroblasts and shows a significant fibroblast-stimulating effect. Fibrin clots are therefore believed to provide ideal conditions for the migration of fibroblasts and capillary vessels and may contribute to faster and less complicated healing of burn wounds.

Conclusion

Some endolaryngeal procedures can be simplified by the use of fibrin glue [8, 11, 15, 18, 19, 21] or their functional results may be improved [3, 5]. The application of fibrin sealant is easy to accomplish and reliable. Adverse reactions have so far not been observed. The risk of spreading HIV or hepatitis viruses is believed to be nonexistant [12]. In our own experience, fibrin sealant has good adhesive properties and the sealed wounds have shown an optimal healing tendency (Fig. 4; endolaryngeal aspect following endolaryngeal resection type II). Primary wound healing was found to be both superior to and more rapid than the healing of endolaryngeal wounds managed without fibrin sealant.

References

1. Brändstedt S, Frank F, Olson PS (1980) The fibrin net formed in a wound appears to act as a scaffold for migrating fibroblasts. Eur Surg Res 12: 18–21
2. Burian K, Höfler H (1979) Zur mikrochirurgischen Therapie von Stimmband-Karzinomen mit dem CO_2-Laser. Laryngol Rhinol Otol 58: 551–556
3. Eckel HE (1991) Die laserchirurgische mikrolaryngoskopische Glottiserweiterung zur Behandlung der beidseitigen Recurrensparese – Operationstechnik und Ergebnisse. Laryngol Rhinol Otol 70: 17–20
4. Eckel HE, Dollinger K, Feaux de la Croix G, Reidenbach HD, Thumfart WF (1992) An electrohydrothermosation system for application in endolaryngeal and enoral surgery. Eur Surg Res 132: 302–308
5. Eckel HE, Thumfart WF (1988) Synechieprophylaxe und -therapie nach Laserresektion von Kehlkopftumoren. Laryng Rhinol Otol 67: 116–117
6. Eckel HE, Thumfart WF (1992) Laser surgery for the treatment of larynx carcinoma. Indications, techniques and preliminary results. Ann Otol Rhinol Laryngol 101: 113–118
7. Elner A, Fex S (1988) Carbon dioxide laser as a primary treatment of glottic T1S and T1A tumours. Acta Otolaryngol (Stockh) 449: 135–139
8. Gastpar H, Kastenbauer ER, Bebehani H (1979) Erfahrungen mit einem humanen Fibrinkleber bei operativen Eingriffen im Kopf-Halsbereich. Laryngol Rhinol 58: 389–399
9. Hirano M, Hirade Y, Kawasaki H (1985) Vocal function following carbon dioxide laser surgery for glottic carcinoma. Ann Otol Rhinol Laryngol 94: 232–235
10. Hoefler H (1983) Ergebnisse der CO_2-Laserbehandlung von Larynxmalignomen. Wien Klin Wochenschr 95: 545–547
11. Isshiki N, Taira T, Nose K, Kojima H (1991) Surgical treatment of laryngeal web with mucosa graft. Ann Otol Rhinol Laryngol 100: 95–100
12. Kaeser A, Dum N (1988) Grundlegende Aspekte des Fibrinklebers. In: Zellner PR (ed) Fibrinklebung in der Verbrennungschirurgie/Plastischen Chirurgie. Springer, Berlin Heidelberg New York
13. Koufman JA (1986) The endoscopic management of early squamous carcinoma of the vocal cord with the carbon dioxide surgical laser: clinical experience and a proposed subclassification. Otolaryngol Head Neck Surg 95: 531–537
14. Krespi YP, Meltzer CJ (1989) Laser surgery for vocal cord carcinoma involving the anterior commissure. Ann Otol Rhinol Laryngol 98: 105–109
15. Martin F, Spitzner H, Gastpar H (1981) Endolaryngeale Eingriffe unter Verwendung hochkonzentrierten humanen Fibrinogens als Gewebekleber. Laryngol Rhinol 60: 368–372
16. McGuirt WF, Koufman JA (1987) Endoscopic laser surgery. An alternative in laryngeal cancer treatment. Arch Otolaryngol Head Neck Surg 113: 501–505
17. Motta G, Villari G, Motta G Jr, Ripa G, Salerno G (1986) The CO_2 laser in the laryngeal microsurgery. Acta Otolaryngol (Stockh) 433 [Suppl]: 1–30
18. Naumann C (1989) Der Einsatz von Fibrinklebern in der Kehlkopf-Chirurgie. In: Gosepath J (ed) Aktuelle Methoden der Gewebeklebung im Kopf-Hals-Bereich. Urban and Schwarzenberg, Baltimore
19. Naumann C (1984) Fibrinklebung in der Larynxchirurgie. In: Scheele J (ed) Fibrinklebung. Springer, Berlin Heidelberg New York, pp 238–242
20. Redl H, Schlag G, Dinges HP (1985) Vergleich zweier Fibrinkleber. Einfluß ionischer Zusätze auf Fibrinstruktur sowie Morphologie und Wachstum menschlicher Fibroblasten. Med Welt 36: 769–776

21. Romeo G (1989) Applications of Tissucol in larynx, trachea and neck surgery. Rev Laryngol (Bordeaux) 110: 121–122
22. Rudert H (1988) Laser-Chirurgie in der HNO-Heilkunde. Laryngol Rhinol Otol 67: 261–268
23. Schlag G, Redl H, Thurnher M, Dinges HP (1986) The importance of fibrin in wound repair. In: Schlag G, Redl H (eds) Otorhinolaryngology. Springer, Berlin Heidelberg New York (Fibrin sealant in operative medicine, vol I), pp 3–12
24. Steiner W (1987) Laserchirurgie im HNO-Bereich (Laserchirurgie zur Behandlung maligner Tumoren des oberen Aerodigestivtraktes). Arch Oto Rhinol Laryngol [Suppl] II: 8–18
25. Steiner W (1988) Experience in endoscopic laser surgery of malignant tumours of the upper aero-digestive tract. Adv Oto Rhinol Laryngol 39: 135–144
26. Steiner W, Aurbach G, Ambrosch P (1991) Minimally invasive therapy in otorhinolaryngology and head and neck surgery. Minim Invas Ther 1: 57–70
27. Strong MS, Jako GJ (1972) Laser surgery in the larynx. Early clinical experiences with continuous CO_2 laser. Ann Otol 81: 791–798
28. Thumfart WF, Eckel HE (1990) Endolaryngeale Laser-Chirurgie zur Behandlung von Kehlkopfkarzinomen. Das aktuelle Kölner-Konzept. HNO 38: 174–178.
29. Wetmore SJ, Key JM, Suen JY (1986) Laser therapy for T1 glottic carcinoma of the larynx. Arch Otolaryngol Head Neck Surg 112: 853–855

Use of Tissucol in Laryngology and in Head and Neck Surgery

M. REMACLE and G. LAWSON

Abstract

We use Tissucol in microsurgery of the larynx either after dissection of the mucosa or following mucosal resection with extensive stripping of the vocal fold or neighboring structures.

- Dissection: wide sulcus, furrows, Reinke's edema, scars
- Resection: cysts, resection of epithelium for keratosis, cordectomies I to III, arytenoidectomy, resection of ventricular folds, resection of laryngocele, granuloma

For microsurgery of the pharynx:
- Vaporization of lymphoid tissue at the base of tongue
- Resection of uncovered epithelial surface
- Zenker's diverticulum

In the head and neck:
- Strengthening and covering of pharyngoesophageal sutures after total laryngectomy or after reconstruction by means of flaps
- Covering of microsutures in blood vessels and nerves

During microsurgery, fibrin sealant is applied through a catheter guided by microforceps. Small quantities are used, from 0.2–0.3 to 2 ml. Quantities can be greater in arytenoidectomy or cordectomy.

The aim is, above all, to apply a protective dressing that will decrease diffuse postoperative bleeding and guide cicatrization, while avoiding the risk of granulomatous formations or regrowths.

The technique is the same as that for microsurgery of the pharynx. In cases of Zenker's diverticulum, when the diverticuloesophageal wall is laid flat, Tissucol provides an additional precaution against the risk of fistula formation and mediastinitis.

The administration of Tissucol in head and neck surgery is carried out in the classic manner by syringe, with the quantities used being, of course, greater (4 to 5 ml).

Is the administration of Tissucol truly indispensable in these indications? One cannot claim that to be so, since such techniques were already practiced before Tissucol was developed. Nevertheless, it does present a useful additional means of promoting good healing through its protection of exposed areas or by strengthening sutures.

Introduction

Fibrin sealant plays a twofold role in laryngology: it can be used both as protective dressing and as glue [1]. As protective dressing, it reduces postoperative bleeding and edema, prevents pyogenic granulomatous formations, guides cicatrization and covers and strengthens the tissues. Used as an adhesive, it glues in place the microflaps and strengthens the sutures.

We use it for various purposes in phonosurgery and for other indications in laryngeal microsurgery, as well as in hypopharyngeal microsurgery and head and neck surgery by external approach.

Materials and Method

Whether for microsurgery by endoscopic approach or for surgery by external approach, a clear distinction can be made between the use of a fibrin seal as an accessory and its invaluable complementary use, where it proves to be a most useful additional aid. Differences in the indications result from the extent of the surface microsurgically resected or dissected, as well as from the tissue quality and the solidity of surgery performed by external approach.

Fibrin sealant is used in phonosurgery when treatment requires dissection of the lesion: wide sulcus or furrows, Reinke's edema, scars, microwebs. It is an accessory in cases of nodule resections, polyps, cysts, small sulci etc.

It is systematically used for other indications in laryngeal microsurgery, whether involving dissection or resection, according to the extent of the area treated. The indications for dissection essentially concern the creation of surgical flaps (synechiae, webs). The indications for resection are represented by endoscopic cordectomies of types I–III [4], arytenoidectomies or posterior enlargements of the respiratory tract, resections of the ventricular folds, laryngoceles, granulomas etc.

The essential indication in cases of hypopharyngeal microsurgery is Zenker's diverticulum [3]. Fibrin sealant can also be used to vaporize lingual tonsillitis or for coating a stripped surface following resection of the mucosa.

In head and neck surgery where it is essential to coat and to reinforce the tissues, fibrin sealant is to be recommended for strengthening the sutures of the pharyngoesophageal tube in cases of total (pharyngo)laryngectomy recovery following radiotherapy; for covering mucosal defects after partial and reconstructional laryngectomy; for covering the canal and lymphatic vessel during neck dissections, particularly where these have had to be sutured following an injury; for covering microsutures of veins and nerves, as well as buccopharyngeal mucosal defects in cases of hemostatic affections. Fibrin sealant can be used also for many other conditions, e.g., to coat the sutured areas of musculocutaneous flaps and total or partial (pharyngo)laryngectomies.

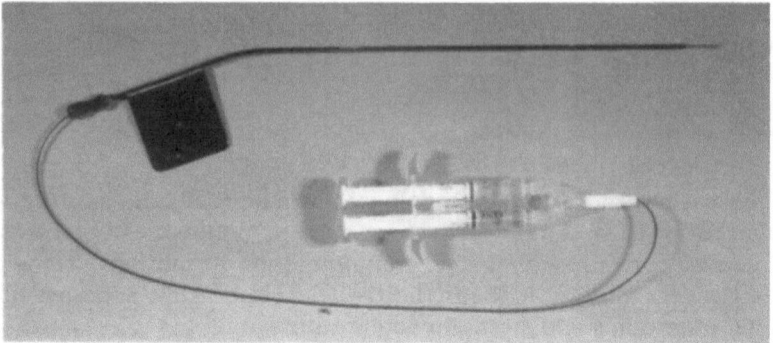

Fig. 1. System for applying fibrin sealant in pharyngolaryngeal microsurgery. The double syringe serving as mixer-injector is connected to a catheter. This catheter is introduced through the suction tube customarily used in microsurgery

In microsurgery, fibrin sealant is applied by means of a catheter (Abbot drum-cartridge catheter) passed through a suction tube of the type generally used in laryngeal microsurgery (Fig. 1) The suction tube enables the catheter to be guided more easily than is possible by means of wide-edged microforceps.

The quantities used are generally small (0.2–2 ml). Fibrin sealant is prepared so as to take effect slowly. The quantities used for surgery by external approach are, of course, greater (2–4 ml or more). Application takes place by an injection system using a device supplied by the maker (Tissucol; Immuno, Vienna). A rapid set is then preferable to a slow one.

Whatever the indication, the surface for application should be dried as thoroughly as possible by an efficient aspiration, otherwise adherence may be inadequate and the fibrin sealant may easily become loose, after a bout of severe coughing, for instance. Application is easy in indications for resection; it suffices for the sealant to be deposited in place and then for its adherence to be verified by observing the whitening that takes place. If high-frequency jet ventilation [2] is used in microsurgery, the anesthetist will be asked to shut off the ventilation during setting, after, of course, having verified that there is adequate oxygenation; otherwise, the fibrin seal might be rejected before having become fixed.

In the case of application after dissection of a microflap (Fig. 2a–c), whether by microinstrument or CO_2 laser micropoint, it is necessary to press the microflap firmly to the zone of adhesion. The pressure thus effected will expulse the excess fibrin sealant.

The purpose of fibrin sealant for the Zenker's diverticulum is to provide an additional precaution against the risk of fistula formation or mediastinitis. It is

---

Fig. 2a–c. Stages of treatment for an extensive sulcus glottidis (furrow). **a** The sulcus ▶ glottidis is explored and smoothed flat. **b** It is then dissected by laser CO_2 micropoint, beam of 280 μ, shoot by shoot, at an intensity of 3 W in superpulse. **c** The fibrin seal is applied afterwards at the level of the dissection zone by means of the catheter inserted into an suction tube

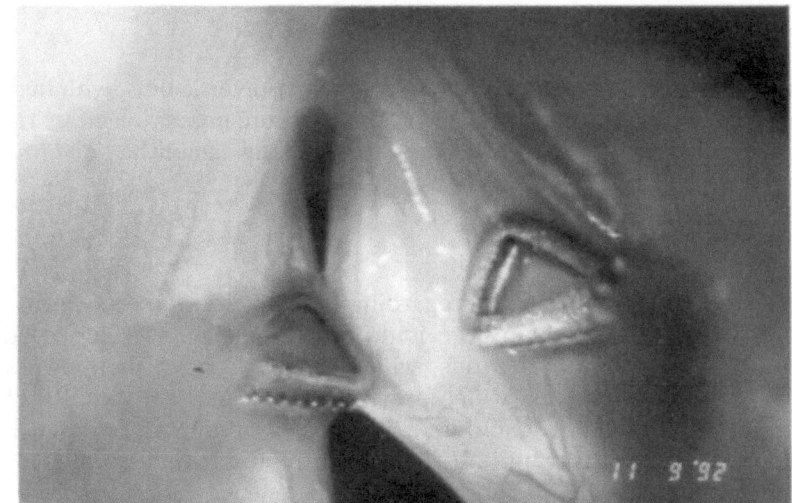

a

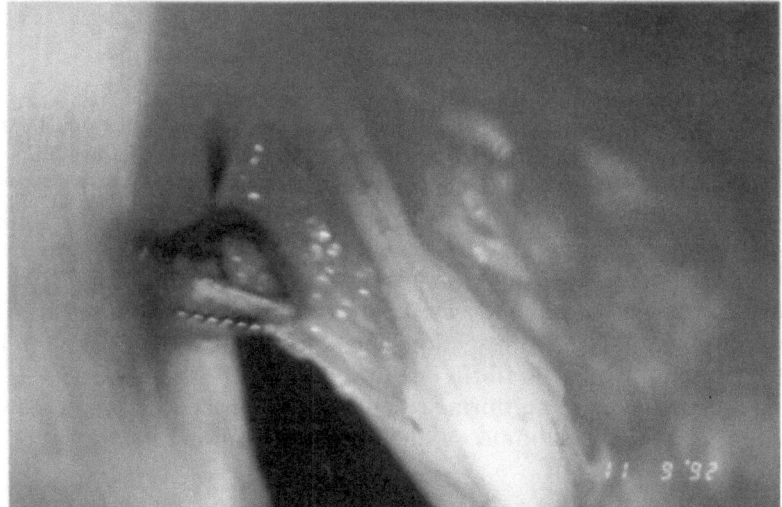

b

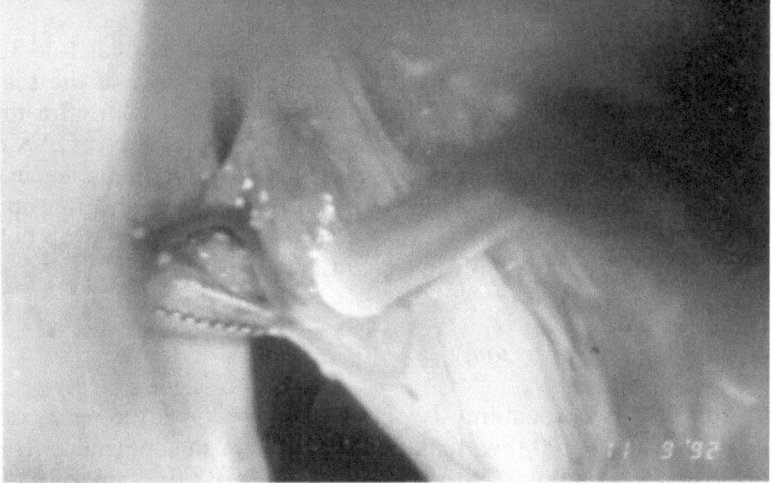

c

indeed known that, in this intervention, it is the peridiverticulitis, with the secondary fibrosis that this entails, which will normally ensure imperviousness. The fibrin seal gives additional security, particularly for less long-established diverticula.

Presentation of Typical Cases

It is difficult to present casuistics regarding the contribution of a fibrin sealant in laryngology. What is given here is no more than an overview of therapy intended to facilitate interventions, which obviously have their own specific levels of failure and success, which previously took place without the help of fibrin glue. That is why it would appear to be of greater interest to describe some representative interventions, illustrating how it is that fibrin sealant can facilitate surgery and the postoperative consequences.

Polyp of the Vocal Fold

Surgery for polyp of the vocal fold takes place under general anesthesia, with direct laryngoscopy and high-frequency jet ventilation. Under microscopic view, the polyp is resected by CO_2 laser micropoint with a beam of 280 μ [5]. Shooting is effected shoot by shoot, with a intensity of 3 W, in superpulse. The polyp is drawn away from the vocal ligament towards the median line by means of a Bouchayer-type wide-edge forceps.

Once the polyp has been resected, a few drops of slow-drying fibrin sealant are deposited on the area of resection. The anesthetist then is asked to turn off the jet ventilation while the fibrin is allowed to set.

The advantage of using fibrin sealant for this procedure is to create a protective dressing for the submucosa and the vocal ligament.

Vocal Fold Scar

A vocal fold scar is a scar in the posterior part of the vocal fold following trauma during intubation. The epithelium coating the zone of the scar is first dissected by micropoint laser using the same parameters as those for the polyp. It is necessary to produce a microflap as thin as possible. Next, GAX collagen is injected into and around the scar to compensate for the deficiency in volume. Then the fibrin sealant is spread over the dissected area and the epithelium replaced. Next, pressure is applied to the area by means of a swab held in microforceps. Lastly, the excess fibrin sealant is aspirated off.

Type III Endoscopic Cordectomy

Type III endoscopic cordectomy is performed by CO_2 laser with continuous shooting by a beam of 700 μ with an intensity of 7 W in superpulse. It removes the vocal process, rejoins the inner surface of the thyroid cartilage, and stops at the anterior commissure. Thus it leaves the arytenoid and thyroid cartilages stripped completely bare. It is therefore wise to coat these with slow-setting fibrin glue in order to avoid granuloma formation and to decrease the risk of postoperative bleeding and edema. After the fibrin has set, a thin white coating can be seen that in no way hampers the respiratory tract.

Zenker's Diverticulum

In surgery for Zenker's diverticulum, the diverticuloesophageal wall is brought into view by means of the Van Overbeek diverticuloscope. It is next cut by CO_2 laser at an intensity of 10 W and with a beam of 700 µ, slightly defocalized in order to promote coagulation. The wall having been cut, only one esophageal opening remains with, at the base of the former wall, a breach in the mucosa and musculature of the esophagus. The placing of fibrin sealant in this breach consolidates the impermeability normally ensured by the fibrosis that is secondary to the peridiverticulitis.

Discussion

It is fortunate that the Belgian social security system has permitted the cost of fibrin sealant to be refunded. All the procedures for which it is now being used had already been successfully practised, but the use of fibrin sealant certainly marks another step towards success.

Tissucol has been in daily use in our department for more than 1 year now, since it became accepted for refund by the social security authorities. No reaction showing any intolerance has been noted among over 100 cases of surgery by endoscopic or external approach. No infection, edema, or allergic reaction has been seen. However, there have been cases where the product was expelled or where the fixing of microflaps has been inadaquate. Such difficulties can arise following efforts to cough on wakening or subsequent to the operation itself.

The advantages of using a slow procedure in laryngeal microsurgery enables there to be better control in the application of the fibrin seal. Less of the product needs to be used and the risk of expulsion by coughing or of inhalation of a large quantity of fibrin sealant can also be avoided. One could regret that there is no specific instrument for applying Tissucol in laryngeal microsurgery, but the use of a simple suction tube is an elementary, low-cost means of overcoming this difficulty by having a catheter passed inside it.

Lastly, using fibrin sealant does not prevent the use of some other substance, such as GAX collagen, for correcting those defects of the vocal fold that are observed in cases of severe sulcus or scar.

Fibrin sealant is a very useful contribution to microsurgery, both of the larynx and of the pharynx as well as for head and neck surgery by external approach. Its role is that of a glue, but at the same time that of a dressing. As a glue, it enables microflaps to be fixed and sutures to be strengthened. As a dressing, it guides the healing process, prevents formation of granulomas, strengthens the suture lines that may, for instance, have been made fragile by radiotherapy, and reduces postoperative bleeding and edema.

In microsurgery, we prefer a slow set to a rapid one in order to have better control of placing the fibrin seal and to avoid excesses, while producing a fine pellicle that does not compromise the respiratory tract, is adherent, and shows little risk of explusion due to coughing or of being inhaled. It is applied by means of a catheter passed through a suction tube of the type generally used in laryngeal microsurgery.

For surgery by external approach, rapid setting can be obtained by making use of the appropriate material supplied with the product.

References

1. De Vincentiis M, Ruoppolo G, Gallo A (1986) The use of fibrin sealant in ear, nose and throat surgery. In: Schlag G, Redl H (eds) Otorhinolaryngology. Springer, Berlin Heidelberg New York, (Fibrin sealant in operative medicine, vol 1) pp 86–90
2. Mayné A, Randour Ph, Joucken K, Gribomont B, Van Boven M, Remacle M (1988) Anesthésie et laser CO_2 en ORL. Louvain Méd 107: 435–441
3. Remacle M, Lawson G, Mayné A (1992) La chirurgie du diverticule pharyngo-oesophagien par voie endoscopique au laser CO_2. Rev Off Soc Fr ORL 15: 21–26
4. Remacle M, Lawson G (1992) Surgery: general aspects. Acta ORL Belg 46: 175–186
5. Shapshay SM, Rebeiz EE, Bohigian RK, Hybells RL (1990) Benign lesions of the larynx: should the laser be used? Laryngoscope 100: 953–957

Subject Index

ACNU 48
acoustic
– nerve 6
– neurinoma 8 ff.
– neuroma surgery 162 ff.
amputation neuroma (*see also* CCA) 76 ff.
anastomosis / anastomoses
– centrocentral (*see* CCA) 76 ff.
– peripheral nerves 5
angiofibroma 32, 38, 40
angiography, substraction (DSA) 34
animal experiments, lens surgery 98, 99
antibiotics 53, 58, 104, 147
– antibiotic solution 53, 58
aprotinin 108, 117, 125
– solution 108, 117
arachnoid cyst, fibrin sealing 59
armamentarium 115
arteriovenous malformation (AVM) 40
arytenoidectomy 212, 219
astigmatism in cataract surgery 116–120, 123, 128, 129
– keratometric 118
– postoperative 118, 119, 123, 128, 129
– preoperative 119
astrocytoma 41
– grade III 41
audiograms 189
auricle reconstruction 169 ff.
autologous tissue 60

bioactive ceramics 175
biological tissue adhesive 42, 43
blowout fracture, medical 144
bone chips 64
bone tissue / bone meal fibrin 52–58
– advantages 58
– disadvantages 58
bovine heterologous cartilage, middle ear reconstructive surgery 193 ff.
brachial plexus, obstetric lesion 68 ff.

– children 71
– etiology 69
– extraplexal neurotizations 72
– follow-up and prognosis 73
– intraplexal neurotizations 72
– multidisziplinary team 74
– recovery signs 73
– secondary surgical interventions 74
– surgical treatment 73
– traumatic origin 69
– upper plexus results 74
brain abscess 52
bronchoscope, fiberoptic 201
Broyle's ligament 212
bulbus olfactorius 53, 54

CaCl$_2$ solution 28, 34
calcium chloride 105, 117
calcium phosphate (CaP) 175
– biphasic 178
canal down techniques 195
canal up techniques 193, 194, 197
canaliculi lacrimales, lacerated 87, 125
canaliculocystostomy 87
canaliculodacryocystorhinostomy 87
capsulorhexis 117
carboanhydrase blockers, systemic 102, 105
cartilage
– bovine heterologous, middle ear reconstructive surgery 193 ff.
– grafts 159 ff., 189 ff., 197
–– cartilage heterografts 194
– layer, reconstructive middle ear surgery 186 ff., 194
– rib 169 ff., 194
– thyroid 222
– xiphoid 194
cartilaginous columella 195
cataract 98 ff., 105, 116 ff., 123 ff.
– surgery, fibrin adhesive for wound closure 105, 116 ff., 123 ff.

-- astigmatism (*see also there*) 116–120, 123, 128, 129
-- conjunctival positioning 124
-- fibrin glue 124, 128
-- fibrin sealant technique 125
-- lens implantation, intraocular 123
-- materials and methods 117, 124
-- results 118
-- scleral flap 126
-- scleral wound 126
-- small-incision technique 116 ff., 123 ff.
-- subconjunctival filtration bleb 126
- traumatic 98–101
catheterization, superselective 40
CCA (centrocentral anastomosis) 76 ff.
- axonal growth inside the graft 79
- definition 78
- end-to-end centrocentral connection 78, 81, 82
- fascicular group 79, 80
- infections 81
- penetrations of axons 79
- second surgery success 82
- surgical steps / technique 77, 79
- vascular disorders 81
ceramic granules, bioactive 175 ff.
- mineralization 177
- mixtue of biphasic ceraic granules and fibrin glue 178
cerebellopontine angle 8 ff.
cerebrocranial injuries 51 ff.
cerebrospinal fluid (see CSF) 3, 59, 60, 135 ff., 145, 147, 162, 163
cervical myelopathy, anterior 3
cesareon section 69
chi-squared test 118, 149
cholesteatoma 8 ff., 164, 175, 184, 189
- petrous 164
cholesterol granuloma 8 ff.
chorioretinal adhesions 114
CO_2-laser surgery 206 ff., 211
coagulation time, fibrin glue 201
cochlear implants 193
collagen gauze as transplant 60, 66
commissure, anterior 210
compound prosthesis, reconstructive middle ear surgery 186 ff.
computer assisted surgery (CAS) 8 ff.
conjunctiva 97 ff., 105, 126–130
- fistulas 97 ff., 105
-- surgical techniques 105
- rupture 105
- subconjunctival injections 128
- surgery 125
cordectomy, endoscopic, type III 222
corneal decompensation 118

cortical bone 53
corticosteroid therapy 204
cranial regions, reconstruction 5 ff.
- cranial fossa surgery, enlarged middle 8 ff.
- cranial orbital fissure 53
craniofacial trauma, fibrin glue 152 ff.
- microsurgical reconstruction techniques 152
craniotomy 141
CSF (cerebrospinal fluid) 3, 59, 60, 135 ff., 145, 147, 162, 163
- cavity 61
- endoscopic repair 135
- fistulas 3, 4, 6, 60, 61, 135, 139, 142, 145
-- repair of 6, 136
-- spinal 59
- leakings 60, 147
- rhinorrhea 26 ff., 162 ff.
-- postoperative rhinorrhea 28
-- prevention and treatment 27, 28, 163
-- radiological checking 29
-- wound sealing 28, 29
cycloplegia 104

dacryocystorhinostomy 87
diastematomyelia 59, 61
digital nerves 79
diverticuloesophageal wall 223
diverticuloscope
- new distending 206 ff.
- Van Overbeek 223
dorsum, remodeling graft of 160
DSA (substraction angiography) 34
dura mater
- lyophilized and fibrin glue 136, 143, 144
- and osseous, double sealing 57
- traumatic and iatrogenic defects 60
dural closure 5, 30
- waterproof closure 30
duroplasty for treatment of defects 59

ear
- bovine heterologous cartilage, middle ear reconstructive surgery 193 ff.
- cancer, external 169
- cartilage with perichondrium 136
- microsurgery of 184
- reconstructive middle ear surgery 186 ff.
eardrum transplant 189
embolization of tumors
- of meningiomas 40
- preoperative 32 ff.
-- capillary embolization 32

– CT after finishing embolization   40
embolization-set for fibrin glue
    injection   33
EMCF (extended middle cranial fossa)
    162, 163
EMG (electromyography)   70, 71
end-to-end coaption   59
endolaryngeal surgery, fibrin sealing
    210 ff.
– adverse reactions   213
– local infections   213
– mucosa   215
– secondary healing   215
endonasal approach, endoscopic   135,
    145
endoscopic
– diverticulotomy   206 ff.
– laser dissection of Zenker's diverticu-
    lum   206 ff.
– rhinologic instruments   136
enlarged middle cranial fossa surgery
    8 ff.
ENT
– departments, interdisciplinary coopera-
    tion between   152
– surgery   133 ff., 147 ff.
enucleation, macroscopic findings after
    111
eosin and Hematoxylin (H & E)   35, 46,
    47
epitympanic wall, reconstruction of   195
Erb's paralysis   69
esophagocutaneous fistula   200
esophagoscope, flexible   201
esophagus cancer, cervical   200
ethmoid microsurgery   150
ethmoidal sinusitis   148
ethmoidectomy, endoscopic   141, 144,
    148
– microsurgical, spray application of fi-
    brin glue   147 ff.
– sphenoethmoidectomy, endoscopic
    141
eustachian tube   188, 189
eye lens, fibrin sealing (see also lens)
    97 ff.
eyelid surgery   87
– skin transplantation   87

F-IFN-β   42–50
– advantages and future possibilities   48
facial
– nerve anastomosis, intracranial
    162–167
–– techniques   166
– nerve reconstruction   162 ff.
– neuroma   164

factor XIII   125
fascia lata   136
fatty tissue, epidural, graft of   65
fiberoptic bronchoscope   201
fibrin
– adhesive, small-incision cataract
    surgery   116 ff., 123 ff.
– glue
–– application in ophthalmology   125
–– coagulation time   201
–– mixture   32, 33, 42, 53
–– rhinologic applications   135 ff., 145
– mass   41
– sealing, endolaryngeal surgery   210 ff.
fibrin-retinopexy in rabbit eyes   107 ff.
– absorption of fibrin sealant   110
– armamentarium   115
– cells of the vitreous base   114
– cyanoacrylate sealants   107
– degenerative reactions   113
– enucleation, macroscopic findings
    after   111
– frozen human fibrin sealant   108
– histological findings   112, 113
– morphological reaction   114
– ophthalmoscopic and histological find-
    ings   107
– postoperative fibrin resorption   110,
    111
– preretinal fibrosis, development of
    112
– results   109
– subretinal fibrin application   107, 109
– transvitreal fibrin sealing   108
– vitrectomy in the rabbit eyes   108
fibrinogen, human   53, 60, 125, 135
– protein   38
– solution   135
fibronectin   125
finger amputation   81
fixation of transplants   61
flaps, auricle reconstruction   169 ff.
fluctuant hearing loss   180 ff.
5-fluorouracil (5-FU)   48
fluorescein injection   135, 136
freeze-dried powder   117
frontal skull base trauma   152 ff.
frontobasal reconstruction using biolo-
    gical material   51 ff.
frontorhinal basis   53

Gadolinium   29
GAX collagen   223
Gelfoam   5
Gersuny technique   169
glaucoma surgery   105, 106
glioblastoma multiforme   41

228   Subject Index

glomus tumors   32, 34
glue-packed IFN-β   41
granulation tissue   210
gutta-percha plate   79

harvested mucosa   136
head
– and neck surgery, use of Tissucol
   218 ff.
– trauma   142
headache   38
hearing loss, fluctuant   180 ff.
hemangioma   32, 38
Hematoxylin and eosin (H & E)   35, 46,
   47
hemifacial spasm   8 ff.
hemorrhages control   59
hemostasis   4, 5, 66, 135, 147, 148, 210
– complex   5
hepatitis   145, 146
– B hepatitis   145
– non-A/non-B hepatitis   145
histoanastomosis   60, 66
HIV (human immunodeficiency)   145,
   146
Horner syndrome   70, 71
hydrochloride   48
hyphema, transient   118
hypoglossal nerve   72
hypoglossal-facial nerve anastomosis
   164, 166

IAC (internal auditory canal)   167
ICCE (intracapsular cataract
   extraction)   120
IFN-(interferon)-β   41 ff.
– concentration in fibrin mass   43
– F-IFN-β   42, 43
– – F used as carrier of IFN-β   48
– histological transition   49
– time course of IFN-β activity in
   tissue   44, 49
indications of fibrin adhesive   59
infections   52, 81, 200, 213
interferon (see IFN)
internal auditory canal   8 ff.
intracranial
– facial nerve anastomosis   162–167
– – techniques   166
– procedures, use of fibrin glue   162 ff.
intracranial-extratemporal anastomosis
   technique   162
intraocular fibrin sealing   110
IOL (intraocular lens)   120
Ionocem   51, 54
iridectomy   99
iris trauma   98

jugular chemodectoma   6

keratometric astigmatism   118
Klumpke's paralysis   68, 70
Krönlein's operation   56

laboratory tests, mixtures   32, 42, 53
lacrimal surgery   87 ff., 125
– indications for fibrin sealing use   87
lamina papyracea   144
laryngeal microsurgery   219
laryngectomy, total   199 ff.
laryngology, use of Tissucol   218 ff.
larynx
– carcinoma   210
– wound healing   210
CO$_2$-laser surgery   206 ff., 211
lens
– astigmatism   100
– saving surgery (see also lens trauma)
   97 ff.
– trauma   97 ff.
– – animal experiments   98
– – cataract, traumatic   98–101
– – clotting   102
– – complications   102
– – conjunctival fistulas (see also there)
   97 ff., 105
– – cycloplegia   104
– – extended rupture of the anterior capsule of the lens   101
– – fibrinogen indications   99
– – fibrinogen-based microsurgery
   99–102
– – fibrinogen-based sealing   100
– – glaucoma surgery   105, 106
– – insufficient sealing   104
– – iridectomy   102
– – perforating injuries   97, 99
– – postoperative care   104
– – posttraumatic fibrinogen   98
– – postraumatic protein levels   99, 100
– – sealing of the lens capsule   98
– – surgical technique   99, 105
– – synechiae, artificial   102
– – thrombin-calcium chloride solution
   105
lipomyelocele   59, 61
lyophilized dura and fibrin glue   143, 144

macroadenomas   30
maladaptation, intrauterine   69
malignant cerebral tumor   41 ff.
– local therapy with interferon-β (see also
   IFN-β)   41 ff.
Mallet score   74
mastoid cavity

– filling with ceramic granules   175, 176
–– mineralization   177
– obliteration   175 ff.
–– fibrin sealant   175 ff.
mastoidectomy, middle ear   189
MBCP (macroporous biphasic calcium
    phosphate) granules   175
meatotomy, middle   147, 148
Menière's disease   8 ff.
meningioma   32, 34, 35
– preoperative treatment   34
meningitis   26, 30, 52, 152
– secondary   152
meningocele   59, 61, 70
meningoencephalocele   135–138, 141, 142
– repair of   136, 138
Methocel   106
micro-otoneurosurgery   8 ff.
microadenomas   28
microlaryngoscopy   213
microsurgery, use of Tissucol   218 ff.
– laryngeal   219
– pharyngeal   219
– pharyngolaryngeal   220
microsurgical
– ethmoidectomy, spray application of
    fibrin glue   147 ff.
– reconstructions, brachial plexus
    lesions   68
minimally invasive surgery   206 ff.
mixtures of fibrin glue   32, 33, 42, 53
Mochida   42
mucosal flaps   210
mucous membrane   57
myelocele   61

nasal
– gauze packing   150
– packing   147
– polyposis   148
– septal perforation (NSP)   135, 136, 145
–– methods   136
–– repair   136
– septoplasy   147, 148
– surgery   147
natrium chloride   106
nausea   38
neck
– dissection, radical   202
– vessels, vascular sutures   6
nerves, peripheral   4, 5
– anastomoses   5
neurinoma of the acoustic nerve   6
neuroma
– facial   164
– neuroma formation results   77
– painful amputation   76 ff.

– surgery, acoustic   162 ff.
– tarsus neuroma   81
– wide-spread   72
– zone of neuroma location   78
neurosurgery   1 ff.
– reconstruction of obstetric brachial
    plexus lesions   68 ff.
– spinal (see also there)   59 ff.
– surgical procedures with human fibrin
    glue   4
nicardipine   48
Nimustine   48
Nippon   42

obliteration   164
obstetric lesions   68 ff.
– brachial plexus lesions, neurosurgical
    reconstruction (see also brachial
    plexus)   68 ff.
–– children   71
–– traumatic origin   69
Ommaya reservoir   48
ophthalmic surgery   87 ff.
– fibrin glue application   125
optic nerve   53, 136, 137
– decompression   135, 136, 141, 144
–– endoscopic   136
– endoscopic view   137
orbital
– decompression   136, 145
– muscle nerve   53
– surgery   87 ff.
–– fixation of secondary orbital
    implant   87
–– postenucleation syndrome   87
–– sclera silicone implant   87
– tumors   51 ff.
–– neoplasms, removal   51
–– procedure after removal   56
–– reconstruction   51 ff.
orbitofrontal basis   51
osseous and dura mater, double sealing   57
ossicular
– chain reconstruction   180 ff., 193 ff.
– replacement prosthesis   188, 194
–– partial (PORP)   188, 194
–– total (TORP)   188, 194
osteoplastic laminotomy   61
otoneurosurgical interventions   8 ff.
otorhinolaryngology   133 ff.
otosclerotic surgery   189
overlay technique   136
Oxycel   137

packing, nasal   147
painful amputation neuromas (see also
    CCA)   76 ff.

panophthalmia 111
paranasal sinus system 57, 137
– sealing of 57, 137
patient comfort, postoperative 147, 150
PCL 117, 118
– biconvex 118
– phacoemulsification 117
percutaneous technique 26
periorbita, reconstruction of 56
periost patches 52
peripheral nerve 76 ff.
petrous cholesteatoma 164
phacoemulsification 116, 117, 121, 123, 128, 130
– with PCL 117
– with scleral tunnel 128
phantom pain / sensations 76 ff.
pharyngeal
– constrictor muscles 200
– fistulas following total laryngectomy 199 ff.
–– infections 200
–– nutrition 200
–– postoperative 200
– microsurgery 219
pharyngoesophagus junction 200
pharyngolaryngeal microsurgery 220
pharyngolaryngectomy 201
pharynx, resection of 199
phonosurgery 219
phrenic nerve palsy, obstetric 70–72
pituitary gland adenoma, transphenoidal surgery 26 ff.
plasminogen 125
plastic and reconstructive surgery 87 ff.
PMMA (polymethyl methacrylate) 120, 121
pneumatocele 52
pneumoencephalitis 26, 30
postenucleation syndrome 87
preoperative tumor embolization, fibrin glue 32 ff.
preretinal fibrosis, development of 112
prolactinomas 28
protein-aprotinin 117
pseudoarthrosis 63, 64
pseudomingocele, fibrin sealing 59, 62, 63
psychosocial problems 152
PVA (polyvinylalcohol) particles 32, 38, 40

rabbit eyes, fibrin-retinopexy (see also there) 107 ff.
recanalization 38
reconstructive surgery 87 ff.
Refobacin-Palacos 51, 54

Reinke's edema 219
repneumatization 57
retinal
– detachment, development of 111
– surgery 125
retinopexy (see fibrin-retinopexy) 107 ff.
rhinologic
– applications of fibrin glue 135 ff., 145
– instruments, endoscopic 136
rhinoplasty, use of fibrin glue 159 ff.
– atraumatic 159
– augmentation rhinoplasty 159
– remodeling graft of the dorsum 160
– reshaping rhinoplasty by open approach 161
– rhinolifting without skin reduction 161
rhinorrhea, CSF (see also there) 26 ff.
– transient rhinorrhea 26
rib cartilage 169 ff., 194
root canal, myelographic CT 65

sacrospinalis muscular system 60
Savary bougie 201
sciatic nerve section 76
sclera silicone implant 87
scleral
– flap technique 125, 129
– pocket technique 116
– surgery 125
sealed dural incision, physiological healing of 60
sinus system
– nasal, surgery of 147
– paranasal 57, 137
skin
– transplantation, eyelid surgery 87
– tumors, malignant 169
skull base trauma, fibrin glue 152 ff.
– microsurgical reconstruction techniques 152
SNAP (sensory nerve action potentials) 70
Spearman rank correlation test 149
Special Reference Laboratory, Inc. 42
sphenoethmoidectomy, endoscopic 141
spinal
– cysts 61
– neurosurgery, fibrin sealing 59 ff.
– subarachnoid space sealing 66
– tumors, hyperemic 59
–– hemostasis 66
spondylosis 3
spongiosa fibrin adhesive graft 64
spray application of fibrin glue 147 ff.
stapedectomy 183
steam-treated 53, 60
stressful psychosocial problems 152

subarachnoid space, sealing of   52, 57, 60
suralis transplantation, autologous   59, 64
Surgigel   5
synechiae, artificial   102

tarsus neuroma   81
TCP (tricalciumphosphat)   175, 176
– bioactivity of   178
team, multidisciplinary   74
tests   118
– *chi*-squared test   118, 149
– *Spearman* rank correlation test   149
– *U*-test   118
– unpaired two-tailed *t* test   118
– *Wilcoxon* rank test   118, 149
thombin, human   33, 42, 53, 60, 125
– solution   99
– trombin S   42
thrombin-CaCl$_2$ solution   105, 117
thyroid cartilage   222
Tisseel   42
Tissomat   53
Tissucol   34, 76, 99, 107, 117, 135, 145,
    146, 148, 175, 176, 189, 201, 218 ff.
Tissucol DuoS   53, 60, 117, 125
tracheostomy   200
traffic accidents   152
transphenoidal surgery
– microscopic surgery   147
– on pituitary gland adenomas   26 ff.
Trasylol   33, 34, 106
Triosite   175
tumors
– glomus tumor   32, 34
– pituitary   26 ff.
– preoperative tumor embolization, fibrin
    glue   32 ff.
– stage I-IV   28
– tympanicum   34

tympanic membrane   186 ff., 193 ff.
– graft   189–197
– perforations   189
tympanicum tumors   34
tympanoplasty surgery   188
– fibrin sealing   180 ff.

U-test   118
Ultravist   33, 34
underly technique   136
unpaired two-tailed *t* test   118

Van Overbeek diverticuloscope   223
vascular
– decompression   8 ff.
– sutures in surgery of neck vessels   6
vascularized lesions   5
veinfascia transplantation   180 ff.
vestibular nerve, neurectomy   8 ff.
vincristine   48
vitrectomy in the rabbit's eye   108
vitreoretinal surgery   107
vitreous cavity, fibrinogen leakage   99
vocal fold
– polyp of   222
– vocal fold scar   222
vocal muscle   211
vomitting   38

webs   210
Wilcoxon rank test   118, 149
wound healing, larynx   210

xiphoid cartilage   194

Zenker's diverticulum, endoscopic laser
    dissection   206 ff.
Zoki   42

Springer-Verlag
and the Environment

We at Springer-Verlag firmly believe that an international science publisher has a special obligation to the environment, and our corporate policies consistently reflect this conviction.

We also expect our business partners – paper mills, printers, packaging manufacturers, etc. – to commit themselves to using environmentally friendly materials and production processes.

The paper in this book is made from low- or no-chlorine pulp and is acid free, in conformance with international standards for paper permanency.